OBESITY
Treatment – Juvenile

Maria Mercedes Rubiano - Vanegas, M.Sc., R.D., CCM

Carmen Macbeth - Vanegas, Executive Chef

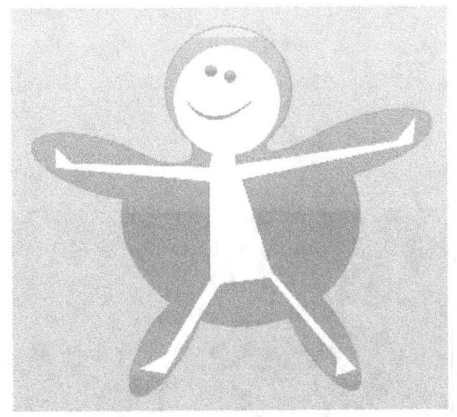

ISBN-10: 1-451-56111-3

EAN-13: 978-1-451-56111-1

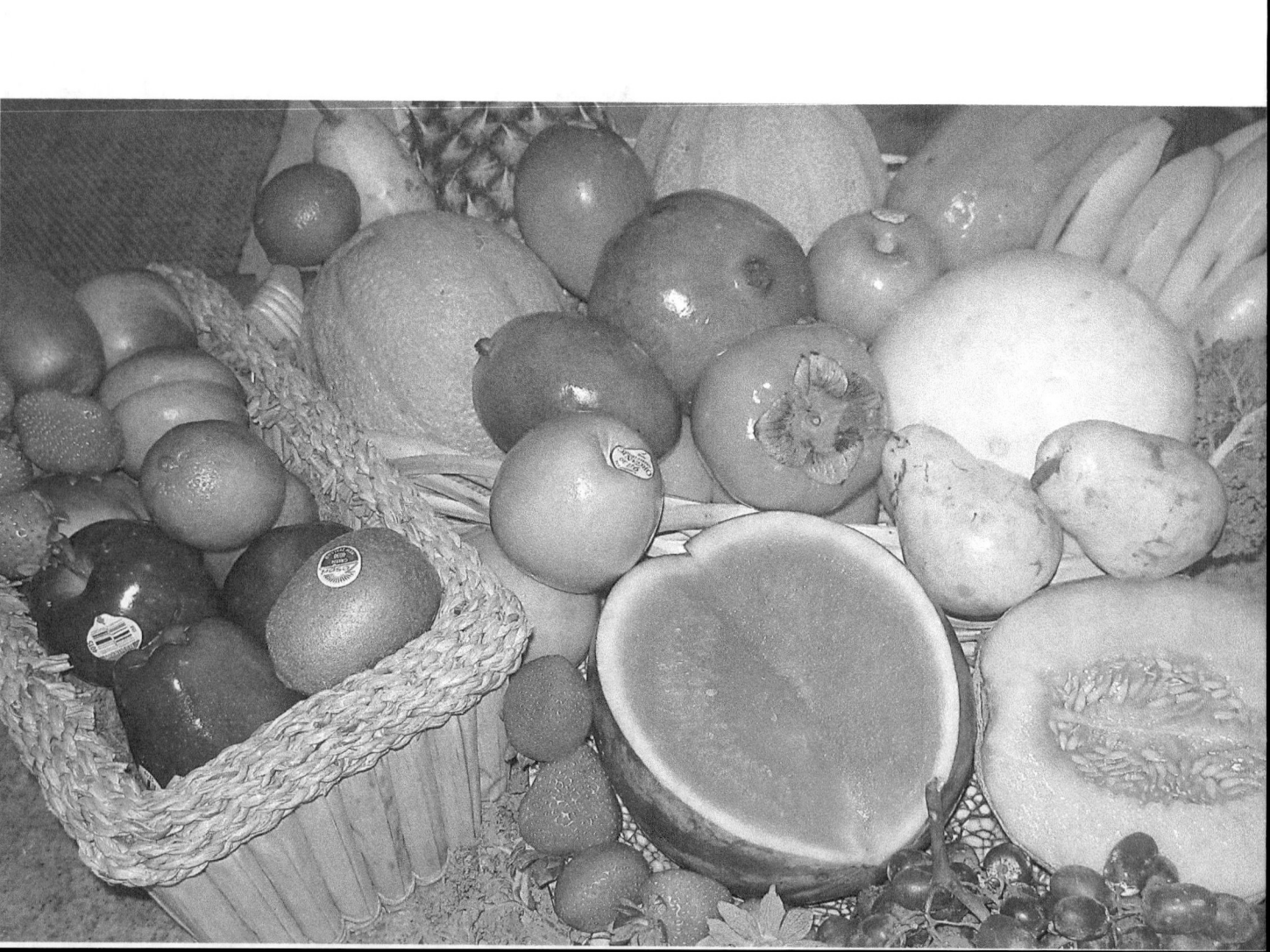

Acknowledgments

We offer our most sincere thanks to the immensely generous collaboration we received from Carmen's husband, Bill Macbeth, whose advice, support and assistance made this book possible.

Our thanks must also go to Laura Burgos, who was in charge of beautifying our book with her wonderful illustrations, and Marcela Camacho, for her magnificent work in the design and coordination of this project.

Finally, our thanks to Carmen's daughter, Sonia Villar, who assisted in the translation of this book into English.

Sincerely,

Maria Mercedes and Carmen

3

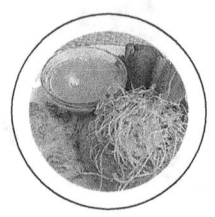

Contents

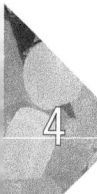

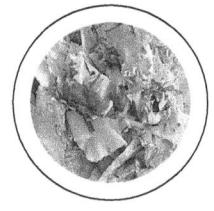
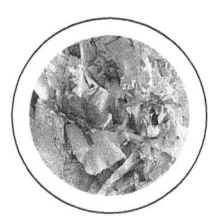
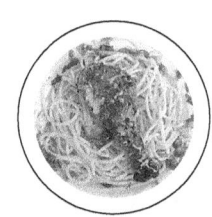

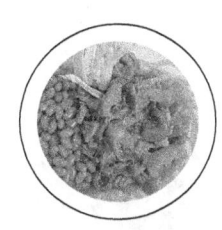
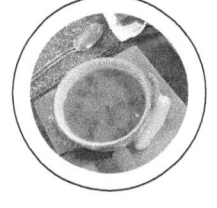
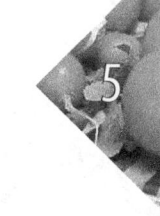
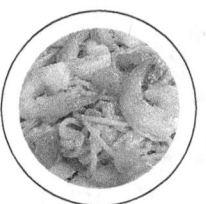
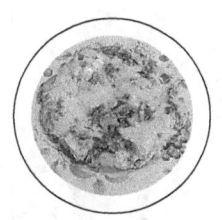
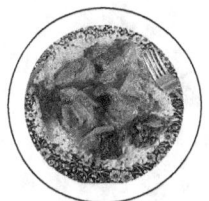
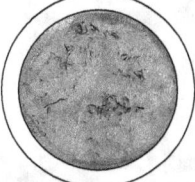

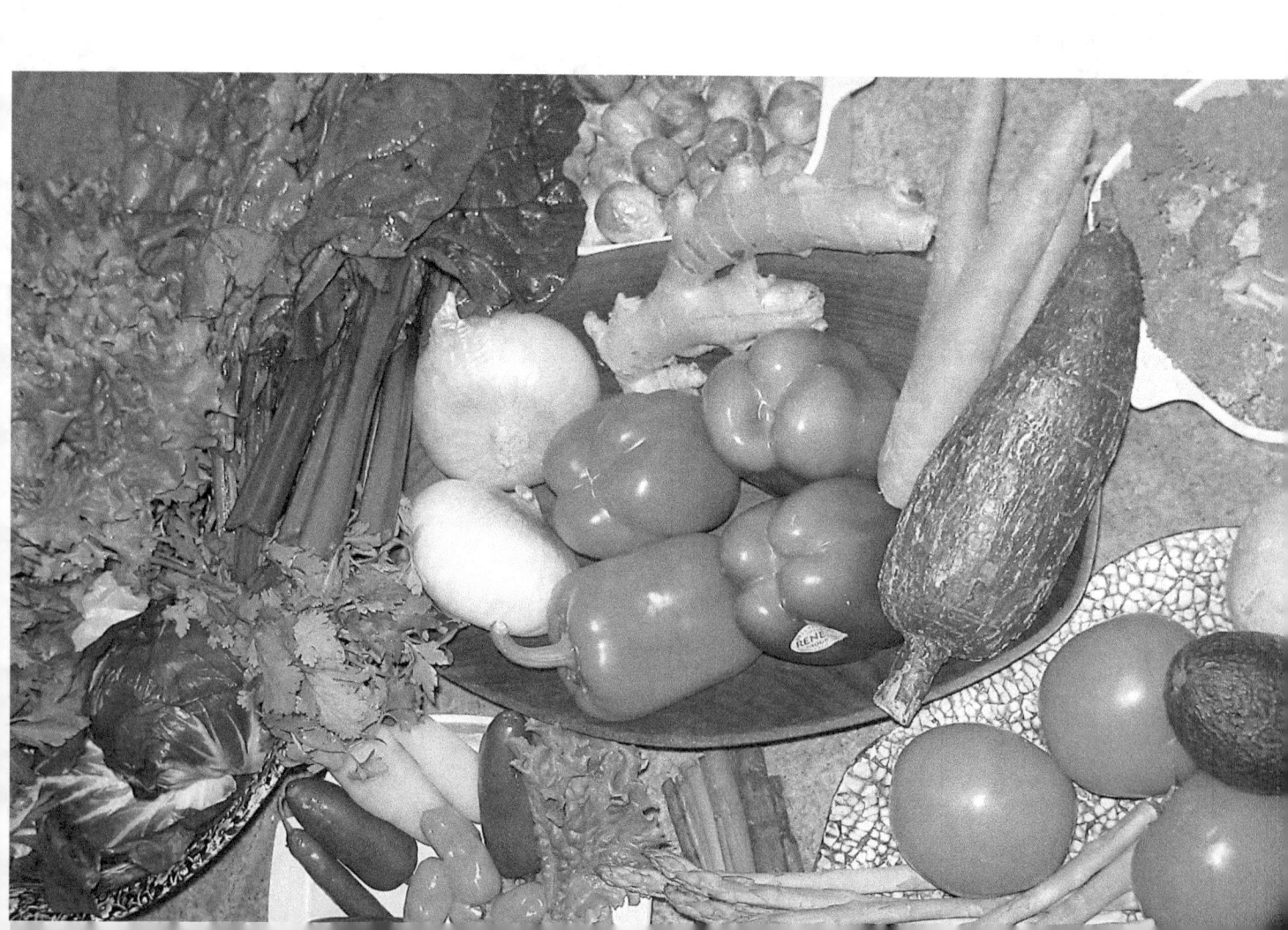

Preface

In this book, the subject of obesity in children is addressed by professionals with vast experience in the treatment of diverse cases of childhood obesity.

To supplement our own knowledge and expertise, we have included several articles that discuss important childhood obesity studies that have been done by public and private institutions in various countries around the world. We also offer our own best advice and solutions based on lessons-learned to combat this worldwide epidemic.

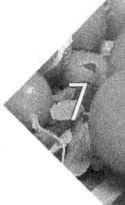

Our goal in sharing this information is to provide families with an aid for the prevention of childhood obesity, as well as solutions for already existing problems. In the second half of the book, we offer recipes for over eighty nutritious and easy to prepare dishes that still keep their delicious flavor. The daily use of these recipes can be an effective means for developing a taste for good nutrition.

We hope this book becomes a valuable resource for many families.

The Authors

María Mercedes Rubiano - Vanegas, M.Sc, R.D., CCM

Maria Mercedes is a licensed nutritionist and registered dietician with a specialization in Clinical Nutrition for over twenty-five years. Currently, she is the medical dietician at the Adventist Hospital and Taams Clinic in Willemstad, Curacao, Netherlands Antilles.

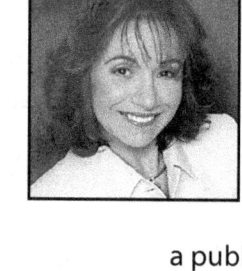

As a nutritionist, she collaborates with the Curacao Cancer Foundation and the Curacao Heart Care Foundation. Both organizations are dedicated to nutritional health and advanced dieting techniques for patients with cancer, vascular problems and other ailments. As an assistant in the Division of Public Health, she helps plan and promote nutrition programs for the Netherlands Antilles.

Maria Mercedes has been a guest nutritional expert on several television and radio programs, and collaborates with local newspapers to provide recommendations on the latest diet and nutrition developments.

For more than a decade, she has served as the official dietician to the Curacao Youth Beauty Contest Organization, which each year selects Curacao's Miss Universe contestant. In this role, she assisted the pageant participants with informative talks regarding nutrition and dieting. She is also a frequent presenter on the television program "A Buena Hora" (In Good Time), a show dedicated to health, therapy, exercise and nutrition that is broadcast throughout the Caribbean Islands.

As a nutritionist and licensed dietician, Maria Mercedes has participated in the creation of educational programs about nutrition for several different organizations in the Netherlands Antilles. She has also written articles for "Super Magazine", a publication dedicated to teens. Most recently, she participated in an epidemiological study of childhood obesity from which sprang her inspiration to write this book.

Maria Mercedes trained with various institutions in Bogota, Colombia, among them San Ignacio University Hospital, Children's University Hospital, Lorencita Villegas de Santos, Central Military Hospital and participated in thesis research of breastfeeding conducted for the Nestle company.

Born in Bogota, Colombia of French and Spanish descent, Maria Mercedes Rubiano-Vanegas has a Master of Science degree with specialization in Nutrition and Dietician from the University Javeriana of Bogota, and a graduate degree in Orthomolecular Nutrition from Baarn, Holland. She speaks Spanish, English, Papiamento, and understands Dutch and French.

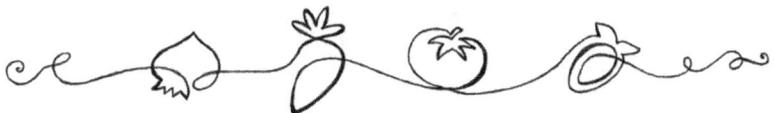

Carmen Macbeth - Vanegas, Chef

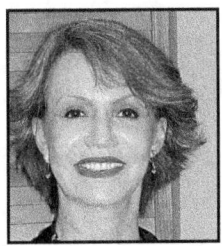

As an adolescent, Carmen enjoyed cooking different dishes for the many gatherings of friends and family at her home, which they all loved. This experience inspired her interest to enroll in the academy of Segundo Cabezas, a Chef Cordon Bleu, where she learned the art of preparing exquisite meals and the knowledge to become an Executive Chef.

After the birth of her children, Carmen further pursued her studies with the Spanish International Atelier, Marco Antonio, who taught her the fine art of preparing cakes and pastries in Australian-style laminated paste, as well as the way to delicately decorate with flowers elaborated in a natural refined sugar.

With this knowledge and experience, Carmen began catering for weddings and other special occasions at private clubs and exclusive events. She offered complete menus that included her cakes and pastries but found her customers wanted something special and unique to taste and admire. That is when she became known for her "garnishing" style, which she developed through the decoration of her dishes, trays, floral arrangements, fruit baskets, candles and ice figures along with the lighting she arranged to create spectacular ambiance.

The taste for fine cooking was inherited from Carmen's paternal grandmother, a French lady with an exquisite taste for gourmet food. Back in her day, she had an exclusive tearoom, Terraza

Pasteur, which was known as the afternoon meeting place for society ladies from Bogota to gather. Today, due to the fame of her tearoom and its location as a point of reference for gatherings, there is a shopping mall with the name Terraza Pasteur.

Carmen has resided in the United States for over twenty years and is now a U.S. citizen. She started preparing food for the diets of several Hollywood celebrities a few years after her arrival. Those celebrities included; Mel Brooks and Ann Bancroft, Victoria Principal, Warren Beatty, Jane Seymour, Rod Stewart, Sheila and Joe Barbera, Roy Schneider, Eriq La Salle, and many other celebrities and artists.

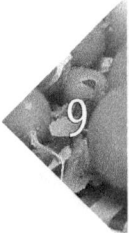

At that time she specialized in macrobiotic diets, which aid in the process of rejuvenating the body and preserving psychophysical stability and is often recommended for people with digestive problems, cancer or heart disease.

Carmen wanted to join her sister, Maria Mercedes, in creating this book to assist families in need of information about the prevention and treatment of childhood obesity. Utilizing her experience as a chef, she has provided easy to prepare recipes for flavourful, low calorie meals. It is her hope these recipes will aid families as they adapt their eating habits to those recommended in this book for improved nutrition, better health and lifestyles.

1. Introduction

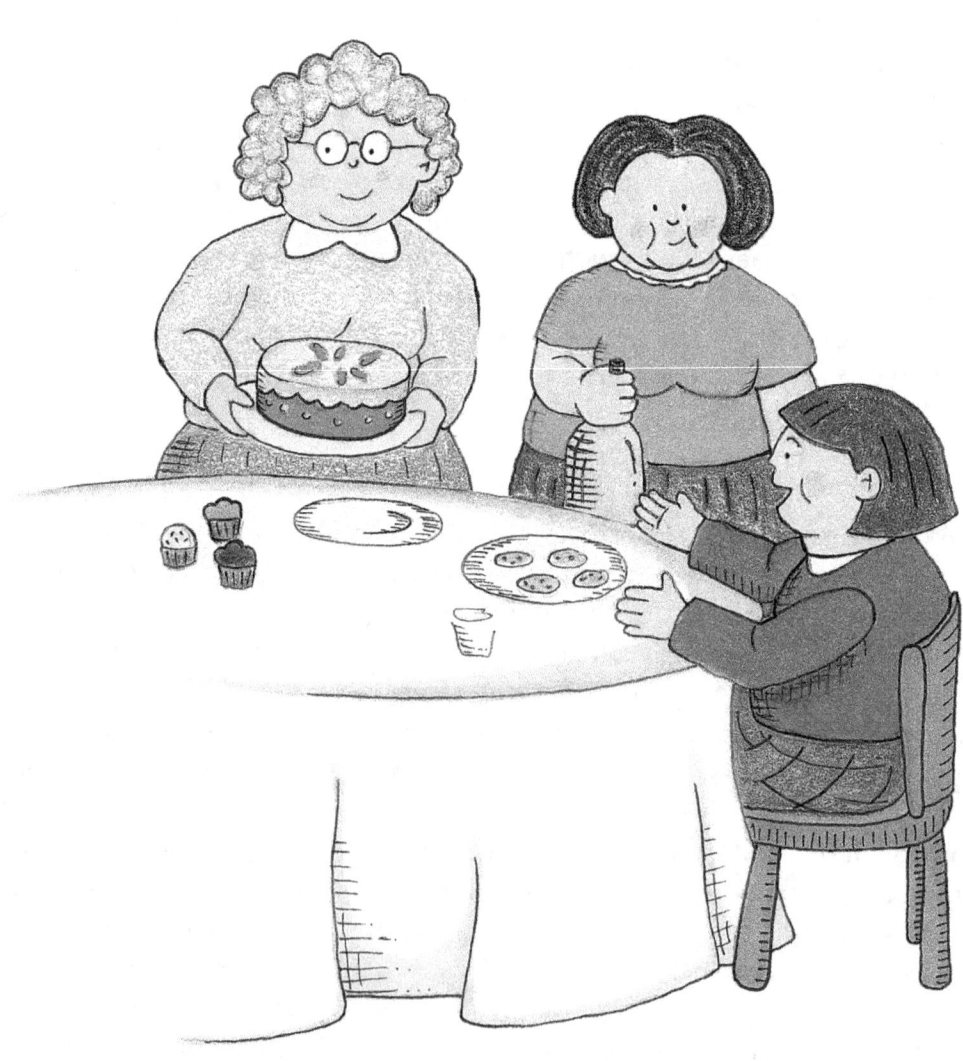

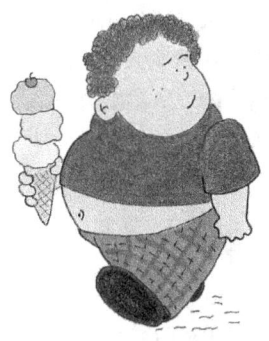

A FUNDAMENTAL MOTIVATION for this book arose from research on childhood obesity, which highlighted the urgent need to help resolve a problem that afflicts far too many children, causing them both suffering as well as reduced life expectancies.

I have received recognition as a dietician and nutritionist for my achievements in successfully treating multiple cases of severe childhood obesity in hospitals and private practice. Now with the support of my sister, Carmen, a chef experienced in the preparation of well-balanced and nutritious meals for families with obese children, we have the expertise required to assist families dealing with the problems of childhood obesity. For this reason, Carmen and I decided to share our combined experiences with people interested in receiving professional advice that will aid in the recovery of their children.

One of the most important motivations to write a book on the treatment of childhood obesity is the knowledge that if the necessary behavioral changes are not made during childhood, it will be much more difficult to make them in the later stages of life. When obesity occurs in childhood and is not treated early, it will persist into adolescence and then usually progress into adulthood.

Childhood is a stage in which almost any change in the establishment of healthy habits and behaviors is possible. At this stage, the personality and patterns formed will become the basis of a child's behavior in adulthood. Therefore, it is necessary to prevent the problem of overweight and obesity from developing from the earliest stage of childhood.

All of society needs to focus their attention on nutritional education. But it is especially important for those who are involved in the sphere of children, either directly or indirectly, to concentrate their efforts on educating children about good nutrition and healthy eating habits. For it is this nutritional education that will help provide them with a healthy foundation for the rest of their lives.

Obesity is a disease caused by an excessive accumulation of body fat, especially in the adipose tissue. It can be detected when the change in body weight exceeds 20% over the "ideal weight" established in relation to a child's age, size and sex. To calculate the approximate ideal weight of a child between ages two to five years, multiply the child's age by two and then add eight. For example, for an average five year old child: $5 \times 2 = 10 + 8 = 18$ kg (kilograms). This method, however, is only an approximation. A pediatrician should be consulted to more accurately determine a child's ideal weight.

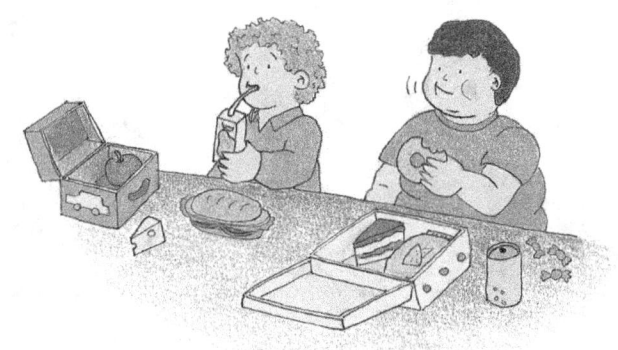

For many families, having an chubby child is a sign of good health, strength and prosperity, though healthcare professionals would not agree. Some parents believe the most important measure of their children's health is that they don't get sick, viewing their increasing weight as much less important. In reality, childhood obesity is a harbinger of disease to come.

The incidence of childhood obesity has doubled in the last ten years. In some places, even five years ago, only 5% of minors were obese. Currently, in the United States, 32% of the school-age population is overweight or obese. In some countries, half of al children are overweight. These are alarming statistic in societies where there is an abundance and wide variety of nutritious foods and no unusually significant economic deterrents to establishing and maintaining a healthy diet.

According to the World Health Organization (WHO), overweight and obesity have reached epidemic proportions worldwide. The figures are frightening. More than one billion adults are overweight and of these at least 300 million are obese. And if parents awareness is not raised, the statistics for overweight and obese children will continue to rise.

It is not possible to state the exact amount of food a child needs to consume daily. Each child's needs and requirements are different. Therefore, we must allow children to decide for themselves how much to eat, without forcing them to eat more, since they instinctively know what they require. Normally, boys will eat more than girls, but when it comes to appetite, we cannot and must not generalize.

Many parents must divide their limited time between home and work, and understandably, think it is easier to offer fast food to their children than a homemade balanced meal. They start with fried foods (e.g., pork chops with fried potatoes), then commercial foods, then processed foods that are microwave safe, and finish with a variety of deserts such as ice cream or sugar cookies. Day after day this becomes a way of life and develops into a bad habit of consuming foods that are fast, attractive and easy to access. But these foods lack the nutrients and vitamins necessary for their children's growth and health and are known by nutritionists and dieticians as "empty calories". To parents, who believe they do not have time to think about nutrition, their primary goal is to satisfy their children's hunger, without understanding their choices are compromising their children's long-term health.

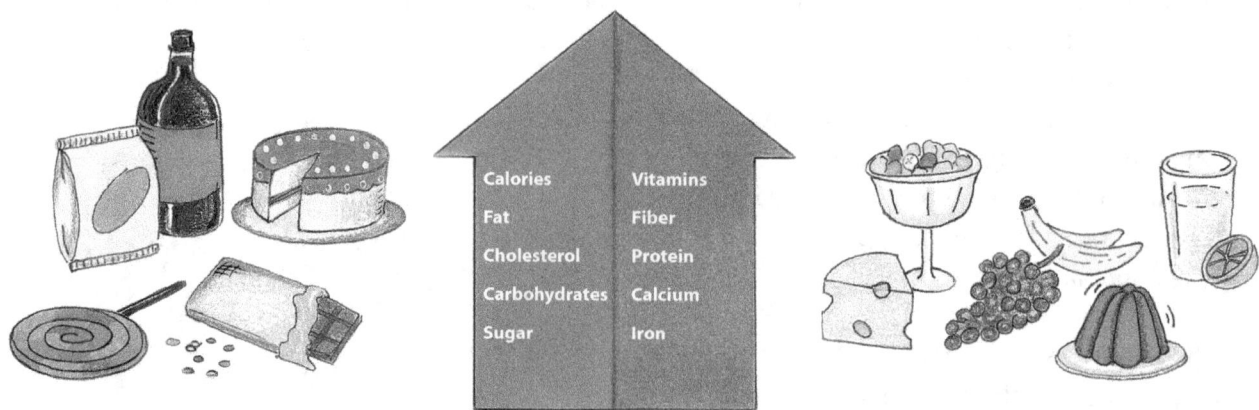

Calories	Vitamins
Fat	Fiber
Cholesterol	Protein
Carbohydrates	Calcium
Sugar	Iron

Parents, as well as grandparents, often fixate over the quantity of food children should consume rather then the food's quality. Menus are offered without consideration or control of its content, such as the high percentage of fat and sugar that causes weight gain. So instead of being offered healthy food choices like vegetables, rice and greens, children eat fatty fast foods full of empty calories along with sugary sodas and candy.

In addition to the consumption of foods with high fat and sugar content, the lack of daily exercise and physical activities cause children to become sedentary which contributes to their weight gain. Establishing a routine of daily physical activity is essential for the healthy growth and weight management of children.

The lifestyle of today's children has changed greatly from that of previous generations. A great majority of their activities are performed sitting in front of a television, computer or videogame.

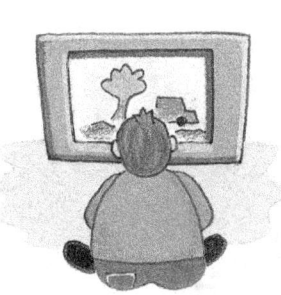

Many parents, for a number of reasons including comfort and convenience, allow their children to play indoors all day, rather than push them to play outdoors or take them to a park. Outdoor games, excursions, sports, etc. are easily substituted by sedentary indoor activities. On daily average, children spend over two-and-a-half hours watching television, and an additional hour playing videogames or on the web.

Bad nutritional habits and lack of physical activity are the leading causes of child obesity. Other contributors may be social influence as well as physiological, metabolic and genetic factors. A child of obese parents, for example, is more predisposed to be obese. Obesity may also result from a psychological disorder.

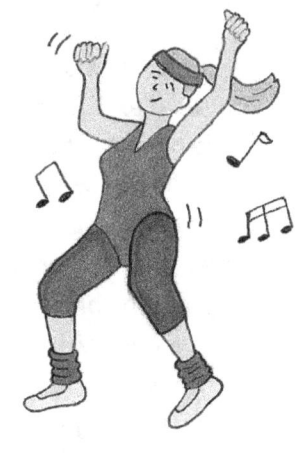

One way to prevent obesity in children is to create the habit of eating well. Giving them proper nutrition from birth is the best way to keep them healthy. It all begins with breastmilk, nursing when possible, then with porridge and then a full menu. It is recommended that children be given the opportunity to taste a little of everything, so their diet should contain plenty of variety, until at least two years of age.

Besides establishing the habit of selecting nutritious foods for our children to eat, it is also necessary to develop in parallel the good habit of sharing meals together and making them pleasant encounters. For example, never eat in front of the television, especially in view of your children. Parents are often the worst example for their children and the primary promoters of bad habits. Case in point, if one or both parents eat large quantities of food and are obese, it is statistically certain their child will acquire this bad habit. In such a case, it would be necessary to modify the entire family's eating habits while simultaneously encouraging outdoor physical activities such as bike riding, ball games, dancing, and swimming.

Many bad habits acquired during childhood can lead to severe consequences later in adulthood. The risk of developing disorders during adolescence is an example of what can happen if a child's nutritional and lifestyle needs do not receive the adequate care and appropriate attention they require.

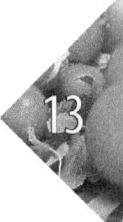

A few years ago, obesity was a problem almost exclusively for adults. Today, many of the complications resulting from obesity affect children as well. Childhood obesity compromises a child's life-long health. It can generate physical problems like type II diabetes, arterial hypertension and high cholesterol levels, while some children may also develop psychological problems. Obese children subjected to bullying, teasing or rejection from their peers may develop low self-esteem. They may become isolated due to their appearance, which can lead to other disorders such as bulimia, anorexia and depression. Tragically, it may even cause some children to develop extremely bad habits like drug or other harmful substance abuse.

The treatment for child obesity is not easy, either for the family or the child. The treatment requires the total modification of a family's lifestyle, including the alteration of their nutritional and physical habits. The older a child is, the harder it will be to achieve a successful treatment, though not impossible. With children under five years old, the parents are responsible for enforcing all aspects of the treatment as well as managing their child's response to therapy. From ages five to nine years, children have more autonomy in their treatment, though close parental supervision is still required. Children nine or ten years of age, for the most part, will be responsible for adhering to the treatment plan and may respond with almost total freedom.

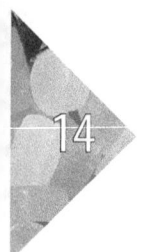

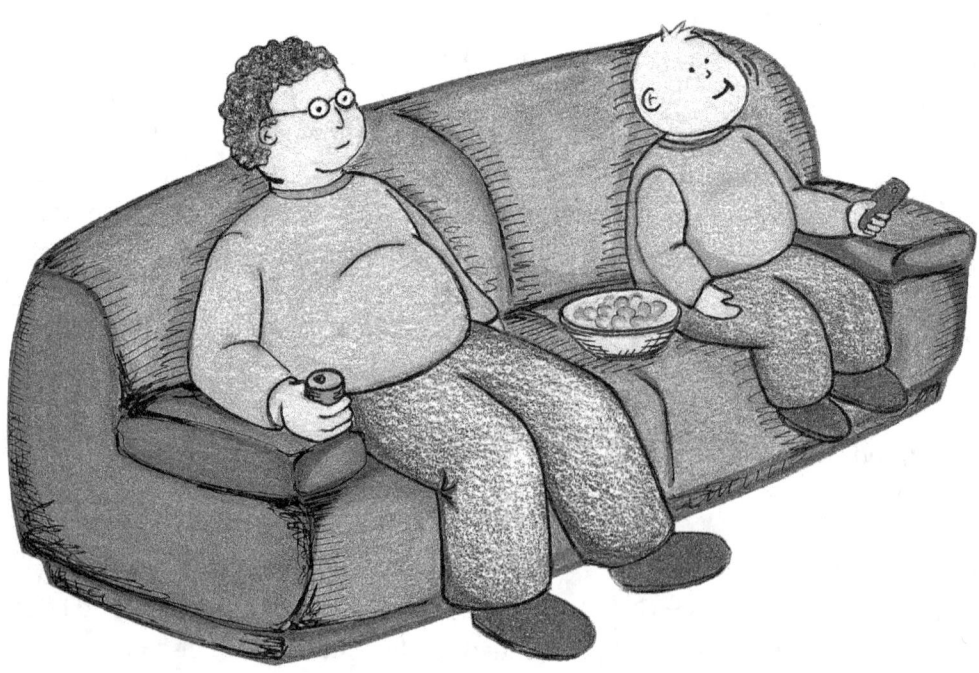

2. What Is Nutrition?

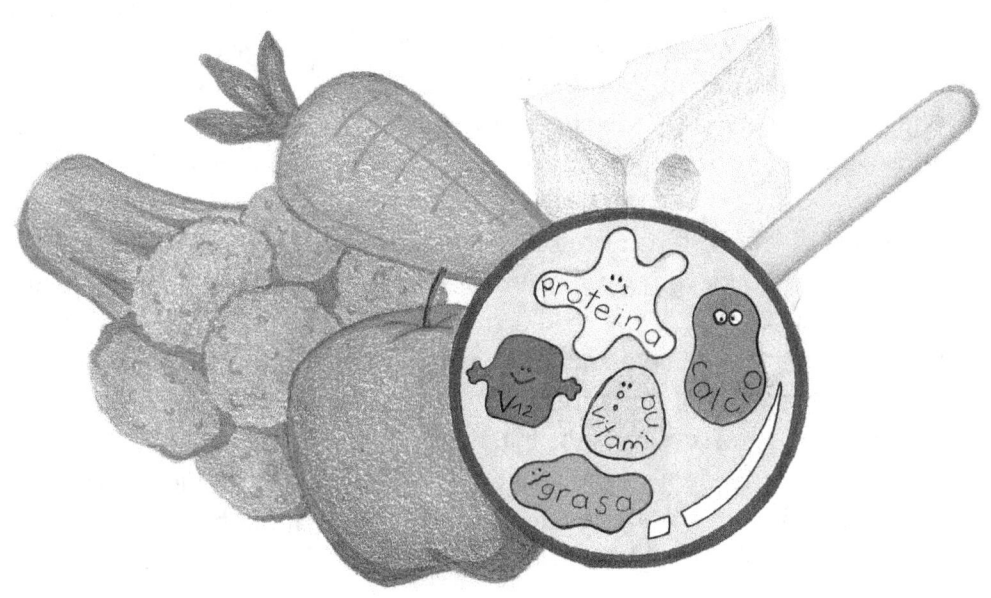

NUTRITION IS THE STUDY of foods and the way they work in our body. Good nutrition is comprised of elements found in food such as vitamins, proteins and fats, which are important nutrients needed for the body's growth and good health. It is important to maintain a balanced diet by consuming nutrient rich foods such as fruits, vegetables, cereals and dairy products, with proteins like lean meats, fish, chicken and turkey. Always remember to read the nutritional value label found on most packaged foods to ensure the food contains the nutrients essential for a good diet.

After the 1970s, the number of children and adolescents with weight problems in the U.S. began to increase. Today, it is estimated, more than nine million children between the ages of five and fifteen are overweight. More than half of adults are either overweight or obese. For children and adults, excess weight can be both a physical and psychological burden that damages their wellbeing and causes many diseases, some of which are life threatening.

A person's weight is the result of a balance between the daily number of calories consumed versus the number of calories burned. If more calories are consumed in one day than are burned, the body will gain weight. If a balance is achieved between the number of calories consumed and the number of calories burned with physical activity and exercise, the ideal weight will be maintained along with healthy growth. In this way, lifestyle changes can demonstrably be shown to improve physical appearance, which in turn may provide for better personal satisfaction.

The Basis Of Treatment

The method used in the treatment of childhood obesity is fundamentally based on the combination of a limited diet, an increase in physical activity, nutritional education and changes in behavior. Treatment will only be effective, however, if the child has the support and encouragement of their family.

Behavior therapy starts by the child learning self-control. To achieve and maintain self-control, it is necessary to provide the child with positive messages of reinforcement and support that will help improve their self-esteem and confidence. In other words, the success of the initial treatment is dependent on alleviating the child's negative feelings of anxiety and depression, which can provoke weight gain.

Prior to treatment, it is important to know the eating habits and behavior of both the child and their family. What, when, where and how often they eat, what kind and how often they exercise and their daily activities. From this analysis the causes of the child's obesity can usually be detected. Changing negative habits through behavior therapy is an essential component to the treatment of a child with excess weight.

Children's behavior is dependent on and responsive to their environment. Parents need to be patient and maintain constant discipline and vigilance so their child does not change the rules and take over management of their treatment. Parents must recognize their child is surrounded by non-stop propaganda on television, billboards, magazines and the internet, most of which is designed to influence what they eat and drink. Unfortunately, their child may also have "sabotaging" friends who pressure them to eat foods that are unhealthy. As a counter-balance, parents need to establish good communications

with their children and clearly explain the reasons why weight loss is so important.

The options available for the treatment of child obesity are limited. For adults with obesity, medications are available that help suppress the appetite or interfere with fat absorption. However, these medicines have not been studied for pediatric usage. Therefore, the primary basis for the treatment of obese children remains diet and exercise, both of which are important to successful weight control.

As mentioned, behavior therapies are useful in the treatment of childhood obesity. The best techniques include establishing a close vigil of the child and maintaining a daily dairy of food their consumption and exercise. Because parents cannot control the access an older child has to food outside the home, the plan usually fails unless a teacher in the child's school is made aware of the treatment and agrees to assist in monitoring what the child eats. For the same reason, parents should also talk to close relatives and friends so they won't unknowingly undermine the child's diet.

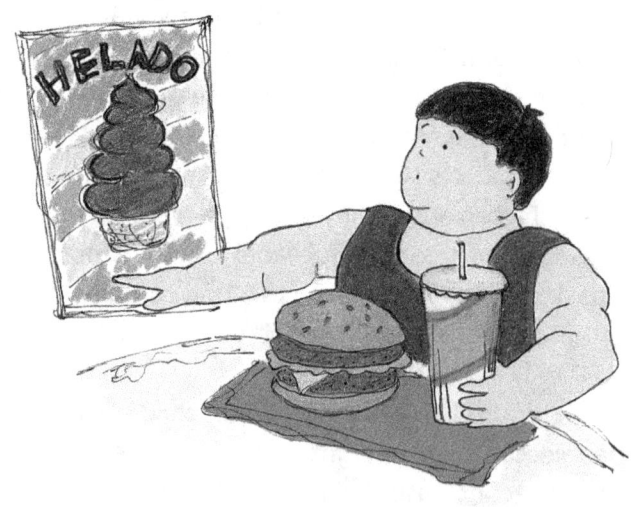

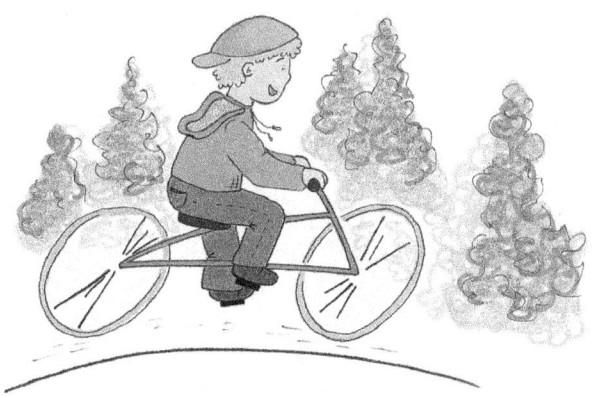

One of the more important behavioral changes requires the child to sit and eat at the table, never in front of the television. Several studies have shown that children who eat in front of a television are more likely to consume a greater number of calories. The child's meals should also be served at regularly scheduled times to minimize any additional food consumption. Strengthening the child's self-esteem and encouraging the child to control his weight with a positive attitude will also contribute to the child's successful treatment.

Obesity is a major problem in our society. Especially since obese children are inclined to be obese adults, with all the associated complications including cardiovascular disease, type II diabetes, arterial hypertension and high cholesterol. Preventive care should include the identification of obesity and any associated complications then the initiation of treatment. It is recommended each child's treatment be personalized with a professional diagnosis.

In summary, the basics of treatment are:
• Change habitual behavior and lifestyle
• Establish and maintain a proper diet
• Perform sufficient daily exercise to burn the daily calories consumed
• Support medical treatment if a specific pathology is found
• Submit to surgical treatment in cases adverse to other medical treatment

With a growing child, the objective of weight control is to maintain their current weight while the child increases in height. This way the child grows into a more appropriate Body Mass Index (BMI). Parents should consult a nutritionist or dietician if they need to know the exact number of calories their child requires. Either professional can help choose the right foods, determine portion sizes, and select exercise routines that should include at least 30 minutes of daily aerobic exercise (walking fast, swimming or riding a bicycle).

To determine if a child is overweight, a Body Mass Index (BMI) calculator can be used. The BMI calculator is a valuable tool widely used to diagnose the development of obesity in children. It has the advantage of counting the height and weight of a child. In practice, the BMI calculator can detect if a child is gaining excessive weight for their height. Unlike adults, the amount of fat in a child varies physiologically with their growth.

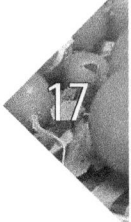

A child with a BMI over 95% is considered overweight. The BMI calculator uses a person's height and weight measurements to estimate their body fat. To calculate the BMI of a child, divide their weight by their height (weight/height). Once the BMI of the child is determined, it can be plotted on a standard BMI chart.

The child will fall into one of four categories:
• Weight below normal: BMI below 5%
• Normal weight: BMI between 5% and 85%
• Overweight: BMI between 85% and 95%
• Obese: BMI over 95%.

The BMI chart will show the weight x height:
• Increases during the first year of life
• Decreases around the age of 6, this is period of maximum growth
• Increases again between the ages of 6 and 8, often recognized as the fat rebound

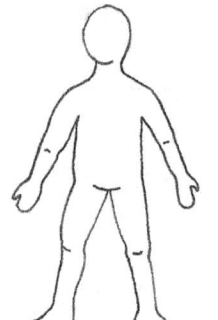 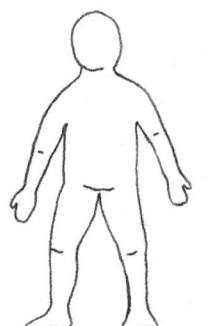 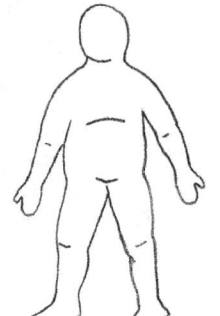 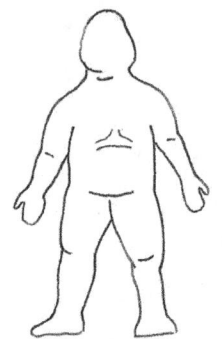 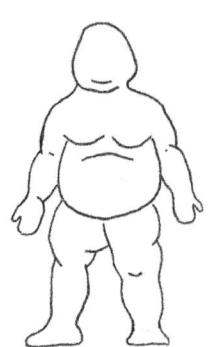

Today, approximately 25% to 28% of children are obese, of even more concern, this is an increased ratio of more than 60% in twenty years.

The problem starts with the form and type of maternal nutrition before conception, through pregnancy until the baby's birth, then continues through breastfeeding, and then into the introduction of solid foods to the child. Because of this, the potential problem of obesity needs to be addressed from the time of expectancy, with

parents taking early responsibility to ensure their child does not become obese.

On the following webpage you will be able to easily calculate a child's body mass index (BMI):

Center for Disease Control and Prevention (CDC)

BMI Calculator for Child and Teen:

http://apps.nccd.cdc.gov/dnpabmi/calculator.aspx

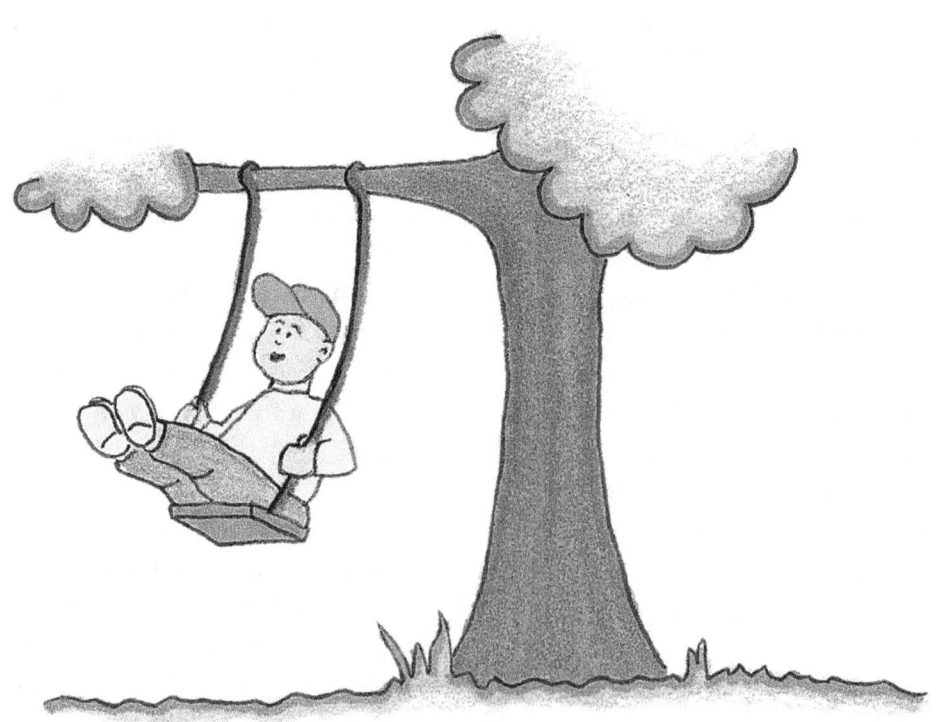

Body Mass Index (IMC/BMI) For Girls

Body Mass Index according to the child's age.

Calculate IMC/BMI first.

Age	IMC/BMI - Low Weight	IMC/BMI - Normal Weight	IMC/BMI - Overweight	IMC/BMI - Obesity
2	less than 13.09	13.09 - 18.08	18.08 - 19.81	more than 19.81
3	less than 13.60	13.60 - 17.56	17.56 - 19.36	more than 19.36
4	less than 13.30	13.30 - 17.28	17.28 - 19.15	more than 19.15
5	less than 13.00	13.00 - 17.15	17.15 - 19.17	more than 19.17
6	less than 13.00	13.00 - 17.34	17.34 - 19.65	more than 19.65
7	less than 13.00	13.00 - 17.75	17.75 - 20.51	more than 20.51
8	less than 13.10	13.10 - 18.35	18.35 - 21.57	more than 21.57
9	less than 13.30	13.30 - 19.07	19.07 - 22.81	more than 22.81
10	less than 13.60	13.60 - 19.86	19.86 - 24.11	more than 24.11
11	less than 13.90	13.90 - 20.74	20.74 - 25.42	more than 25.42
12	less than 14.40	14.40 - 21.68	21.68 - 26.67	more than 26.67
13	less than 15.00	15.00 - 22.58	22.58 - 27.76	more than 27.76
14	less than 15.60	15.60 - 23.34	23.34 - 28.57	more than 28.57
15	less than 16.10	16.10 - 23.94	23.94 - 29.11	more than 29.11
16	less than 16.60	16.60 - 24.37	24.37 - 29.43	more than 29.43
17	less than 17.00	17.00 - 24.70	24.70 - 29.69	more than 29.69
18	less than 17.40	17.40 - 25.00	25.00 - 30.00	more than 30.00

Body Mass Index (IMC/BMI) For Girls

Body Mass Index according to the child's age.

Calculate IMC/BMI first.

Age	IMC/BMI - Low Weight	IMC/BMI - Normal Weight	IMC/BMI - Overweight	IMC/BMI - Obesity
2	less than 14.00	14.00 - 18.41	18.41 - 20.09	more than 20.09
3	less than 13.50	13.50 - 17.89	17.89 - 19.57	more than 19.57
4	less than 13.20	13.20 - 17.55	17.55 - 19.29	more than 19.29
5	less than 13.10	13.10 - 17.42	17.42 - 19.30	more than 19.30
6	less than 13.10	13.10 - 17.55	17.44 - 19.78	more than 19.78
7	less than 13.10	13.10 - 17.92	17.92 - 20.63	more than 20.63
8	less than 13.30	13.30 - 18.44	18.44 - 21.60	more than 21.60
9	less than 13.50	13.50 - 19.10	19.10 - 22.77	more than 22.77
10	less than 13.70	13.70 - 19.84	19.84 - 24.00	more than 24.00
11	less than 14.00	14.00 - 20.55	20.55 - 2510	more than 25.10
12	less than 14.40	14.40 - 21.22	21.22 - 26.02	more than 26.02
13	less than 14.80	14.80 - 21.91	21.91 - 26.84	more than 26.84
14	less than 15.30	15.30 - 22.62	22.62 - 27.63	more than 27.63
15	less than 15.80	1 5.80 - 23.29	23.29 - 28.30	more than 28.30
16	less than 16.30	16.30 - 23.90	23.29 - 28.88	more than 28.88
17	less than 16.80	16.80 - 24.46	24.46 - 29.41	more than 29.41
18	less than 17.10	17.10 - 25.00	25.00 - 30.00	more than 30.00

Defining The Problem

To evaluate the nutritional status of a child, we have provided two "Body Mass Index" (BMI) tables, one for boys and one for girls, based on their age, height and current weight; as related to patterns of growth. These tables will allow parents to classify their children's BMI so they may better understand the state of their children's health and thus better manage the problems of overweight and obesity. Calculating BMI is done in the following ways:

A. Metric Method:

1. Determine the child's current weight. If they are beginning the weight reduction process, it is important to measure them at the same time each week, wearing the same type of clothing and without shoes.

2. Measure the child's height against a wall using a ruler to indicate exactly where to mark height. Make sure the child stands against the wall with feet together and knees straight to avoid mistakes.

3. With these two measurements, use the following mathematical formula:

$$BMI = Weight / (Height)2$$

Example: A 7 year old girl of 1.37 meters height with a body weight of 42 kilograms:

42 / (1.37) 2   then   42 / 1.877 = 22.37 BMI

4. Using this BMI calculation, look on the BMI table that corresponds to the child's sex and age to determine their nutritional classification. Each age and sex has a "healthy weight" value.

In the example, the seven year old girl has a BMI of 22.37 which classifies her as: **Obese**.

Once a problem is defined, proceed accordingly and follow the appropriate diet to achieve a progressive weight loss which will allow the parents and child to develop healthy eating habits. Then set a goal to get the child to their normal weight, understanding the child must not view their goal as being too far away. So do not demand a large weight loss in a single week. One pound or 400 grams per week is more than enough. Remember the child is growing, and sometimes a change in the scale may not be seen. In this case, measure the child's height again and readjust the goal, making sure to reinforce positive motivations so the child does not become discouraged and continues with the treatment.

B. English Unit System:

1. Same as prior "Metric Method" number 1.

2. Same as prior "Metric Method" number 2.

3. With these two measurements use the following mathematical formula: Divide weight by height. Divide the result again by the height. Multiply that result by 703 to get the result.

$$BMI = \left\{ \frac{Weight\ (pounds)}{Height\ (inches)} \right\} X\ 703$$

Example: A boy 6 years of age, 54 inches in height (4.5 feet) and 70 pounds in weight:

70 / 54 = 1.296   then   1.296 / 54 = 0.024
then   0.024 x 703 = 16.87 BMI

4. Using this BMI calculation, look on the BMI table that corresponds to the child's sex and age to determine their nutritional classification. Each age and sex has a "healthy weight" value.

In the example, the six year old boy has a BMI of 16.87 which classifies him as: **Normal**.

Note:

It is important for parents to be aware that in assessing the BMI of their children, they cannot use the same BMI equivalent value as used for adults. Thus, the classification of a "healthy weight" as a BMI of ≤ 25 in adults does not apply to children, as seen by the previous examples.

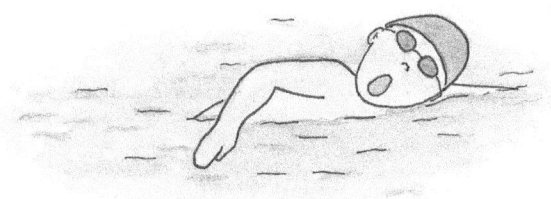

Physical Exercise

Physical activities and diet routines should be planned simultaneously. Initially, an appealing activity should be found that suits the interests and capabilities of the child. Begin with simple movements to which the child can easily become accustomed. If they begin with a strenuous activity it may scare or tire them into rejecting it. Exercise should be done daily, be simple and fun, while also continuously increased. The child should also share their activity with two or three other people.

Important Tips:

• The use of medications in the treatment of childhood obesity has been demonstrated to be mostly ineffective. The primary basis for the treatment of obese children, therefore, remains diet and exercise.

• The earlier a child's weight problem is identified and treated, the better their treatment results will be.

• Treatment is only effective when the obese child has the support and encouragement of their family.

• It is easier to change a child's behavior than that of parents, but achieving parental change benefits everyone.

• Treatment plans are not the same for all obese children. Each child's character, disposition, interests and capabilities are different so treatment must be personalized to meet their individual needs.

• While introducing physical activity into a child's life, also reduce the time they engage in sedentary activities such as watching television.

• The benefit of exercise is directly related to the number of calories burned. During exercise, the stimulation of the thermogenic response rate increases the body's resting metabolic rate.

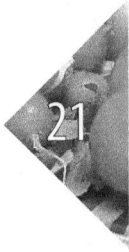

21

• Physical activity increases the capacity for mobilization and fat oxidation. This reduction of body fat can increase muscle mass.

• Regular exercise reduces the body's resistance to insulin, because it increases the transporters of Glut 4 in cells.

• Exercise reduces the levels of bad cholesterol (LDL), at the same time it raises the levels of good cholesterol (HDL)

• There is evidence that aerobic exercise improves cardiopulmonary capacity.

• Exercise and physical activity help to lower level of high blood pressure.

Estimate Of Calories Required

(In kilograms) In groups, by sex and age in three levels of Physical Activity, to lose or maintain a healthy weight

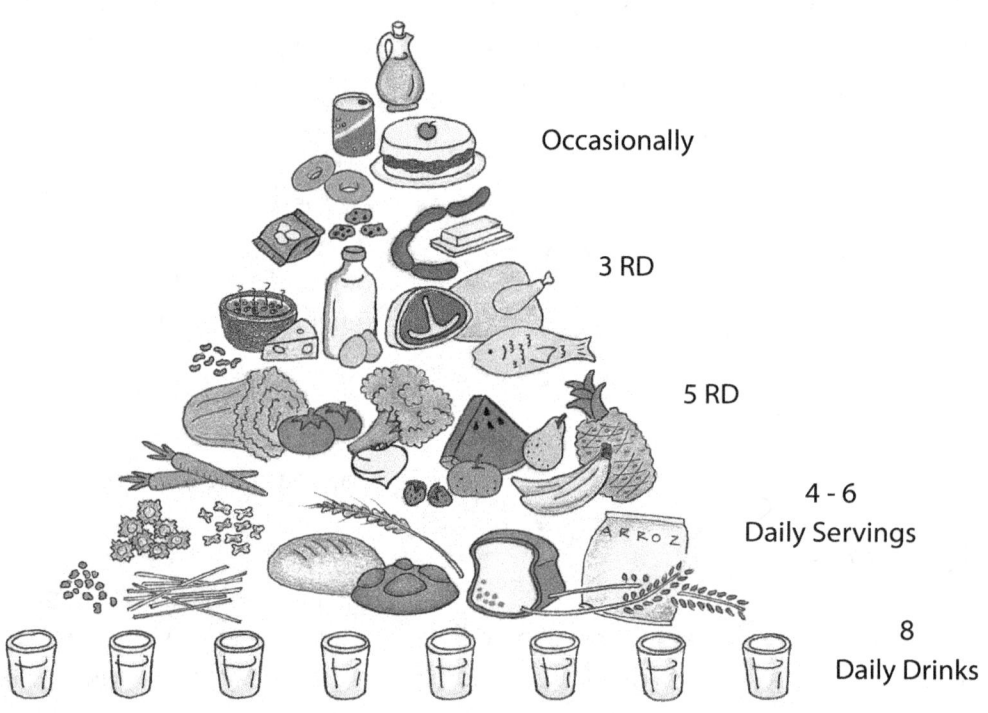

Occasionally

3 RD

5 RD

4 - 6
Daily Servings

8
Daily Drinks

ACTIVITY LEVELS				
SEX	**AGE**	**INACTIVE (b)**	**MODERATELY ACTIVE (c)**	**HIGHLY ACTIVE (d)**
Infant	2 - 3	1.000	1.000 - 1.400	1.000 - 1.400
Girl	4 – 8	1.200	1.400 - 1.600	1.400 - 1.800
	9 - 13	1.600	1.600 - 2.000	1.800 - 2.200
	14 - 18	1.800	2.000	2.400
Boy	4 - 8	1.400	1.400 - 1.600	1.600 - 2.000
	9 - 13	1.800	1.800 - 2.200	2.200 - 2.600
	14 - 18	2.200	2.400 - 2.800	2.800 - 3.200

Fuente: HHS/USDA Dietary Guidelines 2006.

a. These levels are based on estimated energy requirements (EER).
b. Inactive means a lifestyle that contains very little physical activity.
c. Moderately Activity is equivalent to 1.5 to 3 miles of physical activity per day.
d. Highly Active is equivalent to 3 to 4 miles of physical activity per day.

The different levels of calories shown are listed according to age within the corresponding group. Children require more calories than adults.

Guide To Calculate Calories Burned During Normal Activities

SOURCE: www.surgeongeneral.gov/topics/obesity
Sample of the calories burned in 30 minutes

ACTIVITY	CALORIES (burned)
Walking — 2 miles per hour	85
Jogging	170
Gardening	135
Raking leaves	145
Dancing	190
Riding a bicycle — 10 miles per hour	205
Swimming — medium level	240
Running — 5 miles per hour	275

*A person weighing 150 pounds.

 Less weight burns fewer calories and more weight burns more calories.

Each of these activities burns approximately 150 calories.*

REGULAR ACTIVITIES	Less Strength More Time	SPORT ACTIVITIES	Less Strength More Time
Wash & polish car 45 to 60 min.	|	Play volleyball 45 to 60 min.	|
Wash windows & floors 45 to 60 min.	|	Play football 45 min.	|
Garden 30 to 45 min.	|	Walk 1½ miles in 35 min.	|
Drive wheelchair 30 to 40 min.	|	Basketball (shoot hoops) 30 min.	|
Push walker 1½ miles in 30 min.	|	Dancing fast (social) 30 min.	|
Shovel snow 15 min.	|	Water aerobics 30 min.	|
Walk up stairs	|	Swim (hard) 20 min.	|
		Jump rope 15 min.	|
	More Strength Less Time	Run 1½ miles in 15 min.	More Strength Less Time

It is a good idea to vary exercise routines with different types for more effectiveness weight loss.

Calorie Measure vs. Physical Activity

Potato Chips (1 bag, 150 grams)
- 400 cal, 20 g of fat, 5 g of saturated fat.
- Can be burned:
  walking . . . . 93 min.
  swimming. . . . . 33 min.
  bicycle riding. . . . . . . 54 min.

Sausage (1)
- 210 cal, 16 g of fat, 5 g of saturated fat.
- Can be burned:
  walking . . . . 37 min.
  swimming. . . . . 13 min.
  bicycle riding. . . . . . . 28 min.

Mini Pizza (100 grams)
- 290 cal, 11 g of fat, 2 g of saturated fat.
- Can be burned:
  walking . . . . 67 min.
  swimming. . . . . 24 min.
  bicycle riding. . . . . . . 39 min.

Hot Dog on a Bun (1)
- 310 cal, 21 g of fat and 2 g of saturated fat.
- Can be burned:
  walking . . . . 72 min.
  swimming. . . . . 25 min.
  bicycle riding. . . . . . . 42 min.

Meatball (1)
- 60 cal. 4 g of fat and 2 g of saturated fat.
- Can be burned:
  walking . . . . 14 min.
  swimming. . . . . 5 min.
  bicycle riding. . . . . . . 8 min.

Nuts (1 spoon of 20 grams)
- 130 cal, 11 g of fat and 2 g of saturated fat.
- Can be burned:
  walking . . . . 30 min.
  swimming. . . . . 11 min.
  bicycle riding. . . . . . . 18 min.

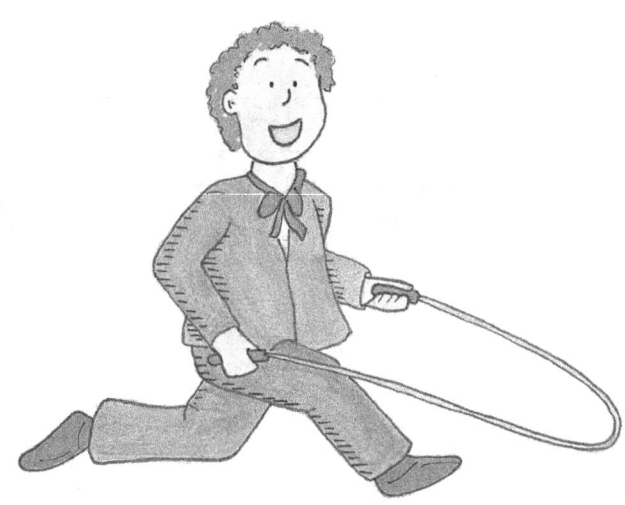

Mayonnaise, (1 tablespoon, 15 grams)
- 110 cal, 12 g fat and 2 g of saturated fat.
- Can be burned:
  walking . . . . 26 min.
  swimming. . . . . 9 min.
  bicycle riding. . . . . . . 15 min.

Empanadas (1)
- 150 cal, 9 g of fat and 4 g of saturated fat.
- Can be burned:
  walking . . . . 35 min.
  swimming. . . . . 12 min.
  bicycle riding. . . . . . . 20 min.

Hamburger (1 regular)
- 230 cal, 8 g of fat and 2 g of saturated fat.
- Can be burned:
  walking . . . . 14 min.
  swimming. . . . . 5 min.
  bicycle riding. . . . . . . 8 min.

Chips, (3, 10 g)
- 55 cal, 4 g of fat, 1 g of saturated fat.
- Can be burned:
  walking . . . . 13 min.
  swimming. . . . . 4 min
  bicycle riding. . . . . . . 7 min.

Peanuts, (1 tablespoon of 20 grams)
- 120 cal, 1 g of fat, 2 g of saturated fat.
- Can be burned:
  walking . . . . 28 min.
  swimming. . . . . 10 min.
  bicycle riding. . . . . . . 16 min.

Waffle, (1 portion of 25 grams)
- 65 cal, 0 g fat and 0 g of saturated fat.
- Can be burned:
  walking . . . . 15 min.
  swimming. . . . . 5 min.
  bicycle riding. . . . . . . 9 min.

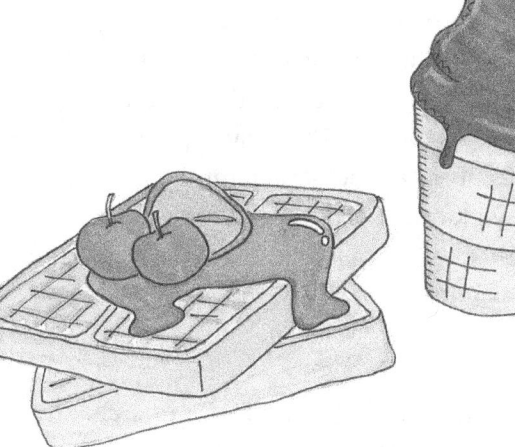

Filled cookies, (2 portions of 60 grams)
- 260 cal, 11 g of fat and 4 g of saturated fat.
- Can be burned:
  walking . . . . 60 min.
  swimming. . . . . 21 min.
  bicycle riding. . . . . . . 35 min.

Ice Cream, (1 scoop)
- 100 cal, 5 g of fat, 3 g of saturated fat.
- Can be burned:
  walking . . . . 23 min.
  swimming. . . . . 8 min.
  bicycle riding. . . . . . . 14 min.

White Cake, (1 slice of 30 grams)
- 130 cal, 7 g of fat and 2 g of saturated fat.
- Can be burned:
  walking . . . . 40 min.
  swimming. . . . . 11 min.
  bicycle riding. . . . . . . 18 min.

Chocolate Covered Ice Cream Bar (1)
- 260 cal, 14 g of fat and 11 g of saturated fat.
- Can be burned:
  walking . . . . 60 min.
  swimming. . . . . 21 min.
  bicycle riding. . . . . . . 35 min.

Fruit Pie, (1 portion of 75 grams)
- 170 cal. 16 g of fat and 10 g of saturated fat.
- Can be burned:
  walking . . . . 40 min.
  swimming. . . . . 14 min.
  bicycle riding. . . . . . . 23 min.

Chocolate, (1 bar of 10 cms)
- 240 cal, 15 g of fat and 9 g of saturated fat.
- Can be burned:
  walking . . . . 56 min.
  swimming. . . . . 19 min.
  bicycle riding. . . . . . . 32 min.

Cream Pie, (1 portion of 90 grams)
- 270 cal, 16 g of fat and 10 g of saturated fat.
- Can be burned:
  walking . . . . 63 min.
  swimming. . . . . 14 min.
  bicycle riding. . . . . . . 37 min.

Candy, (5 units)
- 150 cal, 0 g of fat, 0 gram of saturated fat.
- Can be burned:
  walking . . . . 35 min.
  swimming. . . . . 12 min.
  bicycle riding. . . . . . . 20 min.

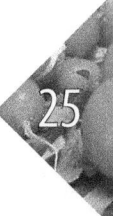

Vary Different Types Of Exercise For More Effective Weight Loss

Even with regular exercise, sometimes immediate results will be difficult to see and a child will complain that their time and effort has not been worthwhile. This may appear true since exercise causes an increase in muscle mass and muscle weighs more than fat, but this weight is healthier. To avoid falling into a routine that uses the same muscles each time, occasionally vary the type of exercise.

It is important for the child to participate in a variety of sports to exercise all the muscles in his body, and allow new targets to be created within the treatment. If the child becomes bored with walking, introduce swimming three times a week instead. If the results from aerobic classes are not good, try another type of exercise such as salsa dancing, or exercises with gym equipment. If bike riding gets old, try running, rope jumping, or playing ball. Even if the child uses the same group of muscles, they will be used in a different way and the change in exercise will burn more calories than usual.

Another important consideration is the inclusion of group sports such as basketball, football and tennis. Group activities can help prevent boredom that can arise over time from repetitious activities. In some cases, if a child is already practicing a sport, there is no need to change to a different one, just vary the activity's routine instead. For example, if they enjoy bike riding, take them to group spinning classes.

Changing sports is also a good way to avoid injuries. Frequently, injuries are the consequence of repeating the same movement, using the same muscles, over and over again, which can cause muscle damage. Varying the physical activity to involve different parts of the body reduces the risk of damaging muscles and joints. Also, if a child in treatment suffers an injury, the whole weight loss process could become endangered. The treatment itself would be delayed, while any immobility caused by the injury could result in the child regaining lost weight and then losing interest in restarting the weight loss process.

Parental Intervention

Obesity is not just a problem of excess weight, but can also cause many illnesses that threaten the well being of the obese child as well as everyone in the family circle.

Many parents "sin" by:
- Pressuring a child to eat more that they need or want.
- Rewarding good behavior with candy and high-calorie snacks.
- Punishing bad behavior by withholding food.
- Celebrating an important event by offering "junk food".
- Providing meals without considering the way they are cooked; in general, fried foods are the easiest option, but the highest in calories.
- Frequently serving pre-cooked "fast food" to save time.
- Allowing the daily casual consumption of "junk food" such as cakes, soda with sugar.

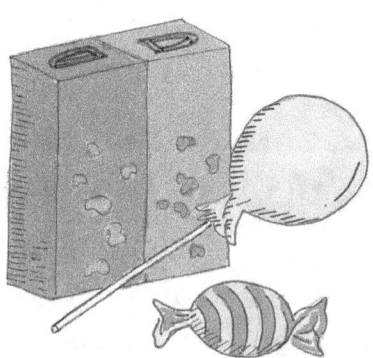

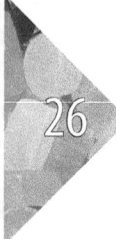

26

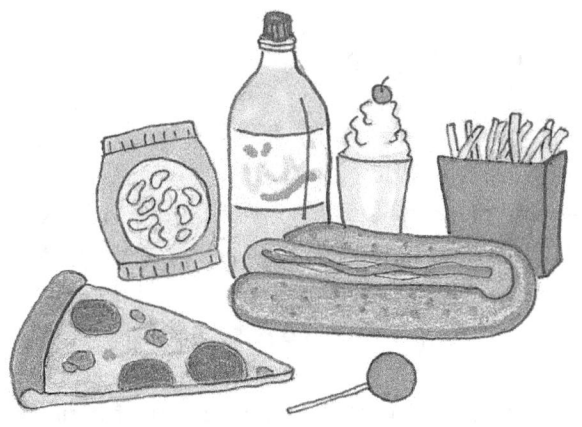

There have also been cases of babies who are born obese. In these cases, a diet appropriate for their nutritional needs should be followed continuously to avoid negative future consequences.

Just because a baby looks "chubby" or is above the recommended weight limit for their age, they will not automatically grow up to be an obese adult. If the parent's manage to keep their baby's weight within the recommended parameters according to age, the baby will develop normally. As the infant grows, naturally so will the number of calories needed and, therefore, consumed though their weight can still remain within their age limit. Once the infant begins to walk, run and become interested in exploring their new world, eating may hold less interest for them. If this happens, the baby should not be forced to eat or given supplements to increase their appetite. These actions would make it impossible for the baby to maintain a normal weight.

Children are born with their own individual tastes and preferences. Some are ready for their first spoonful of cereal at four months of age, while others are not ready until six months. Parents, with their pediatrician's advice, are responsible for making the best nutritional decisions for their child including when to gradually introduce new foods like fruit, vegetables and meats.

Nutrition tips after six months:
The two food groups that can increase a baby's weight:

1. Fruits and cooked vegetables, mashed or pureed (pre-made). It's best to serve vegetables before fruit since children naturally prefer sweets.

2. Fish, chicken and beef, which are protein foods, should be boiled in water or broth.

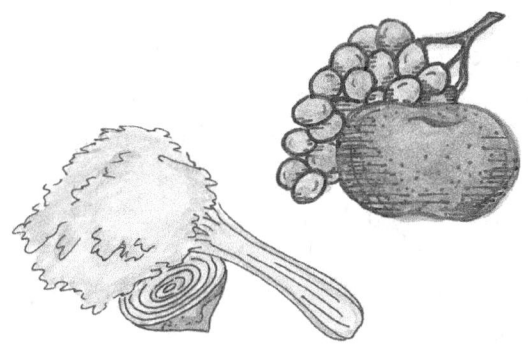

Nutrition tips after nine months:

1. Cut food into small portions so the child does not choke. Offer a good selection of various fruits and vegetables. Adopt a healthy attitude toward meal preparation and make them as attractive and nutritious as possible.

2. Serve soft meats like chicken and fish, (always ensure all bones are removed). Allow the child to eat with their fingers until they develop the ability to hold silverware.

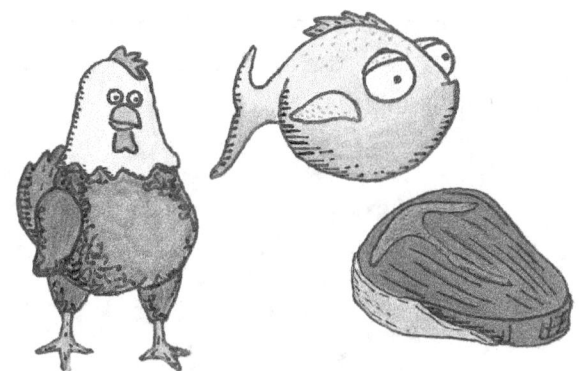

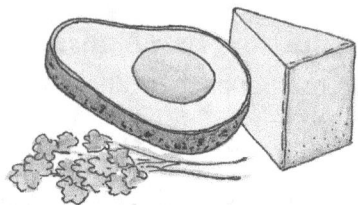

Nutritional tips after eleven months:

1. Always serve the largest possible variety of nutritious foods so the child grows up to eat healthfully as an adult.

2. Do not abuse spices; it is better for the child not to become used to heavily seasoned meals. The more natural the meal, the better. New flavors and textures should be added to the child's diet through the variety of foods offered.

3. Avoid adding salt to meals until the child is at least one year of age.

Factors That Influence Childhood Obesity

Among the many factors that influence childhood obesity:

1. Psychosocial factors:
Environment and lifestyle can significantly influence obesity in children.

a. By relationship between food and affection: the child directly associates the consumption of food with their parents' affection for them.

b. By association: if the child's parents or relatives are obese, the child will perceive being overweight as normal.

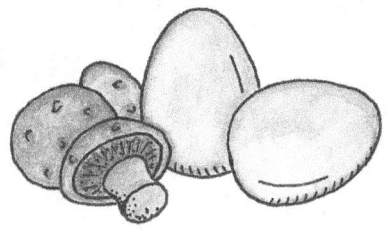

2. Energy burning:

a. Each child in a family does not consume the same amount of food. And while some of the children may maintain a normal weight, others may be overweight. In this case, their differences should be discussed with them at an early age and the consequences of overeating explained.

b. Food portions should not be equal for all school-age children since an elementary child requires less food than a high school teenager.

c. When determining the number of calories a child requires, include in the calculations that child's daily physical activities.

3. Genetic factors:

a. Hereditary: obesity is frequently diagnosed as a hereditary condition within a family.

b. Cushing Syndrome: This is a disorder of the adrenal gland that causes an increase in the production of cortisol and leads to obesity.

4. Hormonal factors:

a. Insulinoma: a rare tumor in the pancreas that secretes insulin and can lead to obesity.

b. Hypothyroidism: decreased thyroid hormone secretion that can lead to obesity.

c. Hypogonadism: a decrease in production of the hormone testosterone in men that causes an increase in fat tissue and can lead to obesity.

5. Pathological factors:

a. Cardiovascular Disease: pulmonary or certain cancer that occur in a family's medical history can be the cause of obesity.

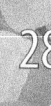

b. Polycystic Ovary Syndrome: the most common cause of obesity in young women, it's associated with menstrual cycle irregularities, acne, hirsutism and insulin resistance syndrome.

c. Hypothalamic Disorders: certain tumors, inflammation or trauma of the central nervous system can cause changes in the regulatory centers that control satisfaction.

Healthy Nutrition For Adolescents

Balancing nutrition and recreation

You have decided to take care of yourself by eating healthy. Congratulations!

Eating healthy is the best way to:
- Have energy throughout the day.
- Get the vitamins and minerals needed daily.
- Maintain strength to perform sports and other activities.
- Reach a maximum height.
- Maintain an optimal weight.
- Prevent unhealthy eating habits.

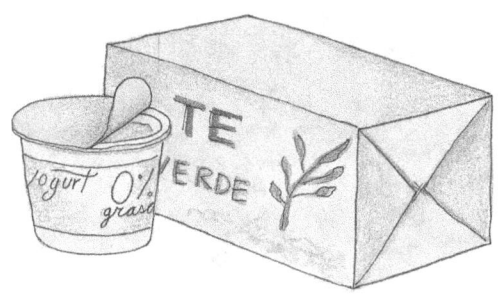

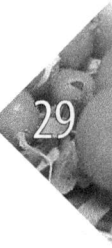

What does eating healthy mean?

- Eating meals and snacks at the proper time.

- Eating a selection from all the food groups to fulfill growth and health needs.

- Balancing high nutrition foods with moderate to small quantities of other foods such as candy and fast food.

- Eating when hungry and stopping when full.

- Learning more about nutrition and making it an important part of daily life.

Tips For Healthy Eating

1. Don't skip meals – plan meals and snacks.

- Surprisingly, eating 3 meals and 2 snacks per day is a better way to maintain higher levels of energy and a healthy weight. Excess hunger makes you more inclined to overeat or select foods low in nutrition.

- Are you eating out? Don't feel left out. Either take foods with you or find places where you can order food that is healthy and satisfying.

2. Learn to prepare simple, healthy foods.

- Instead of frying, try baking, boiling, grilling and microwave cooking as healthier alternatives.

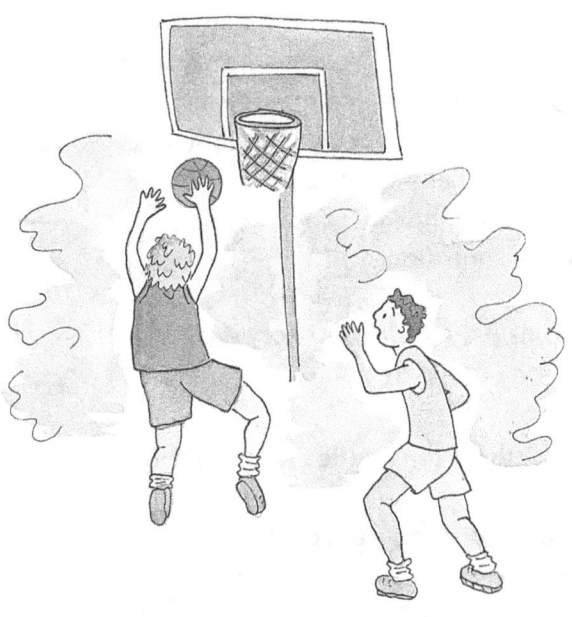

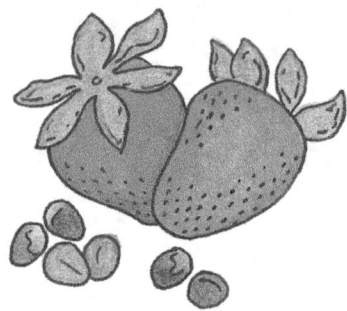

• Use dry herbs (basil, oregano, parsley) and spices (lemon pepper, chili powder, and garlic salt) to flavor food, instead of adding butter, margarine and heavy sauces.

• Remove the skin and fat from your meats. It will retain the nutrition you need and rich flavor you enjoy, but it will be healthier for your heart!

3. Sugar is "empty energy" – avoid eating too much.

• Carbonated drinks and refreshments are a big source of empty energy. This means they contain a large amount of nutritionally unnecessary sugar and very few vitamins, minerals, proteins or fiber. Even unsweetened juices contain a lot of sugar. Instead of sodas and juices, drink diet beverages or sugar free powder drinks and water. But don't exaggerate, it is acceptable to have two small glasses of regular soda or juice a day.

• Sugar is found in desserts, cookies and candy. Occasionally, allow these foods in your diet, but do not let them replace nutritious foods.

4. Pay attention to your body and what you eat.

• Eat slowly. It takes your body a minimum, of 20 minutes to feel satisfied, so try to relax, chew slowly and stretch out your meal.

• Listen to your body. Eat when you are hungry, stop eating when you are full. This will help your body balance its energy needs and feel comfortable. Ask yourself: Am I eating because I am hungry, or because I am anxious or bored?

• Eat foods that are hot (soups, porridge,) and foods high in fiber (whole grains, vegetables, beans) to make you feel full.

5. Stay healthy and happy – avoid thinking about diets.

• There is no such thing as good or bad food. All food consumed in moderation can be part of a healthy diet.

• You do not need to purchase diet or fat free food. Fat free or dietetic foods are not necessarily low in calories and some of them have sugar added to replace fat.

• You are more important than your weight or the size of your body – believe it! Your health and happiness can be affected by drastic diets.

• If you have not yet reached your adult height, excessive weight loss could interfere with your growth, even if you are overweight. For youngsters who are still developing, it is more important to maintain a stable weight as you grow than to focus on weight loss. If you are overweight and want to make changes in your food intake and lifestyle, ask your doctor to refer you to a nutritionist.

Support For Adolescents With Eating Disorders

A Guide For Families And Close Friends

Eating disorders affect millions of children. If you are reading this book, more than likely you are a relative or friend of an adolescent suffering from an eating disorder. It is normal to feel helpless or confused at times. But learning about these disorders can help you provide better support.

Please note that not all suggestions are appropriate for everyone. This guide was created to offer ideas on how to help a child with an eating disorder. It is important to understand this guide does not replace the recommendations and care of a doctor, therapist or nutritionist.

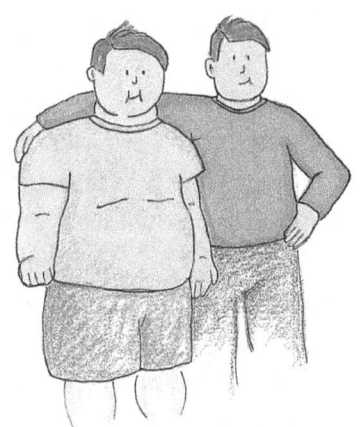

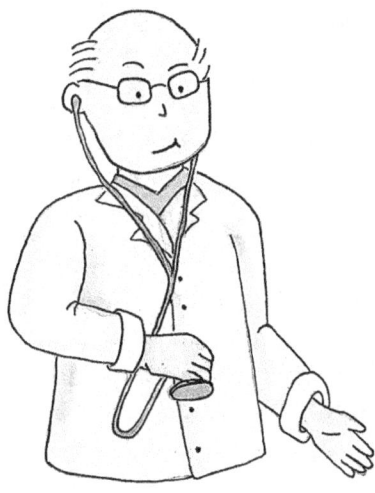

The road to recovery

Be patient. Try to find progress on a weekly not daily basis. Remember, it takes a long time to develop an eating disorder.

They can be triggered by multiple events. Years of messages from the media, food industry and peer groups contribute to shaping eating behavior and perceptions of body image. These negative messages affect the thoughts of adolescents with eating disorders.

There is no fast treatment or cure. It takes time to recover from these disorders because the treatment involves changing both the way of thinking and behavior. Expect the road to recovery to take time.

Offer support during meal and snack times

Eat together. Meal and snack times are the most difficult of the day. Eating can be a source of anxiety for them, and usually requires support and supervision. Generally, these teens feel very guilty about eating. If someone they trust eats with them, it can make the eating experience more enjoyable.

Keep conversations positive. Engage in neutral topics during meals and do not focus on the food or its calories or fat content. Try to talk about fun things instead, like their favorite sports teams, music, or hobbies.

Establish an eating pact. Agree before not to discuss eating disorder issues, like the size of food portions, calories or fat content. Many adolescents with eating disorders have continuously negative thoughts about food. An eating pact may reduce the tension and stress they usually associate with food.

Plan ahead as a family and agree on the structure of meals; the time, menu selection and who will be present during the meal.

Food shopping: new food

Go food shopping together. Explore a favorite market or visit a new one. Seek out new products and set an objective to try a new item each week. Often adolescents with eating disorders create a list of "safe" foods they are permitted to eat. Generally, these foods are low in fat, calories and carbohydrates. During their recovery, it is important to increase their selection of foods. A nutritionist can help establish these goals.

Make sure all these foods are readily available. This will help reduce their stress at mealtime. Sometimes, if a food is missing from the meal, the teen may panic and limit their food intake.

Cook together and try new recipes

Many adolescents enjoy cooking with someone they trust. Learning to cook is another recovery skill. Trying new recipes also helps to increase their list of "safe" foods.

Healthy attitude

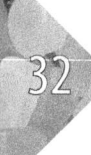

Encourage new interests. Propose activities such as art classes, volunteer service, music or yoga. It is important to replace disordered eating behaviors (excessive exercise, restrictive diets, etc.) with new behaviors and interests. Generally, these adolescents' interests are very limited, since they are obsessed with the idea of losing weight, dieting and ritualistic exercises. It is difficult for them to break their patterns of behavior, however, trying new activities can help replace disordered behavior and eventually improve their self-esteem.

Organize a special event

Make an appointment at a hair or nail salon or to have a massage. While recovering from an eating disorder, important changes in body, face, hair and general appearance occur. Often teenagers do not feel deserving of good things. Planning a special event can provide a positive

way for your teen or friend to adjust to their new image. It is a way of showing them they are deserving of a special and enjoyable event..

Plan a shopping trip

While recovering, their body will transform. Buy some new clothes, but not a whole wardrobe. Going shopping together in a new store or at a new shopping center can be fun.

Talking to teens

Try not to make direct commentary about a teenager's physical appearance or body shape. Comments like: "How many pounds did you gain?" Or "You look better, you've gained weight," or "You look wonderful!" or "Have you lost weight? What's happening? "make them feel very uncomfortable. Even though adolescents usually look healthier, brighter, stronger and better nourished during recovery, they frequently interpret such comments in a negative way. The comment, "You look much better now that you're not only skin and bones." will be interpreted as "I'm fat!" by a teenager with an eating disorder.

Comment on their health and energy level

Comments that acknowledge their improved health but do not focus on their size or shape are more appropriate, (such as "You look full of energy!" or "You look rested.") and make them feel supported in their journey of recovery.

Smile! Joy is contagious

A happy, cheerful and optimistic attitude creates wonders! It is very difficult to watch someone you love struggle with an illness. But your tears and worry can increase an adolescent's feelings of guilt about their disease, which adds to their anguish, anxiety, self-despair and depression. Therefore, it is very important to project optimism. A simple smile can transmit a message of hope and joy to adolescents with eating disorders.

Stay positive!

Sharing a positive attitude can be of great help to a loved one struggling with an eating disorder and body image concerns.

Go to www.nationaleatingdisorders.org to find "Ten Steps To Positive Body Image" and for suggestions on how to fight negative thoughts.

Remember

"You, as parents, are a key factor in your children's education about eating habits."

Summary Of Obesity Complications

There is a danger that a childhood obesity may cause other complications and problems that can reduce a child's life expectancy:

• Psychological problems:
low self-esteem caused by bullying, rejection and teasing from their peers.

• Psychological disorders:
bulimia, anorexia and depression caused by feelings of isolation and which can lead to drug and substances abuse.

• Physical problems:
diabetes type II, arterial hypertension and high levels of cholesterol.

• Orthopedic problems:
arthritis, epiphytical femur and vertebral problems.

• Respiratory problems:
apnea syndrome, aggravated asthma.

• Digestive problems:
gallbladder stones, fatty liver disease.

• Cancer:
some types are associated with obesity and poorly balanced nutrition, such as uterus, breast, and colon cancers.

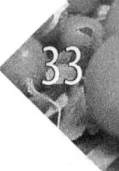

33

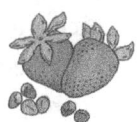

Does Childhood Obesity Have Consequences In Adulthood?

The probability of the persistence of childhood obesity into adulthood increases with the age of the child, (20 to 50% in pre-pubertal, and 50 to 70% in adolescence). The risks associated with a family history of obesity are greater when a child is younger. With the child's increasing age, the degree of their obesity becomes more predictable.

The long-term risks from other pathologies associated with obesity can only be evaluated through epidemiological studies, which relate the degree of obesity in childhood, with diseases or deaths that occurred in a period of prolonged observation. These studies provide our only source of data. These epidemiological studies concluded that obesity in children is associated with a 50% to 80% increase in the adult death risk. In all studies that provided comparison, except for one, the risk was greater in boys.

The majority of deaths presented were of cardiovascular origin. The only study with data regarding body mass index (BMI) in adulthood, suggests that an increase of risk associated with childhood obesity is not entirely explained by the persistence of obesity into adulthood.

Good And Bad Nutrition

To improve nutritional education and achieve goals, mistakes must be recognized and habits changed to rectify them. For clarity, it is always good to verify that correct eating habits are being practiced.

Mistakes In Nutrition

Food isn't a reward, or a punishment and shouldn't be used as an outlet for stress. Food should have its time, place, and be controlled.

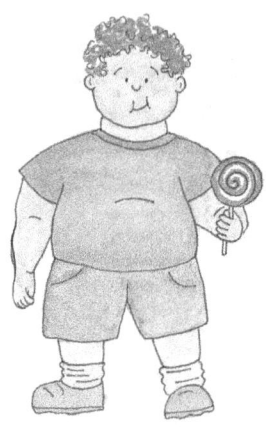

Parents are the most responsible for their children being overweight since they decide and control what is consumed in their home. Either by mistake, obsession or lack of parental knowledge, overweight children often consume large quantities of food: meats, processed foods, snacks and candy, but do not eat vegetables, greens, fruits or fish.

Additionally, many children leave home in the morning without breakfast. The last research regarding overweight children found that 8% of children attended school without breakfast. Yet breakfast is the most important meal of the day and is directly related to weight control.

Truths In Nutrition

When parents provide children and their nutritional needs with the proper care and attention, they lower the probability of excess weight gain. Adult control is fundamental to preventing child obesity, especially since a child's first years of life are crucial in their education. Therefore, it is necessary for parents to observe some dietary guidelines:

• Establish control of food consumption from the beginning of a child's life. Babies do not need to breastfeed on demand. Just like sleeping, infants can be taught a feeding schedule and still be satisfied.

• Understand that babies do not only cry from hunger, but for other reasons as well. So do not automatically offer breastfeeding without first determining the cause of the child's distress and offering alternative comfort. Indiscriminate feeding can lead to life-long consequences if an association with food as an emotional pacifier is carried into adulthood.

• Schedule regular pediatric visits. It has been demonstrated that children who receive regular medical supervision are less likely to suffer from obesity or other diseases.

• Understand and memorize the pediatrician's month-to-month nutritional recommendations for your baby. Respecting guidelines and introducing foods according to a child's age, is a good way of preventing weight problems.

• Select as large a variety of foods as possible until two years of age. This provides a baby with the opportunity to educate their palette by tasting a little bit of everything, as well as gain access to a larger variety of nutrients.

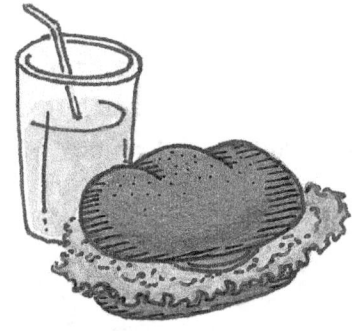

• Establish a consistent routine to ensure children do not skip any meals.

• Prepare meals using fresh and natural ingredients whenever possible, and consider the consumption of "organic" products. Also, do not think of food shopping as "spending" but rather "investing" in a healthier future for your children and their family.

• Consult the graphic of weights and measures provided in this book with your pediatrician. If your child falls outside the normal weight range, discuss with your doctor ways to improve the situation or consult a nutritionist for assistance.

• Offer balanced nutrition by varying meats, pastas, vegetables, fruits, etc. Remember that, "good nutrition begins in the supermarket". What we bring home in our grocery bags is what we will eat throughout the week.

• Provide children with plenty of daily fluids, especially after physical exercise and in extreme heat. Water is a great source without calories.

Reaching The Ideal Weight — How to Keep It Permanently

Once the ideal weight has been reached, how do you maintain it permanently? A great deal of effort has been invested in providing parents with tips, tricks and advice on how to help children lose excess weight. However, the real difficulty is not weight loss, but maintaining a healthy diet and lifestyle once their ideal weight has been achieved. If this is not worked on, children can very quickly and easily regain their lost weight. Many mothers have been heard to lament over this predicament — they do not want their children to remain overweight, and especially not obese.

Keep in mind the following recommendations in which willpower and discipline once again play key roles in achieving this objective:

- Parents and children should remember the mathematical formula that balances the daily amount of calories ingested with the amount of energy expended in daily physical activity. If the former (calories) is greater than the latter (energy), weight increase will occur automatically.

- Teach children that weight loss is not a "temporary change" but a long-term, lifetime achievement necessary for a fuller, healthier life.

- To maintain control of an "ideal" weight, within a margin of two or three kilograms, a child's weight should continue to be measured once a week so their level of physical activity versus food intake can be adjusted. Remember, the child is growing so their weight will gradually increase. For guidance, consult the BMI tables in this book.

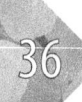

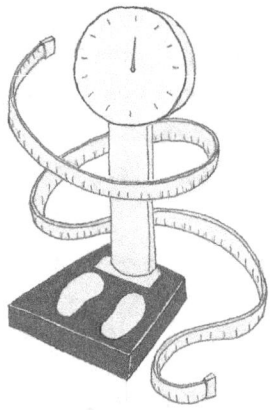

- Regular exercise has been proven to be the key essential to preventing excess weight gain – diet alone is not as effective. Exercise can help children maintain their energy balance, improve muscular function and reduce the risk of depression while also helping them avoid the temptation of overeating.

- Parents should be aware that fats and sweets, while very energizing, do not satisfy the appetite for very long. It is much better to offer children foods that contain fiber in large quantity.

- Since appetite has an important psychological component, it is important for children to feel they've had enough to eat. For example, serve salad as a first course and meals on smaller plates so children think they ate more. Also remind them to chew their food slowly and well so they will remain at the table longer and be more satisfied when they are finished.

- If parents and children recognize during treatment that fruits and vegetables are vital allies to their weight loss effort, it will help them both lose weight and keep it off in the future .

- While on family vacation, plan your child's meals to allow them occasional excess.

- Keep on hand low calorie foods your child is permitted to eat, such as cheese, diet yogurt, baby carrots, and tangerines, etc.

- Ensure children do not have excessive salt in their diets. Salt causes water retention and adds to body weight. Try to avoid pre-packaged foods since they usually contain high levels of salt.

- If your child's weight exceeds their target weight by 5 kilos, return them to the treatment's diet period to prevent the return of obesity.

Teaching Good Nutritional Habits From Infancy

The new arrival of a baby is a joyful event, but can also be a time of doubt and insecurity. In an effort to assist parents, the Spanish Association of Pediatrics in collaboration with Dodot, recently published a **Childcare Manual** to be used as a reference guide for the caring and welfare of infants. With simplified

language and scientific structure it provides answers to parents most common concerns and doubts about their baby's nutrition, hygiene, rest, safety, behavior and development.

The **Childcare Manual** consists of nine chapters, which address a range of issues from childbirth through the first three years of a child's development, and includes aspects related to being a parent. While the manual is a useful tool designed for fast and easy use by parents, it is not intended as a substitute for a child's need of a pediatrician's care.

The manual offers basic recommendations to accompany the changes and novelties of this moment of joy, especially for first time parents. It addresses the simplest subjects, such as preparing the baby's room with necessary items, to the most frequent problems parents face, all with the goal of making them feel more confident and secure when it comes time to meet their baby for the first time.

"The most important thing is to eat and sleep well". These are without doubt, the two main worries for many parents in the first weeks of a baby's life. The merits of breastfeeding, as the best source of nutrition, and its continuation is emphasized to parents, especially mothers. A non-aggressive weight loss program, controlled by the pediatrician, often eases the mother.

In the beginning, breastfeeding needs to be managed according to demand, without a schedule. Progressively, a schedule may be established after the baby's proper weight and nutritional needs have been deemed satisfactory. Sleeping is managed in the same manner. The baby becomes accustomed to daytime and nighttime cycles through good parental habits. During the day, parents allow moderate noise, take rides and interact with the baby; during the night, parents promote silence, tranquility, and use dim lighting. These methods help the baby gradually adapt to the differences between day and night, and is achieved with their parents' patience and pediatrician's advice.

Generally, pediatricians are strong supporters of breastfeeding. Pediatric academies worldwide consider it ideal for infants to be breastfeed for at least six months, and even longer when possible. However, after between four and six months, breastfeeding may become more difficult for mothers, due to external complications like their work schedules. Sometimes, managing to breastfeed for even four months can be an achievement. If for any reason breastfeeding is not possible, artificial milk is a safe and nutritious alternative. Ask your pediatrician to explain the alternatives.

Today, an increased number of children are being diagnosed as allergic to milk, eggs, gluten, etc. This is not due to their parents' error, but because doctors are now better able to diagnose and treat children utilizing new and improved methods. What used to be diagnosed as colic or diarrhea is now attributed to lactose intolerance.

The same is true for gluten, for which celiac disease is diagnosed more often due to more precise analysis. Before, celiac children were only diagnosed once they became ill with diarrhea and other symptoms. Now, thanks to new medical techniques, doctors can diagnose even the mildest cases.

The increasing diagnosis of childhood obesity requires an increased need for nutritional education and good eating habits taught from infancy. In Spain, we are lucky to have the Mediterranean diet, perhaps one of the most important traditions of the country. From the beginning, complementary nutrition includes vegetables, carbohydrates, milk, fruits, proteins in the form of fish, chicken or veal, etc. Following these dietary guidelines helps prevent obesity.

A baby's pacifier is not a tool of convenience but of necessity. When an infant suctions, first its mother's breast then a bottle, it is pacified. The pacifier was made for this function and withdrawal should begin at around two years of age, more or less. However, this can sometimes be difficult to accomplish.

New mothers may feel overwhelmed by the mass of information and opinions offered to her by relatives, friends, books, the internet, etc. But her first visit to the pediatrician, in the first week to ten days (earlier if there appears to be a problem), should help to reassure her. In a way, the doctor acts as an information filter who uses medical knowledge and experience to counter common myths, family lore and advice that is not applicable to the child. It is imperative that parents consult a pediatrician to discuss and alleviate their concerns.

The arrival of a new baby can be complicated if a sibling is already at home. In this case, to promote a healthy atmosphere with normal developmental boundaries, parents should try to retain a feeling of normalcy. Explain to the sibling that all things are better shared, even parents love. Accept this older child will experience moments of frustration, depression, indignation or jealousy. But learning to overcome this first childhood frustration will ultimately contribute to the child's development into a strong self-confident adult. For this reason, it is recommended the child be allowed some leniency in expressing their feelings since suppressing them can lead to emotional disorders and bad eating habits, especially with first-born children.

*Credit for the **Childcare Manual** is given to Valentin Pineda, a pediatric consultant and head of pediatric hospitalization and the Pediatric Infectious Diseases Unit of Sabadell Hospital, Spain.*

Food Portion Measurements

Hand Symbol	Equivalent	Food	Calories
	Fistful (1 cup)	Rice, Pastas Fruits Vegetables	200 75 40
	Open Palm 85 g (3 ounces)	Red Meat Fish Pork	160 160 160
	Handful 28 g (1 ounce)	Nuts Raisins	170 85
	2 Handfuls 56 g (2 ounces)	Potatoes Popcorn Pretzels	150 120 100
	Thumb 28 g (1 ounce)	Peanut Butter Cheese	170 100
	Thumb Tip 1 teaspoon	Oil Mayonnaise, Butter Sugar	40 35 15

Introductory Diet

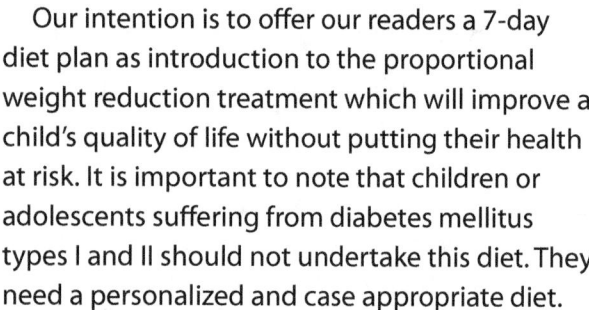

This diet has been tested in the clinic with over a thousand overweight and obese children and adolescents who have verified its functionality.

Our intention is to offer our readers a 7-day diet plan as introduction to the proportional weight reduction treatment which will improve a child's quality of life without putting their health at risk. It is important to note that children or adolescents suffering from diabetes mellitus types I and II should not undertake this diet. They need a personalized and case appropriate diet.

Years ago, fasting was considered one of the most important prescriptions made by a doctor to cure a disease. Fasting is a system used to cleanse the body and mind of impurities. We experience this ourselves when out bodies lose appetite during an illness. Doctors believed an accumulation of "toxins" in the body caused illness and fasting aided in the elimination of these toxins from our bodies.

During the first few days of treatment, physical discomfort such as headaches, dizziness and nausea may occur; these symptoms are normal reactions to the body disposing of its toxic residue. They will disappear in a couple of days.

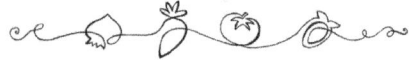

FIRST DAY

BREAKFAST

- 1 glass of mineral water (not carbonated).

- 1 cup of low fat yogurt (no sugar or fruit). (Don't use fat free yogurt; does not provide the same feeling of satisfaction. Don't replace for milk; lactic acid speeds weight loss.)

- 2 spoonfuls of Muesli (without sugar), added to the yogurt.

- Apple and cinnamon tea (without sugar). (See preparation to follow.)

10 A.M.

- 1 fruit.

- 1 glass of mineral water. (To cleanse all the organs, liberate retained water and drain the skin from the inside.)

LUNCH

- Wild rice (without salt).
  Ingredients:
  ½ cup of wild rice
  1 cup of water
  1 spoonful of olive oil "extra virgin"
  Preparation:
  Wash the rice and let it soak in the cup of water for an hour before cooking. Then cook it as any other type of rice with the olive oil.

- Salad with a variety of fresh greens: alfalfa, broccoli, spinach, different kinds of lettuce, cucumber, red or yellow pepper, (no green pepper — they produce gas), radishes and tomato. Squeeze lemon juice on top but no salt, additives or commercial dressing.

- 1 glass of homemade ice fruit tea.
  Preparation:
  To make fruit tea, pour ½ gallon of water into a jar with 4 bags of 100% organic fruit tea.

Place in refrigerator for 1 or 2 hours. Before drinking, add ice and lemon to taste.

Tea with cinnamon sticks
Warm the water until it turns the color of the cinnamon. Pour into jar, then store in refrigerator. Serve with a stick of cinnamon inside of glass. (Helps digestion and activates the metabolism.)

Apple tea with cinnamon
Peel 2 green apples, cut them into fours then cook in 2 liters of water until color appears. Let water cool then store in refrigerator. Can be served hot or cold.

3 P.M.

- 1 glass of homemade vegetable juice with fruit. Use fresh vegetables, preferably organic grown, and a juice processor.
  Slim Combo Preparation:
  Mix ½ cup of carrot juice with
  1 pear and
  1 pink grapefruit. (Acids help digestion and burn calories.)

- Apple and cinnamon tea (without sugar).

- 1 fruit.

DINNER

- Vegetable salad.

- 1 glass of homemade fruit juice (no sugar).

8 P.M.

- Apple and cinnamon tea (without sugar).

- 1 glass of fresh fruit juice.

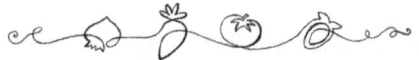

SECOND DAY

BREAKFAST

- 1 glass of mineral water.

- Apple and cinnamon tea (without sugar).

- 1 glass of fresh fruit juice.

- ½ big banana or 1 whole small one. (Bananas contain three different types of natural sugar along with fiber to provide instant energy at breakfast. Athletes recommend them. Remember to follow portion sizes as directed since the goal is to lose weight.)

10 A.M.

- 1 glass of fresh fruit juice.

- Apple and cinnamon tea (without sugar).

- 1 fruit.

LUNCH

- Homemade vegetable soup.
  Ingredients:
  1 medium onion
  1 tomato
  ¼ chicken
  ¼ cup of green peppers cubed
  ½ celery stick
  1 medium carrot
  ½ cup of jams cubed
  2 cups of water
  Preparation:
  Combine all of the ingredients and cook for approximately ½ hour. (Do not add any spices or package soups.)

- 1 slice of whole wheat bread.

3 P.M.

- 1 glass of homemade vegetable juice with fruit.

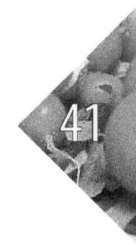

The Fat Burner Preparation:
Mix ¾ cup (6 oz.) of beet juice with ½ cup (4 oz.) of fresh orange juice.
(An extra portion of iron stimulates the metabolism to burn fat and vitamin C strengthens the tissues.)

• 1 fruit.

DINNER

• Homemade vegetable soup (see lunch).

• 1 glass of fresh fruit juice.

8 P.M.

• 1 cup of apple and cinnamon tea (no sugar).

• 1 glass of mineral water.

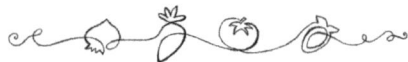

THIRD DAY

DAY OF FASTING

• As discussed before, regular fasting detoxifies the body and releases retained water. (Recommended for a Saturday, when there is no school and you can supervise your child.)

• Consume at least 6 to 8 cups of apple and cinnamon tea or fruit tea, and 6 to 8 glasses of mineral water.

• Refrain from excessive physical activity today.

BREAKFAST

• 2 glasses of fresh squeezed orange juice with pulp.

• 1 cup of apple and cinnamon tea (no sugar).

10 A.M.

• 1 glass of fresh fruit juice prepared in water

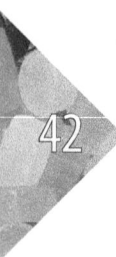

(no milk or sugar). (Watermelon and melon are refreshing fruits that contain 90% water.)

NOON

• 1 glass of vegetable juice.

• 1 cup of vegetable broth.

• 1 glass of fruit ice tea.

4 P.M.

• 1 glass of homemade vegetable juice with fruit.
Vital Shake Preparation:
Mix 1 celery stick, 1 apple and ½ cucumber. (Combines diuretic properties with a high content of mineral to improve organs and accelerate your metabolism.)

7 P.M.

• 1 cup of vegetable broth.

• 1 glass of fresh fruit juice.

FOURTH DAY

BREAKFAST

• 1 glass of mineral water.

• Apple or cinnamon tea (without sugar).

• 1 glass of fresh fruit juice.

10 A.M.

• 1 fruit.

LUNCH

• Fresh vegetable soup.

• 2 whole wheat crackers.

3 P.M.

- 1 fruit.

- 1 glass of homemade vegetable juice with fruit.
  Energetic Preparation:
  Mix ½ small papaya with
  ½ cup carrot extract,
  ½ cup of mineral water and
  2 teaspoons of lemon juice. (Fructose is instant energy, magnesium loosens fat cells and vegetable estrogen is good for the skin.)

DINNER

- Homemade vegetable soup.

- 2 whole wheat crackers.

8 P.M.

- Aromatic tea (fruit tea, without sugar).

- 1 glass of fresh fruit juice.

FIFTH DAY

BREAKFAST

- 1 cup of low fat yogurt (no sugar or fruit).

- Apple and cinnamon tea (without sugar).

10 A.M.

- 1 fruit.

- 1 glass of fresh fruit juice.

LUNCH

- Fresh vegetable salad with dressing of ¼ avocado mashed.

- 1 serving of steamed vegetables

- Wild Rice

- 1 glass of mineral water or fruit tea (no sugar).

3 P.M.

- 1 fruit.

- 1 glass of vegetable juice with fruit.
  Enzyme Wonder Preparation:
  Mash ½ of small papaya, add
  1½ cups of vegetable juice and
  2 teaspoons of chopped basil.
  (Papaya burns albumin faster and helps weight loss.)

- 1 glass of mineral water or fruit tea (no sugar).

DINNER

- Fresh vegetable salad.

- 2 whole wheat crackers.

- Apple and cinnamon tea (without sugar).

8 P.M.

- 1 glass of fresh fruit juice.

- Aromatic tea (fruit tea, without sugar).

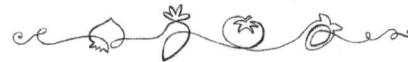

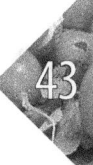

SIXTH DAY

BREAKFAST

- 1 cup of yogurt (unsweetened).

- Two spoonfuls of Muesli.

- Fruit tea (without sugar).

10 A.M.

- 1 fruit.

- 1 glass of fresh fruit juice.

LUNCH

- Fresh vegetable salad.

- Mashed potato with spinach or spinach beet.

- 1 cup of fruit tea (without sugar).

3 P.M.

- 1 fruit.

- 1 glass of vegetable juice with fruit.
  Purifying Power Preparation:
  Mix ¾ cup (6 oz.) of celery juice with
  ½ cup of natural tangerine juice.

- Apple and cinnamon tea (without sugar).

DINNER

- 1 cup of vegetable broth.

- 2 slices of whole wheat bread with
  1 slice of diet cheese, low fat. (The calcium is
  good for the kidneys, an important organ for
  the elimination of excess body fat.)

- Herb or fruit tea (without sugar)/

8 P.M.

- 1 glass of fresh fruit juice.

- Fruit tea (without sugar).

SEVENTH DAY

BREAKFAST

- 2 slices of whole wheat bread.

- Egg Beater
  Preparation:
  1 tomato cut in little pieces with
  1 teaspoon of canola oil. Salt it on a frying
  pan, then add 2 egg whites whipped.

- 1 glass of fresh fruit juice.

10 A.M.

- 1 fruit.

- 1 glass of fresh fruit juice.

LUNCH

- Fresh homemade vegetable salad with
  vinaigrette dressing.

- 1 portion of fish or chicken boiled or grilled.

- 1 glass of ice fruit tea.

3 P.M.

- 1 glass of fresh fruit juice.

- Antacid refreshment
  Preparation:
  Mix ½ cup (4oz) of prune juice with
  ¼ cup (2oz) of grape juice and
  1 teaspoon of lemon juice, then add
  ¼ cup of mineral water.

- 1 fruit.

DINNER

- Fresh vegetable salad.

- 1 cup of yogurt.

- 1 veggie burger on whole wheat bread.

8 P.M.

- 1 glass of fresh fruit juice.

- Fruit tea (without sugar).

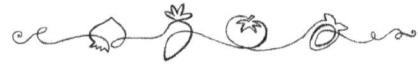

Recommendations

Maintaining a weight loss diet requires changes in lifestyle not big sacrifices or going hungry. It consists of finding nutritional mistakes, correcting them and adopting healthier habits that allow you to stay in shape for a lifetime. This type of treatment demands a lot of discipline and patience, from both the parents and child.

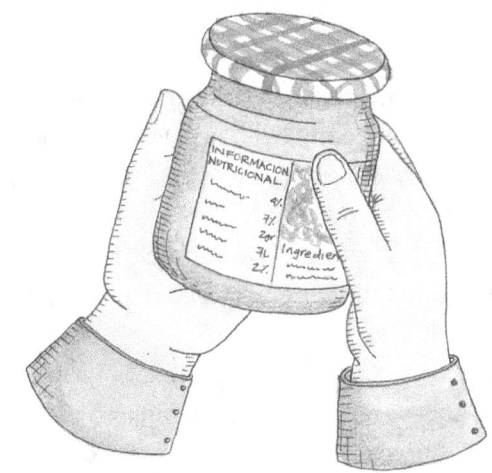

Avoid rushing through the treatment. Remember the child did not gain weight overnight. While it is true that the more overweight, the faster the rate of weight loss, but the ideal weight loss for a child is about one pound per week. This ensures the child is losing body fat not water, or even worse, muscle tissue. Your heart is also a muscle and can be affected by a rigorous weight loss program.

Following the diet is not enough. Though weight loss is associated with dieting, it must be adapted to your child's needs and physical activity. There are genetic factors and health problems that can influence obesity, but in a high percentage of children with excess weight it is the result of poor nutrition and sedentary habits. Considering the increasing number of obese children, this is especially worrisome.

All of the family members need to participate in the treatment. The child's diet necessitates a change in the behaviors and habits of the entire family. For the treatment to succeed, it is important that everyone collaborates and supports the process. It would be pointless to establish a diet regimen without requiring modifications to the family's original habits, which usually helped create the situation in the first place.

Be careful of your child's self-esteem, especially those who dream of attaining a perfect figure. Parents and children can become obsessive and negatively alter the treatment, which can result in disorders like bulimia and anorexia. Parents need to focus on providing the child with accurate information and avoid comparisons with other children their age. Most importantly, encourage the child to understand the main objective to weight loss is to improve their health and wellbeing, which in turn will allow them to participate in more activities and sports from which they may have previously been excluded.

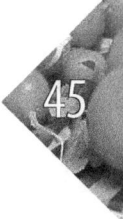

45

Eat slowly, relax and enjoy your food. The foods' flavors will provide more pleasure when they are eaten slower and chewed better. Also, be aware hunger will not feel satisfied until at least 20 minutes after eating has begun; this is the time it takes for the signal of satisfaction to reach the hypothalamus in the brain.

Divide recommended food portions throughout the day. To lose weight, a child in treatment should eat 5 or 6 times a day, not just the standard 3 meals (breakfast, lunch, dinner). This routine helps to regulate the appetite. Do not eliminate recommended refreshments or snacks between meals. Eating reasonable quantities of food regularly aids weight loss by burning the calories while ingesting them.

Do not eat too late in the evening. It is important to teach children the habit of eating during the day and early evening. When eating late, no calories are burned and the degradation process of food is slower. It is better to eat at least 3 to 4 hours before bedtime; a child's last meal of the day should be between 6 and 7 p.m.

Establish the habit of reading the labels on products. Always remember the family's diet starts in the supermarket, so what you take home is what your children will eat. Do not obsess over forbidden foods, since there is no such thing as food that makes you lose or gain weight by itself. The daily diet should be interpreted more universally; nutritious foods must compensate for foods with less nutritional value.

Celebrate your child's accomplishments during the treatment, no matter how small. Each change of improvement achieved should be recognized and, if possible, rewarded. Never use food as a reward, but select something else they've dreamed of such as a book, magazine, movie (without treats), or an article of clothing.

Discover the connection between food and emotions. Adolescents, more than children, will often use food as a source of comfort or immediate gratification. Periods of grief, stress or family difficulties, etc. are compensated for with foods "rich" in calories such as ice cream, chips, chocolates, etc. Try to help your children understand that emotions may trigger the desire to eat, and discuss these feelings and their causes with them so they may recognize this disorder, then help them find other outlets for expression.

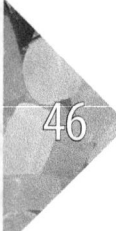

Remember, there are no "miracle diets", or commercial products that reduce weight in a "flash". Even products that do produce fast weight loss do not provide proper treatment, so the weight will return as fast as it was lost. Sometimes, even more weight is regained since muscle mass as well as fat was lost, which can create adiposity (more fat cells).

If after following the recommendations in this book, which include changing nutritional habits and increasing exercise regimens, the child's nutritional status does not achieve sufficient change, a nutritionist should be consulted to help personalize treatment and evaluate the possibility of other complications.

Instructions For The Seven-Day Diet

Do not change any of the products in the menus. After the seventh day, continue with another diet as indicated.

Pay attention to food portions consumed at one time. Do not eat fast. Chew food thoroughly.

Avoid heavy or spicy foods (red meats, curry, hot peppers, etc). Do not use salt or sugar in the preparation of food.

Remember to drink enough fluids to help with the elimination of fat during treatment.

Parents should ensure their children participate in outdoor activities, which will help them feel better.

Best of success with the diet!

Questions or concerns regarding the diet, or for other nutritional information, please contact: **dietista@obesidadtratamiento.com** and the dietitian will respond as soon as possible.

Resources

Public and private health resources for parents and children:

Kaiser Permanente
www.kaiserpermanente.org

Dynamic Kids program
www.dynamickids.org
Program in English and Spanish

University of California, San Francisco (UCSF)
UCSF Children's Hospital
WATCH Clinic
(Weight Assessment for Teen and Child Health)
www.ucsfchildrenshospital.org/clinics/watch/

SHAPEDOWN program
www.shapedown.com

KidShape Foundation
KidShape program
www.kidshape.com

National Institutes of Health
www.nih.gov

National Heart, Lung and Blood Institute
(NHLBI)
www.nhlbi.nih.gov

We Can! program
www.nhlbi.nih.gov/health/public/heart/obesity/wecan

Portion Distortion
http://hp2010.nhlbihin.net/portion

The Nemours Foundation
Center for Children's Health Media
KidsHealth program
http://kidshealth.org

New York Times, Health section
www.nytimes.com/health/guides

Trust for America's Health
http://healthyamericans.org/obesity

CSPI Nutrition Action
(Center for Science in the Public Interest)
www.cspinet.org/new/200808041.html

Weight-control Information Network (WIN)
National Diabetes and Digestive and Kidney
Diseases (NIDDK)
www.win.niddk.nih.gov

Dietary Guidelines for Americans
www.win.niddk.nih.gov/publications

American Academy of Pediatrics (AAP)
http://www.aap.org

Healthy Children parenting site
www.healthychildren.org

Prevention and Treatment of Childhood
Overweight and Obesity
www.aap.org/obesity/about.html

A.D.A.M.
www.adam.com

American Accreditation Healthcare
Commission/URAC
www.urac.org

World Health Organization
www.who.int/en

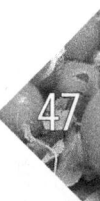

3. Annex

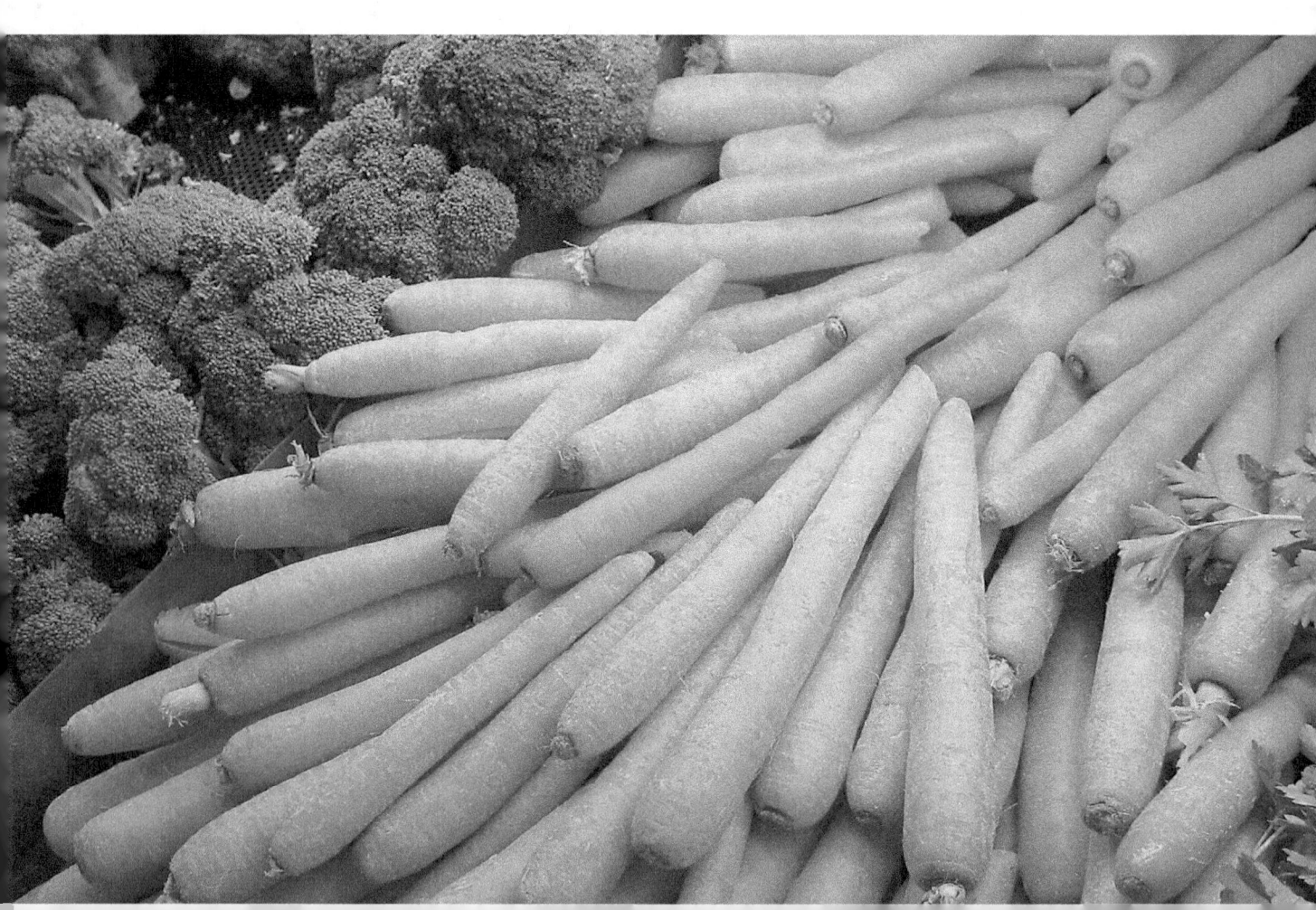

healthy nutrition from infancy to adolescence

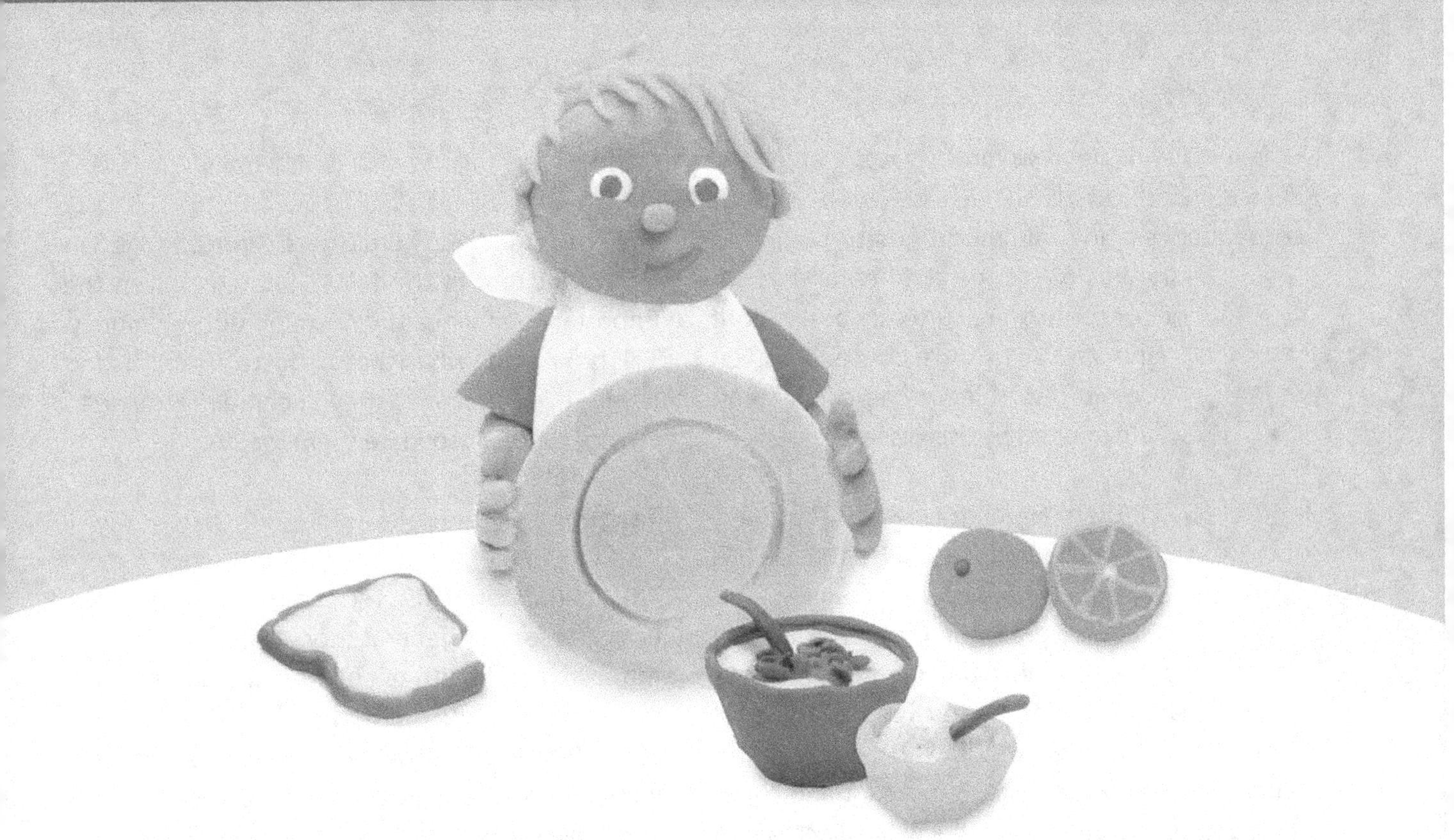

YOUR CHILDREN'S NUTRITION

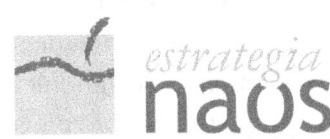

Produced By: Consuelo López Nomdedeu
CORPORACIÓN MULTIMEDIA
Alicia del Real Martín (plastilina y diseño)
Printed By: Rumagraf, S.A.
NIPO: 355-04-003-X
Depósito Legal: M-40742-2007
Reprinted: 2007

estrategia naos

MINISTERIO DE SANIDAD Y CONSUMO

agencia española de seguridad alimentaria y nutrición

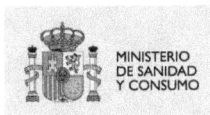

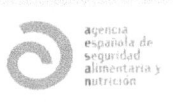

1. Providing health

Obesity and overweight have epidemic characteristics. It is a disease with serious consequences in adulthood that begin in childhood: 26% of the children and youth of our country are currently overweight and almost 14% are obese. But even more disturbing is the rising trend exhibited by this disease.

There are many reasons that have contributed to this situation. In part, because our country has suffered great changes in the last few decades which has greatly impacted the type of food consumed. Traditional diets have been replaced by those with greater energy density, which means more fat and sugar added to our products, together with a decrease in fruit, vegetable, cereal and greens consumption. In addition, these dietary changes combine with lifestyles that reflect a reduction in physical activity at school and during leisure time.

In response to this situation, the Ministry of Health and Consumer Affairs has launched the *Strategy for Nutrition, Physical Activity and Obesity Prevention (NAOS)*, which aims to reverse the rising trend in the prevalence of obesity, especially in children, and fight their impact on health.

Objective

The manual, *Your Children's Nutrition*, is an important tool of the NAOS Strategy, given the importance of a healthy nutrition during infancy. This is the stage when they begin to establish food habits, in adolescence they become resistance to change, and consolidate them for life.

Target

This manual provides, for parents, grandparents, educators and, in general, those responsible for the nutrition and health of children and adolescents, recommendations on food and nutrition to help them develop a varied diet, balanced to their liking, making the meal not only a necessity, but also a pleasure.

If we can get our children to eat a variety of foods in the proper portions, and encourage their regular practice of physical activity and sports, we will have taught them healthy habits that will protect them from obesity and other pathologies that manifest in adulthood.

In the end, we will have given them better health for many years.

Elena Salgado Mendez
Minister of Health and Consumer

2. Nutritional needs

General guidelines exist about the need for energy and nutrients in this stage of life. Translated to frequency of food consumption and portions, it can help us design a healthy diet, taking into account that nutritional recommendations are adapted to each individual.

Respect personal taste as much as possible because there are many ways of eating, **though there is only one way to nourish properly.**

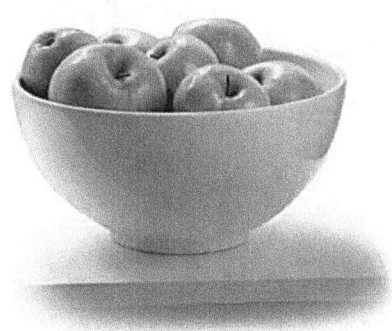

Foods are the "natural packaging" that contain the different nutritive substances our bodies need. Divided into different groups of elements: meats, fish, fruits, vegetables, greens, cereal, dairy... there will always be one, providing the same nutritional value, that responds to the test of the consumer.

Providing Energy and Nutrients

▶ *Energy:*

All foods, depending on their nutritional content, **provide calories in greater or lesser amounts.**

Once foods are consumed they release these calories – energy – that allow us to grow, work, practice sports, etc.

Providing energy – calories – should cover the **needs of your body:**

- **energetic items**, tied to maintaining the body's temperature (37ºc);

- **growth**, very elevated during the first year of life, then decreases sensibly afterward, to increase again in a progressive manner until adolescence.

- **physical activity**, elevated during this period, (especially school-age children practicing sports). It is necessary to fight against a sedentary lifestyle, in order to maintain an adequate weight, because reducing calories without physical activity is not enough.

51

▶ *Proteins:*

Protein requirements are expressed in relation to the correct body weight, which corresponds to height and development. The need for protein is very high in infants, decreasing thereafter then rises once again during puberty. **The maximum need for proteins is between ages 10 and 12 years for girls and between ages 14 to 17 years for boys.**

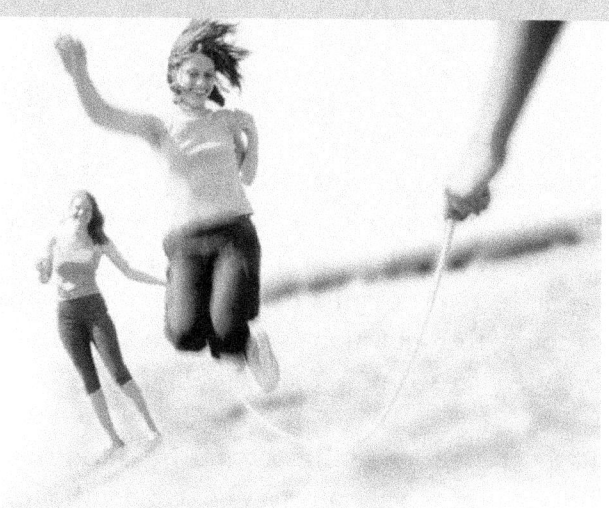

52

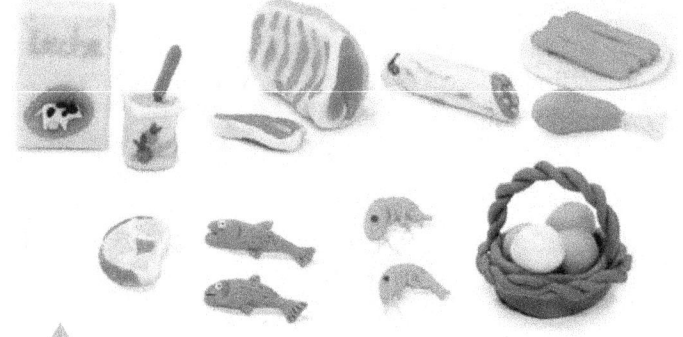

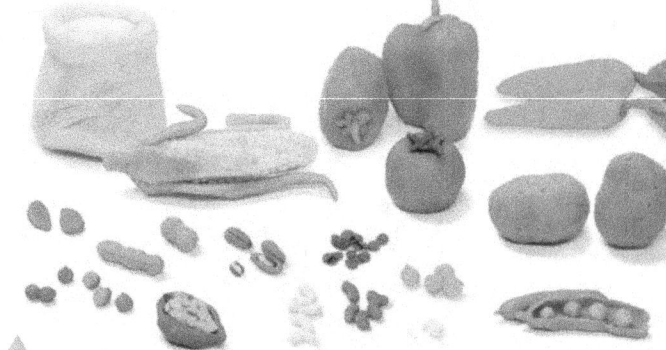

Foods rich in proteins of animal origin	Foods rich in proteins of vegetable origin
• Milk and derivates • Meats: pork, beef, chicken, lamb, rabbit, etc. • Processed meats: hotdogs, sausages, cold cuts • Eggs • Fatty fish (blue): mackerel, salmon, herring…; lean fish (white): filet, sole, flounder, haddock, dabs, hake… shellfish	• Vegetables, chickpeas, beans, lentils • Dry fruits: nuts, almonds, hazelnuts • Cereals: wheat, rice, corn • Potato, carrots, green beans, peas, peppers, tomato *Proteins are a good complement and of great value when consumed along with vegetables, rice and greens.*

▶ *Carbohydrates:*

The presence of carbohydrates in the diet is essential to cover all our energy needs, this is why the consumption of foods that contain them must be encouraged. There are two kinds of carbohydrates: the complex, such as those found in cereals; and the simple, like sugar. A healthy diet must have an adequate quantity of both, with an emphasis on the complex.

▶ *Dietary fiber:*

Dietary fiber is a substance found in foods of vegetable origin.

Fiber is necessary in diets because it constitutes a way to prevent and treat constipation, lower total cholesterol and improve glycemic control in diabetics. It is calculated that a diet must contain, at least, 25 grams of fiber daily.

53

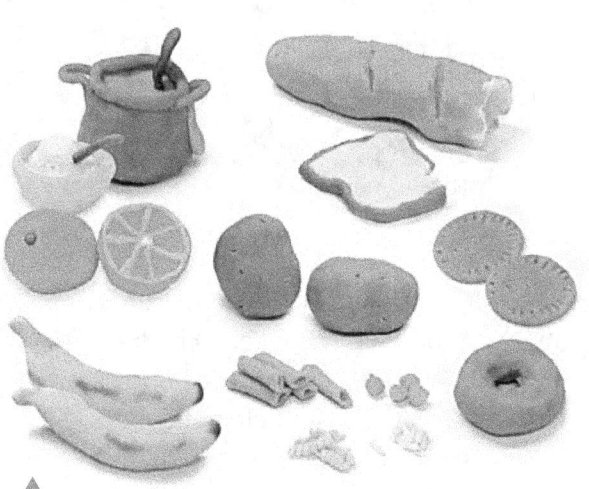

▲
Foods rich in carbohydrates

- Complex: rice, bread, pastas, potatoes, vegetables
- Simple: sugar, marmalade, honey, fruits, sweets in general

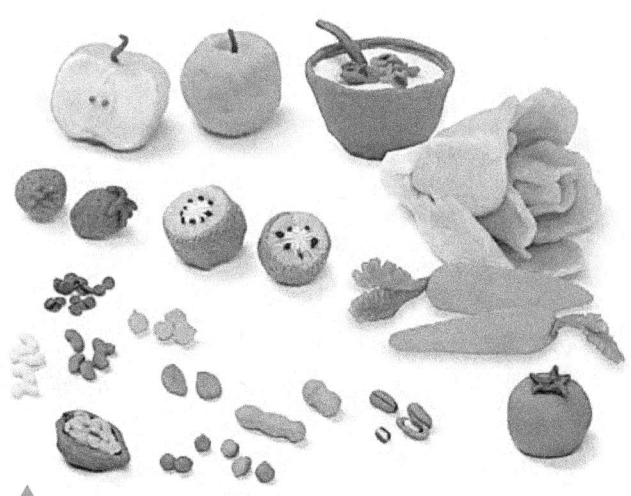

▲
Foods that provide fiber

- Grain cereals
- Vegetables
- Greens, salads, fruits
- Dry fruits

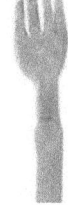

Fats:

The amount of fat consumed in the western world is higher than recommended. Lowering the amount of fat in diets is recommended, especially fats of animal origin (saturated). Conversely, **consuming fats of vegetable origin (unsaturated), especially olive oil,** is advised.

The abuse of fatty and fried foods as standard procedure in the kitchen, increases the caloric value of diets and contributes to obesity.

54

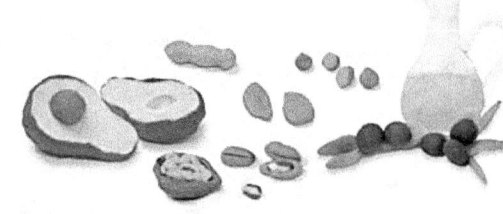

Foods rich in vegetable fat

- Oils (olive, sunflower)
- Dry fruits: walnuts, almonds, hazelnuts and peanuts
- Avocado

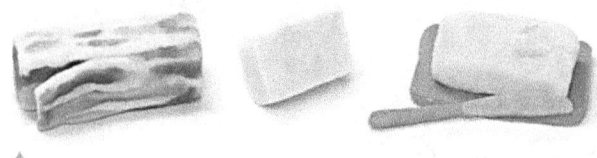

Foods rich in animal fat

- Butter, bacon, shortening, lard

Vitamins:

Vitamins are **nutritious substances essential for life**, which are found dissolved in food, water or fat composition.

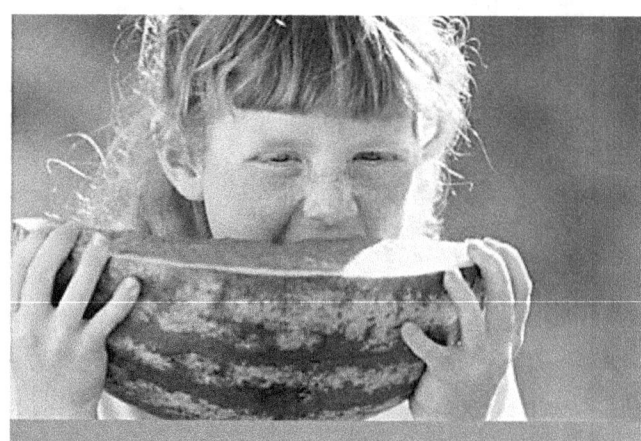

The best way to ensure an adequate supply of all vitamins is to provide school-age children with a variety of foods and increase the concentration of fruits and vegetables in their diets.

The expression, **"5 a day"** summarizes the daily number of recommended servings of fruits and vegetables

Vitamins should be purchased "in the market", buying foods that contain them, while supplements should only be used when advised by a doctor.

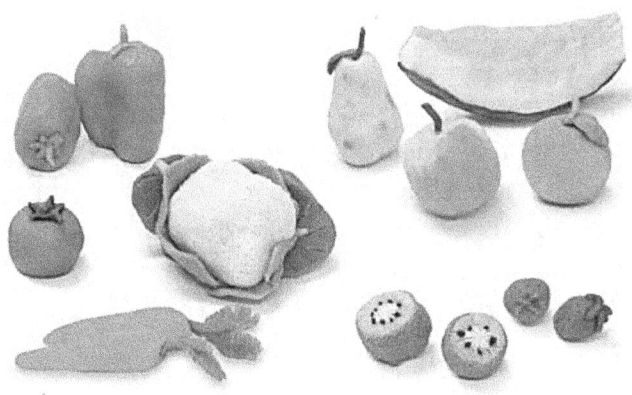

Foods rich in vitamins A & C

- Vegetables: carrots, red and green peppers, tomatoes, cauliflower and cole
- Fruits: oranges, kiwi, strawberries, apricot, peaches, pear, apple, melon

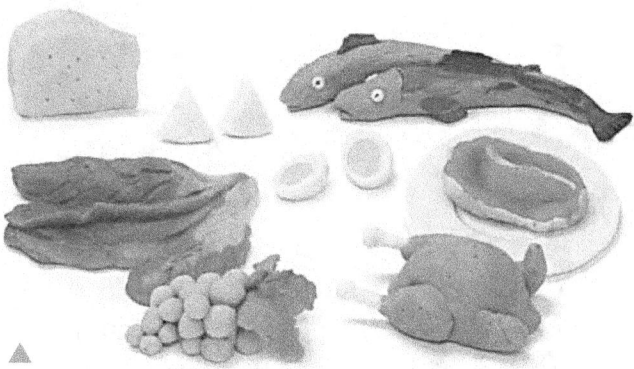

Foods rich in vitamin B complex

- Variety of meats and fish, eggs and dairy products

Folate or folic acid, found in vegetables and fruits, deserves a special mention.

▶ *Minerals:*

Like all the others, **minerals are essential** for life. Some are required in excess of 100 milligrams per day (calcium, phosphorus, sodium and potassium) while others are required in smaller quantities (iron, flour, iodine, copper, zinc, selenium, etc.).

Let's discuss some of them:

Calcium

Calcium needs are high throughout childhood, especially in adolescence, so meals should be rich in products that contain calcium in its most assimilable form.

Calcium is essential for the formation of the skeleton and, on completion of adolescence, good levels of this mineral must be maintained in the diet to repair losses that occur in adulthood. Osteoporosis — loss of bone calcium as an adult — is a major health problem. It is most common in women, so they especially need a good start in bone formation — from infancy through adolescence — which can be derived from a diet rich in calcium and the practice of adequate physical exercise.

55

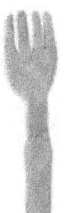

Foods rich in calcium

• Overall, dairy products: milk, cheese, yogurt, shakes, dairy desserts in general
• Fish: especially those varieties that can be eaten with the bones (anchovies, sardines, etc.)

Iron

Iron needs are elevated during periods of fast development, thus this mineral is essential for school-age children. In the case of girls, the start of their menstrual bleeding at puberty constitutes a relatively important iron loss, therefore, the presence of this mineral in their diet should be greater than for boys.

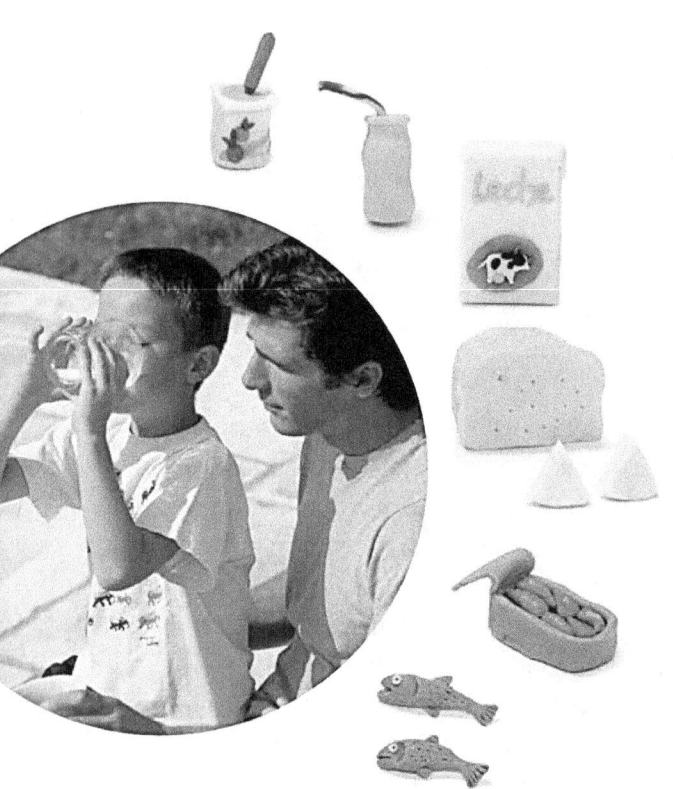

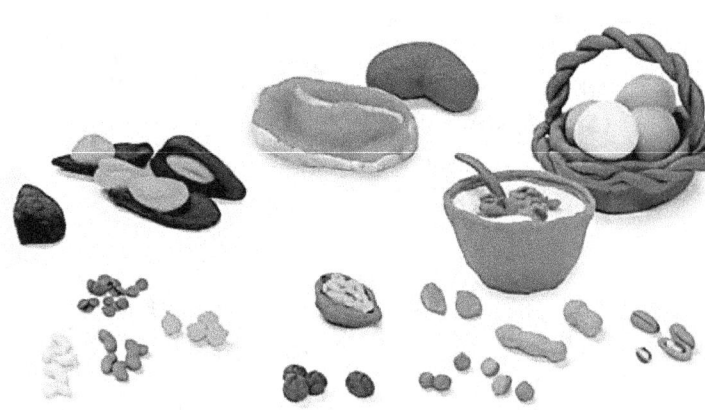

Foods rich in iron

• Liver, kidneys, beef in general, egg yolks, shellfish (mussels), greens, dry fruits, pasta, raisins, prunes and breakfast grain cereals

Calcium derived from foods of vegetable origin is poorly absorbed.

As in the case of calcium, iron derived from food of animal origin is better absorbed.

Iodine

The need for iodine increases moderately during puberty, especially for girls.

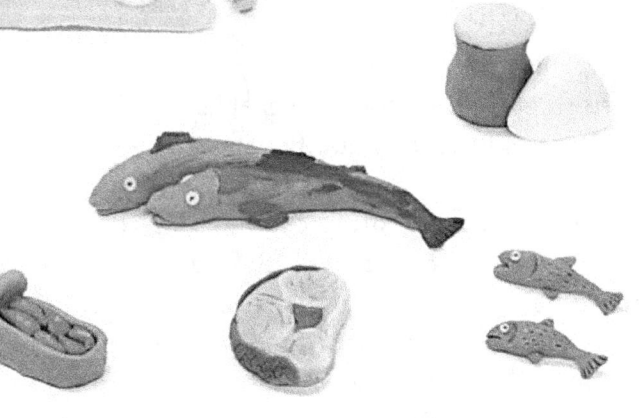

The consumption of iodized salt to season foods is a desirable practice, since it ensures the presence of this important mineral in the diet. This does not mean salt intake should be increased, because its addition must always be moderated.

Foods rich in iodine
- Saltwater fish and iodized salt

Fluoride

Dental cavities are an important public health problem. The favorable action of **fluoride has been proven as a protector** against attacks from the organic acids produced by plaque bacteria and sugars in the mouth.

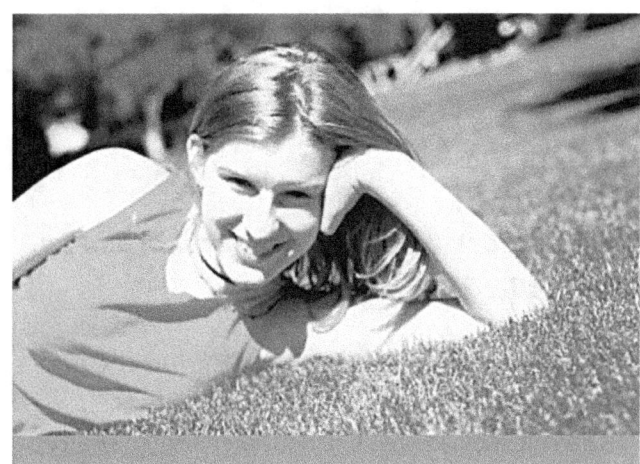

57

Fluoridated salt or sodium fluoride tablets may be used if advised by a doctor. Fluoride toothpaste or fluoride mouthwashes are also excellent ways to combat tooth decay.

The prevention of dental cavities should take place during infancy and adolescence

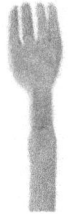

3. *Nutritional rhythm, distribution of food in the daily meals*

As a guideline, it is proposed that the **nutritional needs of school-age children** be distributed throughout the day in the following proportion:

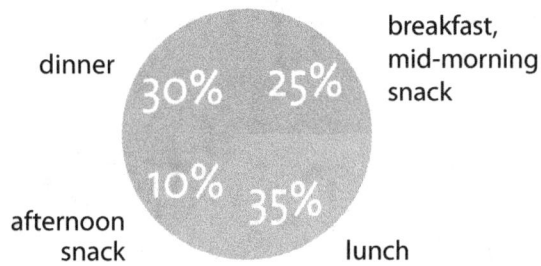

dinner 30% 25% breakfast, mid-morning snack

afternoon snack 10% 35% lunch

58

▶ *Breakfast: before going to school and by mid-morning*

Breakfast is one of the most important meals of the day and should contain at least 25% of the nutritional needs of schoolchildren. The type of foods that comprise breakfast are generally liked by children, making it easier to follow this recommendation.

The rush to get to school, and the drowsiness of the first moments of the morning, sometimes disturbs that first meal of the day, which can cause a decrease in attention span and performance in the first hours of class. The family should try to organize their time to ensure school-age children can enjoy a healthy breakfast.

In Spain, about 10 to 15% of children go without breakfast, and 20 to 30% eat insufficiently; it is, therefore, very important for families to be aware of the problem.

At mid-morning, as reinforcement of the food consumed at breakfast, children should eat a fruit, yogurt or bread snack with cheese. Frequently, children that have a deficient breakfast are hungry by mid-morning break, they then snack excessively on junk food that takes away their appetite at lunchtime. **Children should never be allowed to substitute this type of food for breakfast.**

▶ *Lunch*

In Spanish nutritional habits, lunch is the most consistent meal. It should cover at least 35 to 40% of an individual's daily nutritional needs.

It is becoming increasing common for children to eat at school. **Parents should know the monthly meal plan** and actively collaborate with the management of the school to ensure their children are being offered balanced diets. Parents should also take into account the daily menu and properly it incorporate it into the rest of the day's meals. **Fruit should usually constitute as dessert.**

▶ Afternoon snack

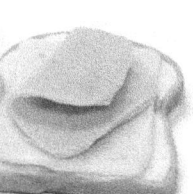

A snack is usually well accepted by children and can supplement the diet, because it allows you to include nutritional products of great interest: dairy products, fresh fruits, different cold cuts...

The snack should not be excessive, so children can maintain their appetite for dinner.

The so-called "snack dinner" is an acceptable option when it is done occasionally and includes nutritious foods with enough variety. For example, a French omelet and cheese with a fruit, and before bed a glass of milk, can be an eventual alternative to a snack and dinner.

▶ Dinner

Dinner is prepared based on the foods already eaten during the day.

It should be consumed in a timely manner, not too close to bedtime, so it does not interfere with the children's sleep.

Appropriate dishes for dinner are purees, soup or salad, and as a complement, meat, eggs or fish depending on what was eaten at mid-day. For dessert: fruit or a dairy product.

▶ A problem: "snacking"

It has been determined that within the diet, the distribution of food throughout the day provides children with healthy nutrition. However, there is a bad habit that, unfortunately, is growing: the "snacking" performed at any time of the day that is usually based on foods containing excessive fat, sugar and excess salt.

59

The school-age children that "snack" consume sweets, juices, soda pop, junk food, pies, pastries, ice cream... This habit contributes to weight gain by adding empty calories to their diet and, ultimately, can cause obesity.

When the caloric value of these foods is studied, it is observed that even if the foods meet a child's energy requirements, they lack the nutrients essential for a balanced diet.

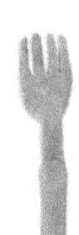

4. Learning to eat

If we want schoolchildren to reach adulthood practicing healthy nutritional habits, aligned to their region's culture and influenced by their own and family tastes, then food must be "introduced" to them.

Food contains nutritional substances in different forms, consistencies, textures, smells, flavors and culinary treatments.

During infancy and adolescence, food and its different combinations become known through gastronomic practices in the family and social experiences (family dinners, friends, school cafeteria, etc.) and each person develops their own preferences. It is difficult for children to learn to eat well if they are not in contact with a wide variety of products. So, like being taught personal hygiene guidelines, the effort should be made to teach them about food and nutrition.

There are children with good appetites, curious to try everything, which makes educating them easier for their parents. Others, by contrast, are indifferent, lazy, or uninterested in food, while some even use it to get what they want (movies, a toy, later bedtime, watch more television, etc.)

Nutritional education by parents requires patience, dedication, and no compromise with unacceptable bargaining by their children, as well as respect for a child's individual appetite, provided their growth and development is considered normal by their pediatrician.

Parents that are overly concerned with food may create in their children an unhealthy dependency on something that should be natural and pleasurable. Children, like adults, may have changes in appetite related to different stages of their development. There are times when growth is stationary or slows down and their nutritional requirements are lower. By contrast, there are times when children eat with pleasure and in abundance in response to their bodies' demand for the nutrients it needs for growth. This situation must be understood by the family.

Height and weight are excellent indicators of nutritional status, and the pediatrician's opinion is essential to evaluate whether the situation qualifies as normal or demands concern.

▶ *Weekly school meal plan*

Breakfast

Breakfast allows for a variety of foods to be offered, but for the best quality nutrition it should include; a dairy product (milk with or without sugar or cocoa, yogurt, cheese — avoiding high-fat), bread (toast, cereal, cookies, muffins, biscuits), a fruit or juice (any variety), jams, honey, a complementary fat (olive oil, butter, margarine) and on occasion, ham or other type of cold cuts.

Mid-morning

A piece of fruit.

Lunch and dinner

Lunch usually provides the highest level of energy and nutrients and should be complemented with a balanced dinner.

As a suggestion, we are proposing **a weekly meal plan** for school-age children. Keep in mind **the following considerations:**

61

- *The proposed meal plan may be modified in conjunction with the family organization and the parents' eating habits.*

- *The proposed diets, in general, can be applied any time of the year. We do recommend making adjustments to use "seasonal" foods, especially for fruits and vegetables.*

- *To facilitate the understanding and application of this meal plan, the table lists foods from all regions. But keep in mind that different communities have their own gastronomy, which should be respected when possible, since it is part of their nutritional culture.*

  - *The suggestions in this table are to encourage the consumption of products from the so-called "Mediterranean diet" as the best example of a guide to healthy food , cooked or seasoned with olive oil (virgin if possible).*

    - *We emphasize "hearty soups" as a main dish, to ensure that products of vegetable origin have a decisive presence in the diet.*

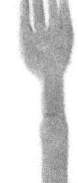

WEEKLY PLAN FOR SCHOOL MEALS

breakfast	*lunch*
MONDAY Milk. Whole wheat bread with honey or jam. Orange juice.	Veal stew with potatoes, carrots and peas. Cheese. Apple.
TUESDAY Milk. Bread with ham, tomato, and olive oil.	Meat cannelloni. Salad of lettuce, tomato, onion, carrot, and pepper. Orange.
WEDNESDAY Milk. Whole wheat cookies with cheese spread. Fruit juice.	Vegetable stew: chickpeas, spinach, potatoes, and carrots. Russian fillet with salad. Yogurt.
THURSDAY Milk. Toast with jam and butter. Fruit juice.	Creamy vegetable soup. White rice with fried egg and tomato sauce. Fruit salad.
FRIDAY Milk. Cereal. Fruit juice 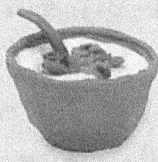	Lentils with rice, potatoes and carrots. Chicken salad. Fruit salad.
SATURDAY Milk. Toasted bread with olive oil. Fruit juice.	Soup medley with noodles, vegetables, greens, meat, and sausage. Pear.
SUNDAY Chocolate (cocoa) with toast. Fruit juice 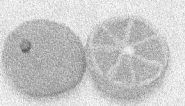	Roast beef with fried potatoes, mushrooms, peas. Salad of lettuce, tomato, asparagus. Baked apple.

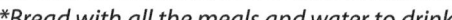

Bread with all the meals and water to drink.

62

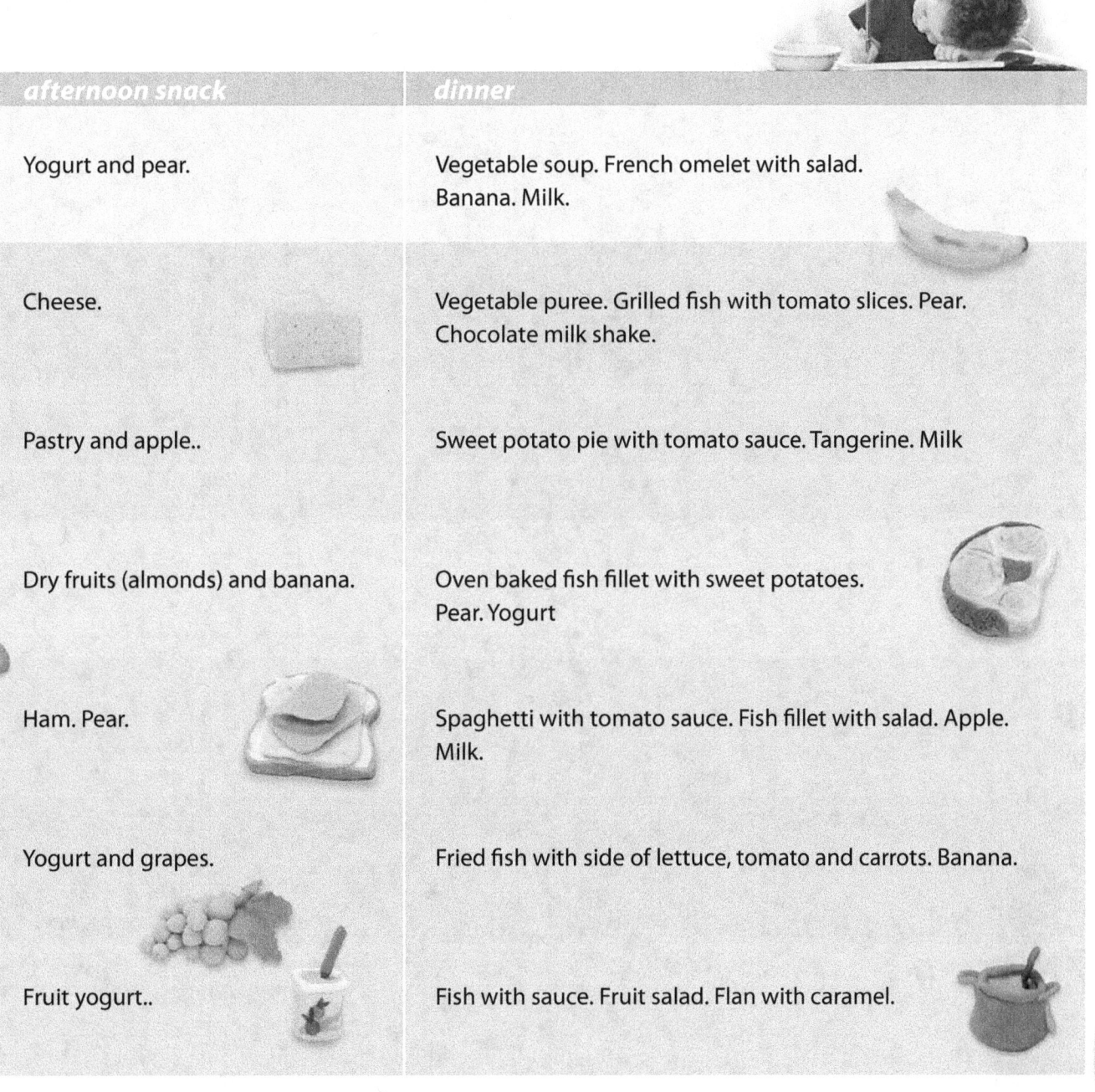

afternoon snack	dinner
Yogurt and pear.	Vegetable soup. French omelet with salad. Banana. Milk.
Cheese.	Vegetable puree. Grilled fish with tomato slices. Pear. Chocolate milk shake.
Pastry and apple..	Sweet potato pie with tomato sauce. Tangerine. Milk
Dry fruits (almonds) and banana.	Oven baked fish fillet with sweet potatoes. Pear. Yogurt
Ham. Pear.	Spaghetti with tomato sauce. Fish fillet with salad. Apple. Milk.
Yogurt and grapes.	Fried fish with side of lettuce, tomato and carrots. Banana.
Fruit yogurt..	Fish with sauce. Fruit salad. Flan with caramel.

▶ *Frequency of food consumption and practice of physical activity*

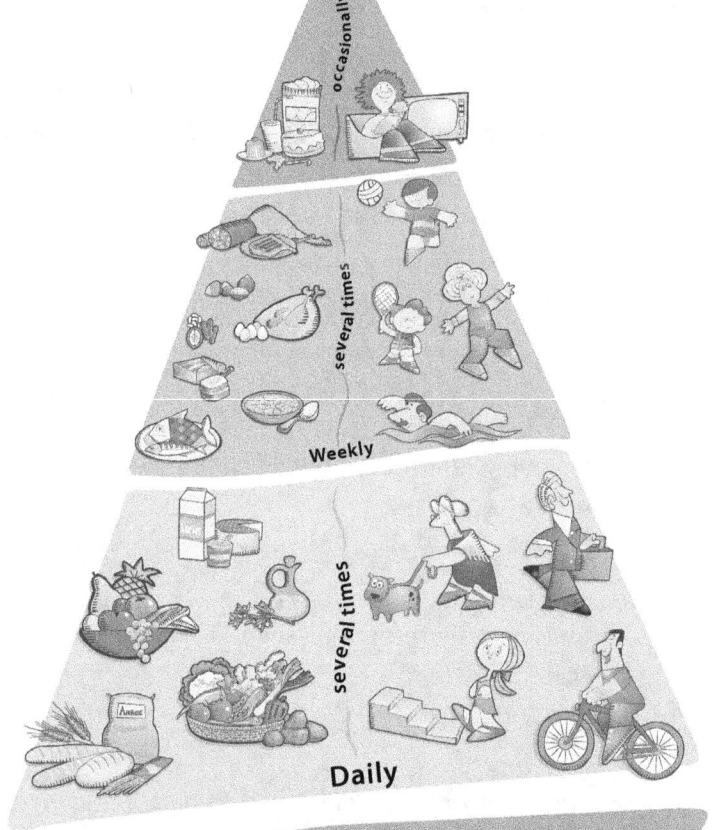

NAOS Pyramid®

occasionally

several times

Weekly

several times

Daily

drink ✚ water

H e a l t h y   L i f e s t y l e

NAOS Pyramid® shows healthy lifestyles from the Spanish Health and Nutritional Safety Agency (AESAN)

64

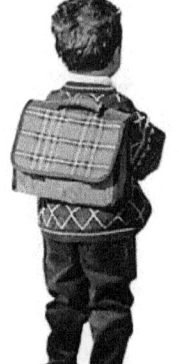

5. Recommendations for healthy nutrition according to school age

▶ *From 3 to 6 years of age*

This is an essential stage in the formation of children's eating habits.

- Teach children to "**eat everything**".
- Tend to their energy needs, since it is an important period of their life for normal growth and development, and a lot of physical activity.
- Provide for **high quality protein intake** (meat, fish, eggs, dairy) because their .... needs are greater proportionally than an adults.
- Create the **habit of a complete breakfast**.
- Avoid abuse of sodas, sweets, and junk food.
- Dedicate the necessary time to **teach children to enjoy eating**. Food should not be perceived as either a treat o

▶ *From 7 to 12 years of age*

Growth needs remain a priority, so their dietary energy intake must be taken care of by **controlling their weight and rate of development**. Their food preferences are becoming established and need to be managed properly so they don't pressure the family to eat only what they want. Frequently, if they handle money or have an allowance, they will buy and select their own food.

65

- **Avoid abuse** of sweet consumption, sodas, fatty cheeses, spreads, or salty foods.
- There are **foods indispensable** for normal growth and development, such as:
  - *Daily*: dairy, fruits, vegetables, salad, and bread.
  - *Alternating*: meat and derivates, fatty and lean fish (white & blue) and eggs.
  - Vegetables, rice, pastas, *combined with meals throughout the week*.

Moderation in the consumption of pastries, candy and refreshments is recommended. **Do not allow alcoholic beverages** even if they have low alcohol content.

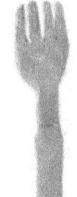

From 13 to 16 years of age

During these years, children will experience growth spurts and attain their full height, which requires very special care of their diet, ensuring it has sufficient calories, and high quality proteins and calcium. Remember, food is the source of the materials that our bodies use to build muscles and bones.

- Watch for food **excesses to avoid** falling into overweight or obesity.
- Parents should **supervise their children's diets** to prevent food combinations they may try on their own to lose weight. These diets can cause significant nutrient deficiencies or irregular eating habits that can lead to dangerous disorders like anorexia.
- Encourage children to **lead active lives** and devote part of their leisure to sports.
- Avoid making meals conflict situations that interfere with relationships.
- **Inform children about proper nutrition** and its importance to their health, appearance and general welfare.

The ideal weight

Families' should supervise children's diets to prevent the abusive over-consumption of calories that cause excessive weight gain. This overweight later turns into a social burden, personal discomfort and, more importantly, a risk factor for many diseases that could occur in adulthood. A doctor should advise on any issues related to the weight (excess/defect), growth and development of children.

Physical exercise

Physical exercise is an essential complement to a healthy diet which promotes wellness and protects infants and adolescents from illnesses that appear in adulthood.

You should encourage participation in sports according to the skills, preferences and abilities of each child. But it is most important to **educate about active lifestyles** that include some type of daily exercise like walking, climbing stairs, etc. Become accustomed to incorporating exercise into leisure activities and avoid a sedentary lifestyle (too much television, computer, etc.). **The practice of physical exercise is very important to combat excess weight and obesity.**

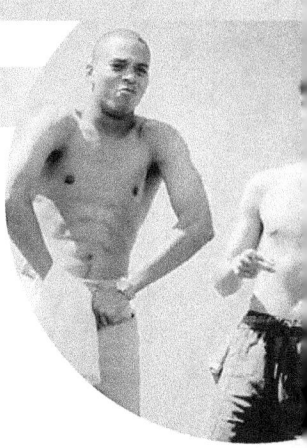

6. Eating behavior disorders

Eating disorder is a term for behaviors that deviate from normal eating patterns and a healthy nutritional diet. Extreme disorders are **anorexia and bulimia**. These diseases have increased in recent years, affecting both sexes and occurring in increasingly early ages.

normal growth. In many cases, anorexia is triggered by these poorly planned starvation diets which are accompanied by intense physical exercise and supplemented with drugs.

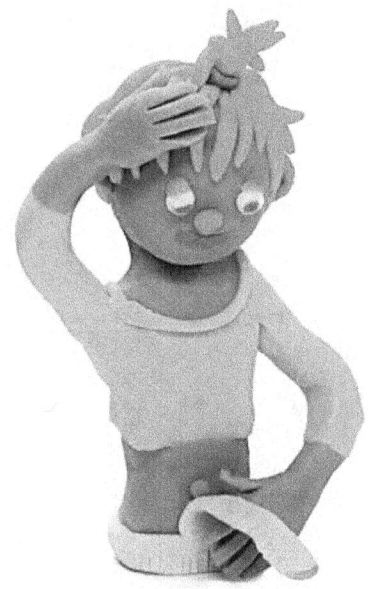

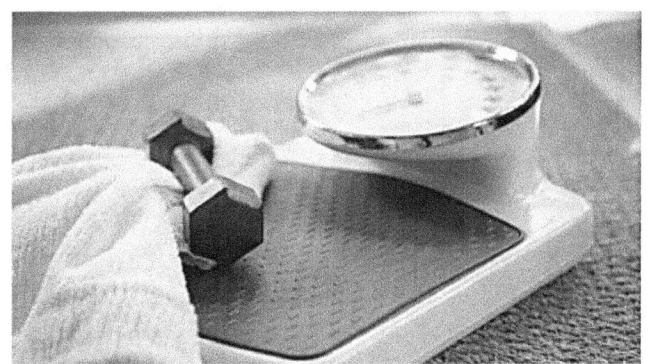

67

Its origin is basically social and fulfills the need of adolescents to emulate the ideal images that fashion imposes.

To achieve this, they submit themselves to very strict diets and stop eating foods that facilitate

The family is the first place to detect behaviors which can lead to dramatic situations.

Also, **school authorities should warn** of abnormal behavior, which can be corrected more efficiently by working in close collaboration with parents.

The **psychologist and pediatrician** are key professionals in the diagnosis and treatment of eating behavior disorders.

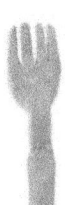

7. Analysis of nutritional habits at school

CONSUMPTION OF	ACTUAL SITUATION	RECOMMENDATIONS
Dairy products	High consumption, especially in products like yogurt, cheese and dairy desserts.	Child should consume milk (at least ½ liter a day). Except by medical prescription, need not be skim. Yogurt or piece of cheese may be used as a complement or substitute for glass of milk.
Meats	Usually consumed every day, abusing pork meat, cold cuts, hotdogs and hamburgers.	Not necessary to eat meat every day. Should alternate with fish and different kinds of meat: beef, pork, chicken, lamb, veal, etc.
Fish	Low consumption.	Should promote consumption, especially "fatty" fish (blue) like sardines, mackerel, anchovy, cod, trout, etc.
Eggs	Appears in two forms: direct (omelets or fried) or indirect (as ingredient in sauces, pudding, custard, cookies, etc.)	Eggs excellent source of protein, comparable to meat or fish. But should not consume more than 4 or 5 eggs a week.
Potatoes	High consumption, especially fried.	Moderate consumption, use in entrees and side dishes with vegetables and salads.
Legumes	Low consumption.	Encourage consumption of vegetables rich in dietary fiber and proteins which have good biological value.
Fruits	Abuse of fruit juices, often commercial-made. Consumption low of whole fruits	Insist children eat naturally fresh fruit.

HEALTHY NUTRITION FROM INFANCY TO ADOLESCENCE

CONSUMPTION OF	ACTUAL SITUATION	RECOMMENDATIONS
vegetables and salads	Some resistance to this type of food, especially vegetables.	Accustom children to consuming vegetables and vegetable-based dishes and as side dish for meats, fish or eggs.
Bread	Moderate consumption with high consumption of specialty types.	Consumption to be maintained as carbohydrate intake contributes to balance of the diet.
Pasta	Heavy consumption of macaroni, spaghettis, pizzas, etc.	Should be moderated to allow for other main dishes that contribute richer nutrition, especially fiber such as legumes, vegetables, greens, etc.
Rice	Well accepted.	Rice and wheat are cereals that combine well with foods, must be alternated with vegetables.
Sweets	Excessive consumption, generally factory-made.	Should consume in moderation.
Refreshments	High consumption.	Causes loss of appetite. Drink only occasionally.
Fats	High consumption in form of fatty cheese, butter, flavored margarine, generally used for breakfast and snacks. Also, in pâtés, spreads, sandwich bread and cakes.	Fat is necessary since it provides the body with essential vitamins and fatty acids, but its abuse causes rapid satiety and prevents intake of more nutritious food necessary for growth and health. Abuse of fat in the diet is not recommended, the percentage of calories from fat should not exceed 30% of the total consumed.

▶ *Recommendations*

Nutritional education, when exercised by a family from infancy, helps to prevent eating disorders, hence it is recommended:

• **Attempt to organize the schedules** of parent and family to include, as much as possible, sharing some meals with the children. This provides an effective way to bond and enjoy some activities together, (shopping, preparation and consumption of food) which should be enjoyable experiences while also teaching proper behavior and eating habits.

• **Avoid eating between meals** and the abuse of snacking.

• Ensure the **diet is varied** and includes the largest diversity of foods possible, as this makes it easier to meet children's nutrient needs.

• Do not use food to solve non-related problems such as boredom, tension, anxiety attacks, etc.

• Parents should monitor their children's meals from a distance, avoiding repetitive continuous recommendations and advice that may create bad feelings and even an aversion to those foods we seek to encourage.

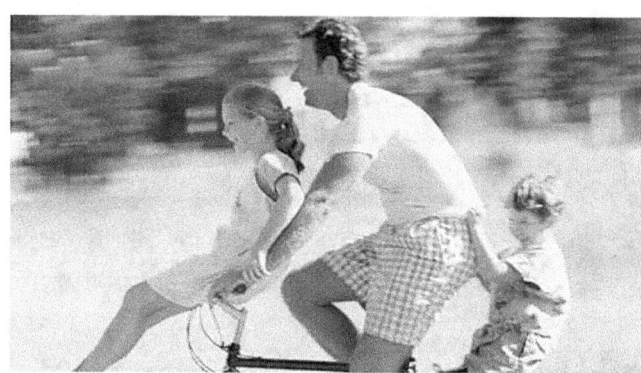

• Ensure the family behavior is consistent with verbal recommendations to children, because it is difficult to instill healthy eating habits that are not practiced by those offering advise.

• Obesity is a disease with serious consequences in adulthood that begin in childhood. In Spain, **16% of schoolchildren aged six to twelve have obesity problems**. In the case of adults, one in two people are overweight. Inadequate eating habits and physical inactivity are responsible for this public health problem.

70

8. *Epilogue: Reminder*

- Children should be taught to **eat all kinds of foods**, for the more variety of foods in the diet, the greater the chance it will be balanced and contain the nutrients they need. Eating only what is liked is a bad nutritional practice.

- Food should be **distributed throughout the day** so the body gets the nutrients it needs, depending on its requirements.

- The **ways of preparing foods** must be changed by using different cooking procedures: baked, boiled, grilled, and stewed, but avoid abusing fried foods. Encourage the consumption of raw foods (salads, gazpacho, cold soups...).

- School meal plans should include the presence of protein-rich foods **of animal origin**: dairy, meat, eggs and fish, **in balance with foods of vegetable origin**: cereals, legumes, vegetables and fruits.

- Foods **rich in carbohydrates** (bread, pasta, rice, vegetables) are needed for their energy supply and should be part of the regular diets of schoolchildren. They introduce gastronomic variety and are essential for good nutrition.

- **Fruits and salads** should be common and abundant in the diet of schoolchildren.

- **Water** is the best beverage and should always accompany meals.

- Alcoholic beverages should never be consumed by school-age **children**.

- The consumption of sweets, sodas and "snacks" should be **moderate**, because, although there are no good or bad foods, restraint should be the norm.

- Control excess fat, sugar and salt.

71

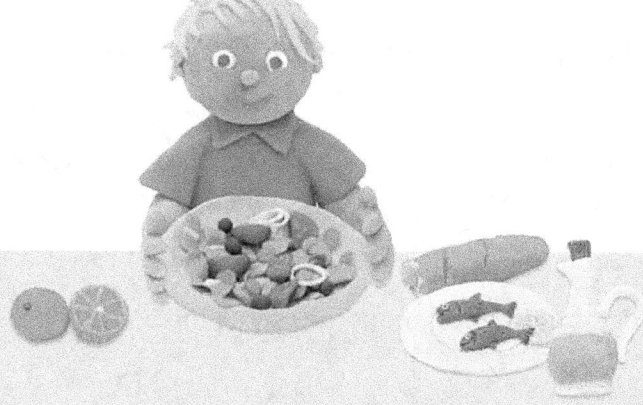

- **The Mediterranean diet is the best example of healthy eating.** In our country its practice is easy because all the necessary ingredients are available and of the highest quality: olive oil, fish, legumes, cereals, breads, fruits, vegetables, yogurt, and dry fruits. Their combinations give rise to numerous gourmet recipes of high nutritive value. Teach schoolchildren to enjoy the benefits of the Mediterranean diet, shopping and cooking.

- **Physical exercise,** supplemented with a healthy diet is essential to prevent disease and promote good health. Children must get used to physical activity and reduce sedentary leisure by avoiding excessive hours of television and video games.

- The role of **parents** in the education of their children's eating habits and a healthy lifestyle is essential. They should encourage them to eat everything and appreciate food, dishes and recipes as a cultural treasure.

- **Eating is a necessity and a pleasure.** Food should supply the quantity of energy and nutrients the body needs, as well as for the psychological welfare brought by a gastronomically well prepared dish consumed in a pleasant environment and good company.

- **The abuse of fast foods** is never advised, since it contributes to the formation of poor eating habits and childhood obesity.

72

The **Spanish Agency for Food Security and Nutrition (AESAN)** is an autonomous body under the Ministry of Health and Consumer Affairs, which is responsible for ensuring the highest standards in food safety and promoting the health of citizens, through the consumption of a healthy balanced diet.

MORE INFORMATION IN:

www.aesan.msc.es

73

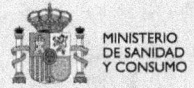

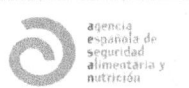

4. Other Published Articles

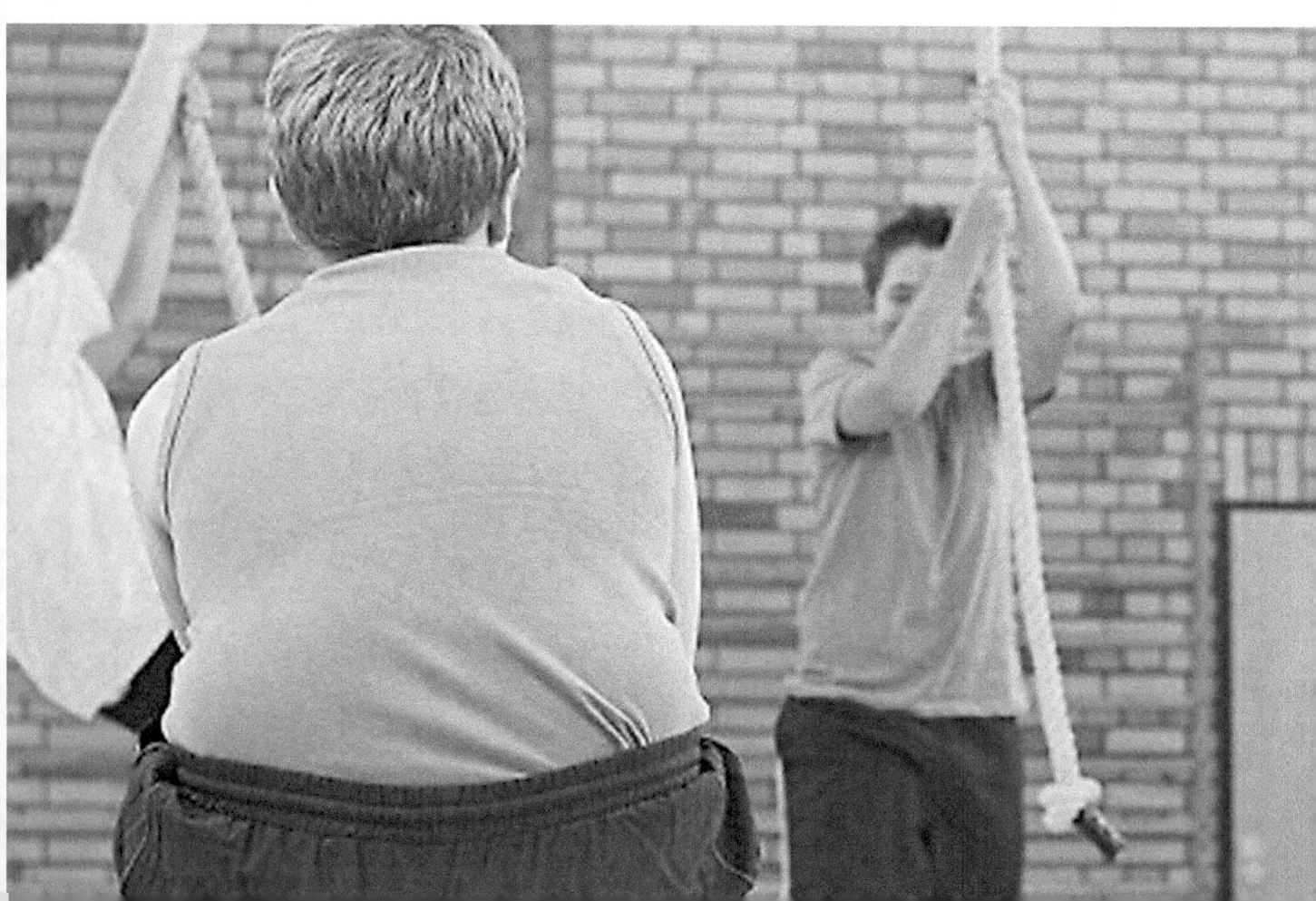

Obese Children – Diabetic Adults

By Carolina Delgado

Nexos Magazine
September 2008

Hours devoted to watching television, computer and video games prevents children from spending their free leisure time playing sports or exercising while obesity creeps into their lives as a silent enemy.

Obese children have some insulin resistance, a disorder that makes the hormone produced by the body not function properly, thus making the pancreas work faster.

Overweight and obesity in children also promotes the inflammation of blood vessels, a key factor in the development of cardiovascular diseases, diabetes mellitus type II and I, that begins abruptly before the third decade of life and is increasing in the pediatric population, especially among children under the age of five years.

These data are based on a study by the Joslin Diabetes Center, associated with the School of Medicine at Harvard University in the United States. The researchers studied 18 Hispanic children and teenagers between the ages of ten and eighteen, 21 of whom were obese but had normal levels of glucose (sugar in blood), thus not yet having developed diabetes. The other participants in the study were much more slender.

The "obese group" had already begun to show some resistance to insulin, a disorder that makes the hormone produced by the body function improperly causing the pancreas to work at a faster pace to maintain the proper insulin levels in the blood.

According to Dr. Enrique Caballero, an endocrinologist at the Joslin Center and director of research, Hispanic children and adolescents that have excess weight, showed signs of poor circulation and evidence of an inflammatory process in their blood vessels.

Vascular inflammation is a key factor in the development of cardiovascular disease and is closely linked to not only excess fat, but also insulin resistance, a disorder that can signal the early development of type II or acquired diabetes.

According to Dr. Caballero, the study indicates that overweight children will not necessarily develop diabetes type II or cardiovascular problems, but that their risk of suffering from them increases, and the problem is serious enough to adopt a strategy of prevention among Hispanics.

Despite significant advances in diabetic treatment, not cures but controls, experts stress the need for improved training of pediatricians to ensure early diagnosis and increase compliance with therapy, to prevent the serious complications children may have with diabetes.

To achieve this, it is essential to closely monitor the child's development, both the physical and psychological adaptation of their diet, treatment and physical exercise.

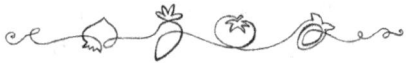

The New York Times – Supplement
"Obesity in Children"
January 2006

The following are excerpts from an article published in January 2006, concerning major studies made by leading institutions in healthcare in the state of California. The University of California, San Francisco (UCSF), the University of California, Los Angeles (UCLA), and Kaiser Permanente, together with other institutions, are engaged in the battle against the scourge of obesity in children.

The alarming obesity epidemic in California and the rest of the nation, has resulted in an emergency for which we, as healthcare leaders, have come together to assume responsibility for and combat.

The battle against the obesity epidemic is on-going with many financial and public health stakeholders providing solutions with senior employees, health plans, and government, community, nonprofit, food and beverage industry representatives, as well as all the experts taking part in achieving short-term solutions.

Due to the high risk involved, experimental medicines for overweight patients and surgeries for children as solutions to obesity can only be considered after all other treatment options have been exhausted.

Amy Porter, MD Pediatrician, who directs the Childhood Obesity program at Kaiser Permanente in the southern California region, says that prevention is the key to success and should be the first, and single most important step. We must raise awareness and move ahead of the problem, because obesity is of increasing concern as it affects many more infants and children daily.

Feeling trapped by the epidemic of childhood obesity demands a reassessment in the health system, to seek the education of patients on its prevention and control, and the urgency to obtain resources to achieve this goal.

If all governments, public entities, private foundations, and other interested organizations, assumed the prevention, information distribution and public education of childhood obesity as a priority, surely in the future we could achieve the eradication of this disease.

In addition, we have the opportunity to improve the lives of future generations, or else the current generation is at risk for more diseases than their parents and prior generations.

Kaiser Permanente has emerged as a leader in this respect, providing stability and synergy through a system of health insurance for their members, bringing national attention to groups of obese children while providing them with the necessary care, ensuring they are both aware of their problem and taught healthy eating habits. Similarly, it offers the children's parents special classes on ways to handle their children's problem and the radical changes needed in the whole family's nutrition. To achieve their objectives, Kaiser Permanente has invested $2.6 million dollars in each one of its hospitals.

Kaiser Permanente's program, Kids in Dynamic Shape (KP KIDS), offers help in both English and Spanish and is one of the largest efforts within all its medical centers and clinics in California, and is based on special weight management strategies for children.

All current programs related to weight management, reach maximum effect in three to twelve months. These programs can be very effective for awhile for some people, but they are limited in effect due to the lack of sufficient funds needed to provide assistance and support to local health centers, schools and community organizations in the district as well as partner organizations throughout the United States.

There are a number of programs to help children lose weight, but few options that assist them in maintaining their new habits and normal weight. Kaiser's KP KIDS program in California is one dedicated to strategies for the management and control of the affected children's weight.

Most weight management programs reach their maximum effectiveness after three to twelve months. The programs are effective for some people, but the impact is limited because they engage the interest of highly motivated patients who have some level of education, and the psychological and economic resources to follow the programs' recommendations.

For its part, UCSF Children's Hospital has offered guidance and counseling on weight issues for children and teens since 2003. Places like their Weight Assessment for Teen and Child Health (WATCH) Clinic are providing some answers, but prevention is the key to change the pace of this disease. According to Dr. Andrea Garber, PhD, RD, coordinator of the WATCH Clinic, to achieve this, more effective public policy decisions and fundamental changes in the habits of today's society are required.

We need to make this battle a priority, in the same way we battled the AIDS epidemic in previous years. Otherwise, our population will have an increasingly shorter life expectancy, and the costs to society in resources and lost opportunities will be huge!

The basic programs offered by communities are struggling to respond to the increasing demands of families and health care providers,

trapped by the epidemic of childhood obesity. Meanwhile, fundraising for this fight is still difficult. While doctors reported progress on some fronts, others expressed frustration at the limited resources allocated to the management of obesity.

We teach our children to understand the importance of not drinking sodas, since they can contribute to obesity. But at school, when thirsty, their options are so limited they are practically forced to purchase them from vending machines.

For the last two years, the WATCH Clinic has assembled specialists in the fields of endocrinology, cardiology, psychology, nutrition and surgery to form a complete team to treat childhood obesity.

This program has a waiting list of five months for new patients. The clinic's organizers are certain the disease is due to biochemical and genetic factors, since much of the food we eat is altered by the hormones in preservatives, which increase the appetite and desire to eat more, thus creating a vicious circle.

Moreover, a recent study by UCLA shows that most children eat fast food at least once a day. Nationally, according to the Department of Agriculture, fast food has grown in total annual sales by 4% from 20 years ago.

Dr. Naomi Neufeld, MD, is clinical professor of pediatricians at the Mattel Children's Hospital UCLA. She says that during her practice, she became frustrated due to the absence of programs dedicated to childhood obesity. This is due to the difficulty in prescribing exercise and medication for obese children and then sending them home. Failure to include adult supervision as part of the solution, ensures they will remain part of the problem.

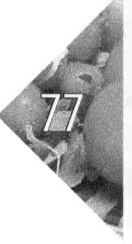

KidShape Foundation, created about 20 years ago, is one of the oldest organizations dedicated to the fight for good childhood nutrition.

Their eight week program is designed to teach the entire family how to eat nutritiously, exercise as a daily routine and form new habits integral to their health.

Similar to KidShape, the Shapedown program is also dedicated to incorporating the entire family in this process, offering instruction about the importance of nutrition, image and stress management.

There are a number of programs that help children to lose weight, but few that help them develop new nutrition and eating habits, and maintain their normal weight.

Schools are a proper venue to teach children the value of good nutrition and adequate exercise, before it is too late! They are necessary for monitoring and support, since it is where children spend most of their day.

To improve the fitness of children, their physical education should include vigorous activities and exercises such as games, sports and recreation, for approximately 60 minutes a day.

This, along with the nutritional and educational support of parents, can provide excellent results. Children who do not exercise at home and spend the majority of their time in front of the television, often develop sedentary lifestyles that eventually lead to weight gain.

The defenders of public opinion are promoting an active role for government, at all levels, in the fight against childhood obesity.

This article also mentions the risks obese children run of developing diabetes type II, cardiovascular conditions, orthopedic problems, depression, low self-esteem, substance abuse, situational pneumonia, asthma and sleep deprivation, which are already an epidemic among obese teenagers.

The preceding is a collection of articles by the University of California, San Francisco, the University of California, Los Angeles, Kaiser Permanente and others, published in the New York Times.

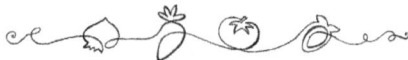

The New York Times
Health Guide
September 8, 2008

The article states that close to two thirds of the United States population is overweight. There are several ways to determine if a person is overweight, but experts believe the body mass (BMI) is the most accurate measurement for children and adults.

A.D.A.M., The American Accreditation Healthcare Commission/URAC, www.urac.org.

This article also offers alternatives treatments for obesity, citing the different forms of surgery such as adjustable gastric bypass, adjustable band "gastroplasty", Roux-En-Y, and biliopancreatic diversion (BPD).

A.D.A.M. warns that the above information should not be used during a medical emergency or for the diagnosis or treatment of a medical condition. Only a licensed medical professional should be consulted for the diagnosis of eligibility for one of these alternative treatments.

Childhood Obesity: Making the Grade

Illustrations

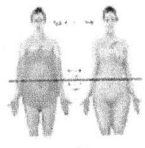
Different Types of Weight Gain

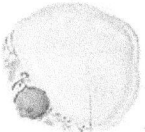
Lipocytes (fat Cells)

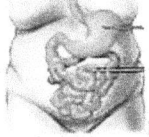
Roux-en-Y Stomach Surgery for Weight Loss

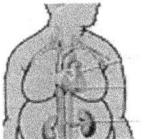
Obesity and Health

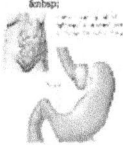

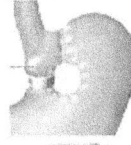
Adjustable Gastric Banding

Vertical Banded Gastroplasty

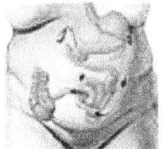
Biliopancreatic Diversion (BPD)

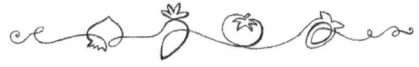

Children's Hospital Of Boston And The University Of Michigan
Make Nutrition Work in Growing Children
April 2008

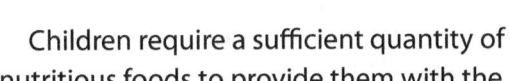

Children require a sufficient quantity of nutritious foods to provide them with the vitamins necessary for their growth. But today, 32% of school-age children in the United States are overweight or obese.

The number of obese children is so extraordinarily high, that the impact of the epidemic will be strongly felt when it increases in the future, says Dr. David Ludwig, MD, PhD, of Children's Hospital of Boston.

How do we ensure children receive the nutrition they need, without gaining additional weight? Dr. Hass says, as added insurance against nutritional deficiencies, many parents give their children supplements: like the chewing kind popular with children, particularly the younger ones; as they grow, capsules, tablets or powder formulas added to food may be administered.

Nutrition And Learning

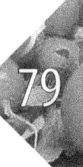

Dr. Patrick Holford says children who eat fish and nuts have superior results in their studies. The best foods are fruits and vegetables, and children that eat them in quantity have been shown to perform better than those who prefer fast or fried foods. A good pure grain-based breakfast cereal (without sugar) with a protein like eggs, and some nuts or seeds, supplies the necessary energy they require for learning.

Dr. Holford adds, that healthful nutrition helps children discover and reach their full potential. For example, researchers at the University of Michigan related iron deficiency in children to poor intelligence until 19 years of age. Coincidentally, experiments conducted in England found that children with early signs of learning difficulties, after taking "Omega – Fatty Acid" for three months, showed significant improvements in their reading, spelling and even behavior.

Do Not Forget Exercise.

Sedentary lifestyles also have a negative impact on behavior and learning ability. According to studies, after performing moderate exercise or being highly active for more than two hours, children show superior improvement in their concentration, creativity, learning, memory and problem solving skills. Physical activity is also an important aid to prevent and relieve obesity.

Currently, many communities are encouraging children to walk or ride their bikes to and from school. Similarly, parents who do not have time to workout, would benefit from taking the time to walk or ride bikes with their children to school, which is good for both communication and the environment.

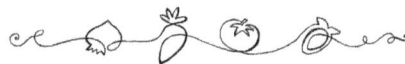

Harvard University, USA
School Of Public Health
Infant Obesity
September 30, 2008

Continuing research into the role of parents in preventing the development of childhood overweight and obesity. Nutrition studies in the NET show the way parents feed their children and schedule their activities, determines the children's nutritional attitudes.

Ana Lindsay, Katarina Sussner, Juhee Kim, and Steven Gortmaker, believe parental involvement is a major force in changing children's attitudes toward food. The authors begin by reviewing evidence on ways parents can help their children to develop and maintain healthy habits, and engage in physical activities that will help prevent overweight and obesity.

They emphasize the need for parents to understand and assume their role in preventing obesity and creating change through the various critical periods of their children's development, from before birth through adolescence. They also note that researchers, teachers and those in charge of establishing standards, could use additional information to provide more effective engagement and educational programs.

This group also conducted an evaluation of school-based obesity prevention programs and found circumstances directly related to the parents involvement with their children's eating and physical activity habits, with the results showing a low quality and limited effectiveness of the programs.

Based on these studies, they concluded that to prevent and control obesity in childhood, parents' knowledge and understanding of obesity must be broadened through multiples community programs community with standards regarding their roles, to learn to properly provide the healthy diets and physical activities that are required to change their children's attitudes.

An assertive intervention should involve direct work by the parents from an early stage in the child's development, and support of healthy practices within and outside of the home.

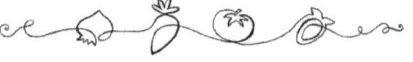

John Hopkins Children's Center, USA
Obesity in Children as a "Way to Satiate",
in Spanish language television
February 19, 2008

According to studies made by pediatricians at John Hopkins Children's Center, Hispanic television is "bombarding" children with such a large number of fast food commercials it has put them in the lead of the obesity epidemic among Latinos. Hispanic children are currently the fifth largest population in the U.S., yet have the highest level of overweight and obesity among all ethnic groups.

A report on the study was published by the Robert Wood Foundation, before being printed in the Journal of Pediatrics.

In another study by pediatricians at John Hopkins Children's Center, Dr. Darcy Thompson, MD, MPH, says: We can not blame overweight and obesity solely on TV commercials, but there is solid evidence that children exposed to such messages tend to eat those unhealthy foods and this is causing them to become overweight.

Another study, conducted among English-speaking children, showed that television commercials also influence their choice of foods, especially younger children.

Other studies following a review of 60 hours of programming between the hours of 3 pm and 9 pm, (hours most schoolchildren watch television), found that the largest Spanish-language channels, reaching 93 to 99% of Latino households in the U.S., show two to three food commercials every hour specifically directed at children with half of them about fast foods and sodas with high sugar content.

To avoid the effects of these commercials, researchers suggest young children have their television time restricted to only two or less hours a day. Parents should also talk to their children about how to prepare healthy meals and teach them to choose nutritious foods. Pediatricians recommend that children under two years of age not watch television.

They also recommend that parents of Latino children take special care to limit their hours in front of the television to avoid any possible adverse effects.

THE PUBLIC HEALTH MEDIA SHOULD INSIST ON ENACTING MEASURES TO LIMIT FAST FOOD COMMERCIALS THAT ARE DIRECTED AT CHILDREN, AS MANY EUROPEAN COUNTRIES HAVE ALREADY DONE.

Yes, We Can!

We Can! is a national movement designed to give parents, caregivers, and entire communities a way to promote sound nutrition and physical exercise for the health of children.

Statistics show that, since 1980, childhood obesity in the U.S. has more than doubled among children ages two to five, and more than tripled among ages six to eleven, as well as between ages twelve to seventeen. Since obesity is the biggest risk factor for diabetes, heart disease, stroke and other serious health problems, there is an urgent need to quickly address this situation.

Fortunately, the National Heart, Lung and Blood Institute (NHLBI) one of the National Institutes of Health (NIHO) is taking the lead in publicizing this epidemic. In 2005, NHLBI launched "We Can!", a national program designed to help children ages eight to thirteen achieve and maintain a healthy weight.

The program gets community organizations, schools and hospitals involved in assisting families to improve their food choices and increase their physical activity which increases their defenses.

The American Academy of Pediatrics (AAP) is among the organizations to partner with the NHLBI to ensure "We can!" works for American children. Across the nation, communities are joining the crusade and to date more than 125 are collaborating.

For more information, "We can!" has a website for parents where you can download guides and forms for tracking your family's progress, get directions and suggestions for physical activities, recipes, cooking tips and much more.

Visit the site **wecan.nhlbi.nih.gov** and make sure to download or order the free booklet, "Families Finding the Balance: a Parent Handbook". It has plenty of easy ideas to help families achieve healthy weights, a goal you all can reach.

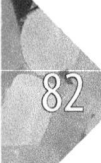

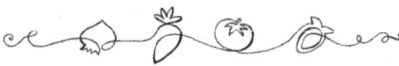

KidsHealth
Overweight and Obesity
Revised by: Mary L. Gavin, M.D.
Revised on: August 2005
First revision by:
Sandra G. Hassink, M.D.
February 12, 2005

Introduction

The percentage of overweight children in the U.S. and industrialized countries is increasing at an alarming rate. Many children are spending less time exercising and more time in front of the TV, computer, or video-game console. And today's busy families have fewer free moments to prepare nutritious, home-cooked meals, each day. From fast food to electronics, quick and easy seems to be the mindset of many people in the new millennium.

Since the seventies, the number of overweight children and adolescents has doubled in the U.S.. Today, 10% of children between ages two and five and more than 15% of between ages six and nineteen are overweight. If the percentage of overweight children is added to those who are at risk of developing it, the figure of overweight is one in three children.

Preventing children from becoming overweight means adapting the way your family eats and exercises, and how you spend time together. Helping children lead healthy lifestyles begins with parents who lead by example.

Overweight And Obesity
Is Your Child Overweight?

A child with a body mass index (BMI) above the 95th percentile, taking into account their sex and age, is considered overweight. BMI uses height and weight measures to estimate how much body fat a person has. To calculate a child's BMI, divide their weight (in kilograms) by the square of their height (in meters), i.e. weight / height. For pounds and inches, divide weight by height squared and multiply the result by the conversion factor 703.

An easier way to measure BMI is to use a BMI calculator. Once you know the child's BMI, it can be plotted on a standard BMI chart.

Children fall into one of four categories:
- Underweight: BMI below the 5th percentile
- Normal weight: BMI at the 5th and less than the 85th percentile
- Overweight: BMI at the 85th and below 95th percentiles
- Obese: BMI at or above 95th percentile

BMI is not a perfect measure of body fat and there are situations where BMI may be misleading. For example, a muscular person may have a high BMI without being overweight (because higher muscles mass increases a body's weight, but not fat). In addition, BMI may be difficult to interpret during puberty when children are experiencing periods of rapid growth. It is important to remember that BMI is usually a good indicator but not a direct measure of body fat.

You may be hearing a lot about BMI lately. Pediatricians now calculate BMI in routine visits and many schools include this measure in their students annual checkup.

If you are worried that your child or teen may be overweight, make an appointment with your doctor, who can assess your child's eating habits and physical activity and offer suggestions on how to make positive changes. The doctor may also screen for some of the medical conditions commonly associated with obesity.

Depending on the child's BMI, age, and health, the doctor may refer you to a registered dietitian for guidance on changes needed in the child's diet. In some cases, your doctor may recommend a comprehensive weight management program.

The Effects Of Obesity

Overweight children are at increased risk for serious health conditions including type II diabetes, hypertension, and high cholesterol; all once considered exclusively adult diseases. Overweight children may also be prone to low self-esteem that stems from being teased, bullied, or rejected by peers.

Children who are unhappy with their weight may be more likely than average-weight children to develop unhealthy eating habits and suffer from eating disorders like anorexia nervosa and bulimia; they are also more likely to become depressed and fall into addictive behaviors such as substance abuse.

Overweight and obese children are at risk for developing medical problems that affect their current and future health with a direct impact on their quality of life, including:

- high blood pressure, high cholesterol and abnormal blood lipid levels, insulin resistance, and type II diabetes.
- bone and joint problems.
- shortness of breath that makes exercise, sports, or any physical activity more difficult and may aggravate the symptoms or increase the chances of developing asthma.
- restless or disordered sleep patterns, such as obstructive sleep apnea.
- tendency to mature earlier (overweight kids may be taller and more sexually mature than their peers, raising expectations that they should act as old as they look, not as old as they are; overweight girls may have irregular menstrual cycles and fertility problems in adulthood).
- liver and gall bladder disease.
- depression.

Cardiovascular risk factors present in childhood due to obesity (including high blood pressure, high cholesterol, and diabetes) can lead to serious medical problems like heart disease, heart failure, and stroke in adulthood. Preventing or treating overweight and obesity in children may reduce the risk of developing these cardiovascular diseases in adulthood.

Causes Of Overweight

A number of factors contribute to becoming overweight. Genetics, lifestyle habits, or a combination of both may be involved. In some instances, endocrine problems, genetic syndromes, and medications can be associated with excessive weight gain.

Much of what we eat is quick and easy, from fat-laden fast food to microwave and prepackaged meals. Daily schedules are so jam-packed there's little time to prepare healthier meals or squeeze in some exercise. Portion sizes, in the home and out, have drastically increased.

Plus, now, more than ever, life is sedentary, children spend more time playing with electronic devices, from computers to handheld video game systems, than actively playing outside. Television is a major culprit.

Children younger than six years of age spend an average of two hours a day in front of a screen, mostly watching television or movies. Older children and teens spend almost four hours a day watching television or videos. When computer use and video games are included, time spent in front of a screen increases to over five-and-a-half hours a day! Children who watch more than four hours a day are more likely to be overweight compared with children who watch two hours or less.

Not surprisingly, TV in the bedroom is also linked to the increased likelihood of becoming overweight. For many children, once they get home from school, virtually all of their free time is spent in front of one screen or another!

The American Academy of Pediatrics (AAP) currently recommends limiting the time kids over two years of age spend in front of a screen to no more than one to two hours; the AAP also discourages any screen time for children younger than two years.

Many children don't get enough physical activity. Although physical education (PE) in

schools can help kids get up and moving, more and more schools are eliminating PE programs or cutting down the time spent on fitness-building activities. One study showed that gym classes offered third-graders just twenty-five minutes of vigorous activity each week.

Current guidelines recommend that children over two years of age should engage in at least sixty minutes of moderate to vigorous physical activity on most, preferably all, days of the week.

Genetics also plays a role; genes help determine body type and how your body stores and burns fat just like they help determine other traits. Genes alone, however, cannot explain the current obesity crisis. Because both genes and habits can be passed down from one generation to the next, multiple members of a family may struggle with weight.

People in the same family tend to have similar eating patterns, maintain the same levels of physical activity, and adopt the same attitudes toward being overweight. Studies have shown that a child's risk of obesity greatly increases if one or more parent is overweight or obese.

Preventing Overweight And Obesity

The key to keeping children of all ages at a healthy weight is taking a whole-family approach. It's the "practice what you preach" mentality. Make healthy eating and exercise a family affair, get your children involved by letting them help you plan and prepare healthy meals, and take them along when you go grocery shopping so they can learn how to make good food choices.

Avoid falling into some common food/eating behavior traps:
  • Don't reward children for good behavior or

punish bad behavior with sweets or treats. Come up with other solutions to modify their behavior.

- Don't maintain a clean-plate policy. Be aware of children's hunger cues. Even babies who turn away from the bottle or breast send signals that they're full. If children are satisfied, don't force them to continue eating.
- Reinforce the idea that they should only eat when they're hungry.
- Don't talk about "bad foods" or completely eliminate all sweets and favorite snacks from their diets. Children may rebel and over-eat these forbidden foods outside the home or sneak them in on their own.

Here are some additional recommendations for children of all ages:

- Birth to age 1: In addition to its many health benefits, breastfeeding may help prevent excessive weight gain. Though the exact mechanism is not known, breastfed babies may be more able to control their own intake and follow their own internal hunger cues.
- Ages 2 to 6: Start good habits early. Help shape food preferences by offering a variety of healthy foods.
- Encourage children's natural tendency to be active and help them build developing skills.
- Ages 7 to 12: Encourage them to be physically active every day, whether it's an organized sports team or a game of soccer during recess. Keep your children active at home too, through everyday activities like walking and playing in the yard. Let them be more involved in making good food choices, such as packing their lunch.
- Ages 13 to 17: Teens like fast food, but try to encourage healthier choices like grilled chicken sandwiches, salads, and smaller portions. Teach them how to prepare healthy meals and snacks at home. Encourage them to be active every day.

Also, cut down on TV, computer, and video game time and discourage eating while watching the tube. Serve a variety of healthy foods and eat meals together as often as possible. Encourage children to have at least five servings of fruits and vegetables a day, limit sugar-sweetened beverages, and eat breakfast every day. If you eat well, exercise regularly, and incorporate healthy habits into your family's daily life, you're modeling a healthy lifestyle for your children that will last. Talk to your children about the importance of eating well and being active, but make it a family affair that will become second nature for everyone.

Most of all let your children know you love them, no matter what their weight, and that you want to help them be happy and healthy.

Reviewed by: Mary L. Gavin, MD
Date reviewed: June 2008

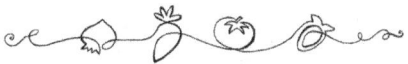

British Medical Association
Report On Child Obesity
2008

The British Medical Association report concludes: The BMA agrees with the Obesity Task Force that in order to halt the obesity epidemic "interventions at the family or school level will need to be matched and changes in the social and cultural context so that the benefits can be sustained and enhanced. Such prevention will require a coordinated effort between the medical community, health administrators, teachers, parents, food producers and processors, retailers and caterers, advertisers and the media, recreation and sport urban architects, city planners, politicians and legislators".

Environments that encourage healthy eating and active living are vitally important. The focus of such strategies should be to make it easier for the public to make healthy choices. Such strategies require funding for, but should ultimately lead to a reduction in, the costs to the NHIS from obesity related to health. Overweight and obesity in children have escalated dramatically in England over the past 20 years.

Nearly 22% of boys and 27.5% of girls aged two to fifteen were found to be overweight, including 5.5% of boys and 1.2% of girls who were obese in 2002. The 1077 analysis indicates a marked acceleration in the trend from the mld-1980s using the national Body Mass Index percentiles approach (adopted by the Department of Health, assuming 15% including 5% obesity in 1990) 20.3% of boys and 30.7% of girls were overweight, including 16% who were obese, by these Department of Health statistics.

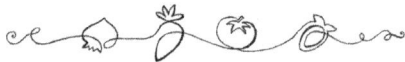

Le Figaro, France
Workshop to Detect Infant Obesity
By: Caroline Petitnicolas
October 1, 2008

The number of obese children has doubled over the past 10 years. The workshop's objective, organized by pediatricians, is to detect and prevent childhood obesity.

"Eat in a balanced, simple and economic way."

One of every six children in France is affected: 14.5% are overweight, 4% are obese; excess weight appears as early as age two years. The age with the highest exposure is seven to twelve years. With a big difference between regions: 22.2% en Corcega, 17.6 in Alsacia, 16.8% in Loira counties, (boys as much as girls).

Pediatricians estimate that, above all, it is necessary to raise awareness and prevention, because the problem is not recognized at an early age. The family only becomes truly conscience of the child's problem around age seven years. To help in the detection of this phenomenon, children's health cards should provide accurate body mass curves, depending on their size and weight, sex and age, which help define the limit of overweight and obesity.

Introducing Better Eating

Many studies show that prevention begins with breastfeeding. At one year of age, the baby nursed by its mother weighs approximately 500 grams less than a baby of equivalent size fed with formula. It is necessary to watch for an excessive protein allowance, and limit the over-consumption of sugars, saturated fats and sugary beverages, following the advice of pediatricians. Also avoid eating between meals.

However, to more easily control excess weight, both the child and their family are advised to not "eat less", but "eat better" and to "move more" with daily physical activity (walking, bike riding, skating, etc.), as well as develop the ability to make smart food choices.

The World Health Organization has established a linked cause — a relationship between the food industry's marketing of its products and the increase in childhood obesity. Overall, the AFPA (French Association of Ambulatory Pediatrics) points to the combination of two factors: sedentary behavior and easy access to high calories foods, to explain this worldwide epidemic, in both wealthy and developing countries.

Approximately 90 communities in France have proposed conferences, activities in schools or gyms, motor courses, "stands" of information, including screening tests (with the health card).

McMaster University, Hamilton, Canada
Population Health Research Institute
The Predominance of Childhood Obesity and its Treatment
September 30, 2008

The childhood obesity epidemic has reached very high levels in developed countries.

In the U.S., 25% of the children are overweight and 11% are obese. Overweight and obesity have a significant impact on a person's physical and psychological health.

The mechanism of obesity development is not completely understood and is believed to be a disorder with multiple causes. Environmental factors and lifestyle preferences play a fundamental role in the continuous growth of obesity in the world.

In general, overweight and obesity is presumed to be the result of an increase in calories and fat in the diet. There is supporting evidence that an excessive amount of sugar in sodas and beverages, an increase in the size of meal portions and lack of physical activity are determining factors in the phenomena of obesity worldwide. Consequently, both the excess consumption of calories and reduction of physical activity contribute to obesity.

Most researchers agree that prevention could be the key strategy to control this epidemic.

Prevention includes avoiding ever developing overweight or obesity, and not gaining weight to then continuously losing it again.

So far, the most attainable goal aims to change the attitude of people with diet and exercise.

However, it appears these strategies have had little impact on the high growth of this epidemic. While nearly 50% of adults are overweight or obese in many countries, it is difficult to reduce excess weight once it is acquired.

Children should be considered a priority in the population. Prevention may include a variety of interventions in the environment of children, promoting physical activity and good diets. Some of these potential strategies may be implemented by institutions in childcare centers, kindergartens, schools and after-school services.

Based on the above, there is an urgent need to initiate campaigns for the prevention and treatment of overweight and obesity in children.

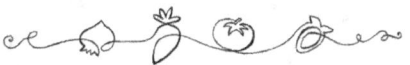

5. Delicious Nutritious Recipes

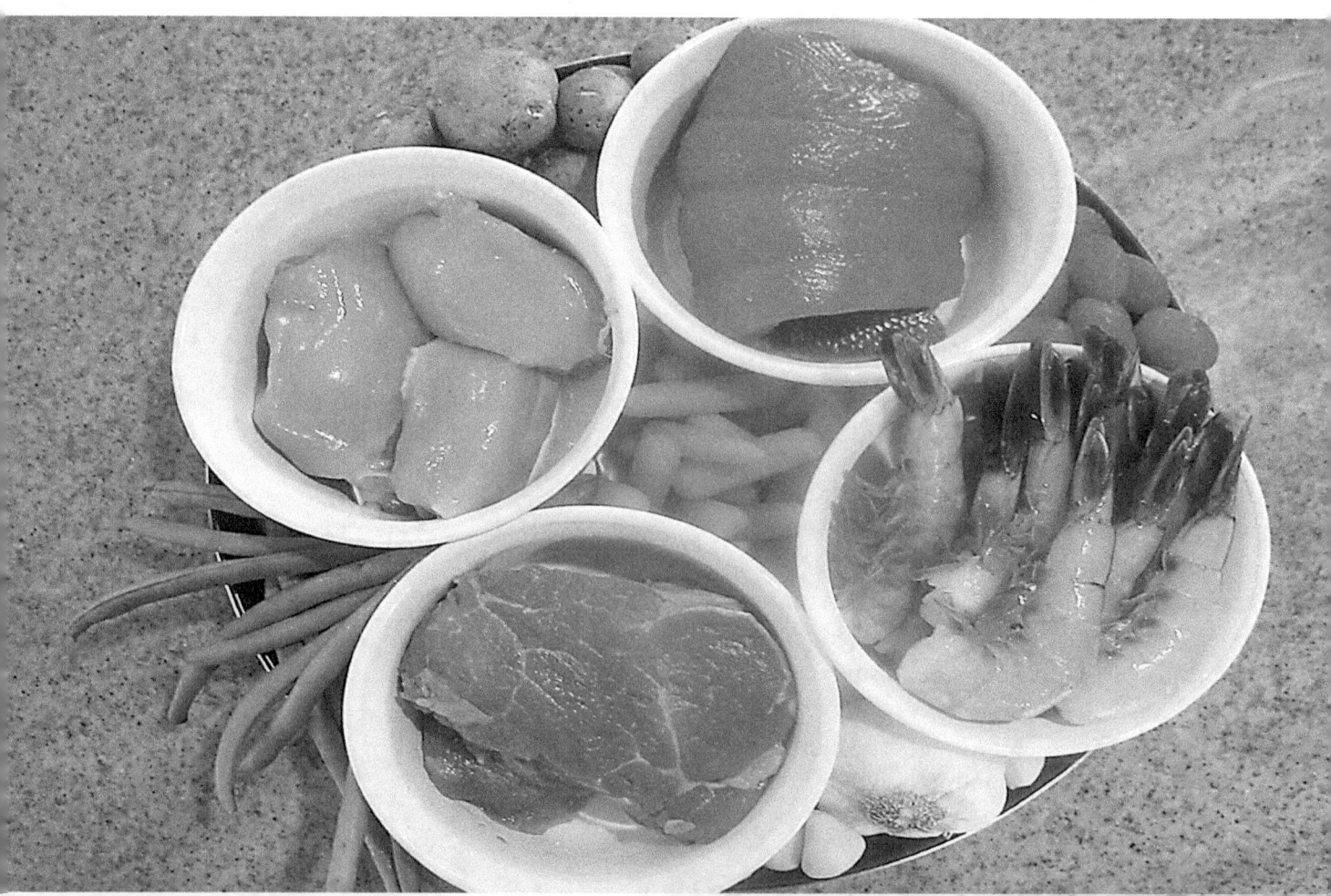

Is It Done Yet? Temperature Rules To Cook Safely

You cannot tell by looking. Use a food thermometer to be sure.

USDA recommends these guidelines for minimum internal temperatures:

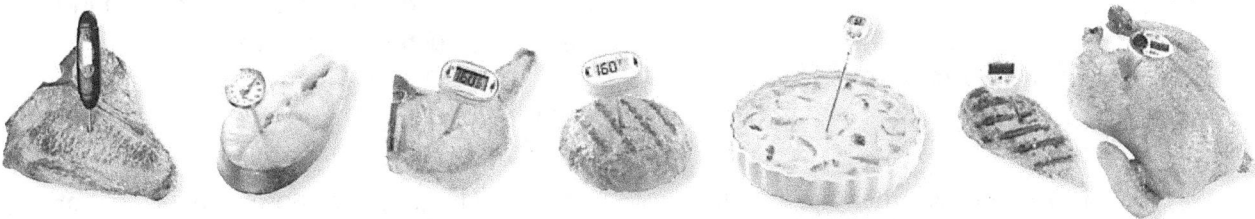

Meat, Lamb, & Duck	Fish	Pork	Meat, Lamb	Pies & Pastries with Egg	Turkey, Chicken
Pork chops or pieces	Roast		Rack of veal		Whole or bag
145°F	145°F	160°F	160°F	160°F	165°F

• Make sure meat, poultry and egg dishes, are cooked with the temperatures shown above to avoid foodborne illness.

• When cooking meals always be careful to use the correct temperature to ensure health. Bacteria can grow in foods between the temperatures 40°F and 140°F.

• To avoid the risk of food bacteria, keep cold the food to be served fresh and hot the food to be served warm.

• Use a clean thermometer every time it is introduced into food. Take the internal temperature of the food to ensure it is properly done.

Visit **www.IsItDoneYet.gov.**

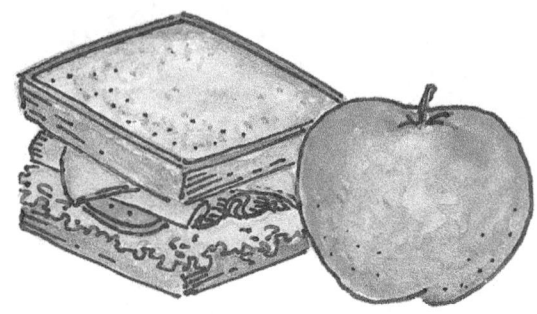

Practical Advice To Make Your Children's Lunches Attractive

Prepare sandwiches and other dishes to look attractive so they won't be swapped or thrown in the trash.

The smell, color, wrapping and presentation of food will affect your children's desire to eat it, which is why it should be packaged in a varied, colorful and attractive way.

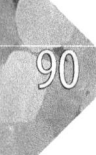

Cut sandwiches in two, three or four parts to make them easier to eat, and always use a clean lunch box as it represents the child's personality.

Know your children's taste, likes and dislikes, in food. If a child prefers heavy or fattening food, find a way to make them but with ingredients that contain fewer calories and fat substitutes.

Always use fresh vegetables and meats.

Before preparing a weekly menu, ask your children for five favorite foods, and then balance them with other foods to provide the necessary nutrition. They can even make up their own menu, ensuring they will eat it.

Encourage your children to participate in the preparation and packaging of their lunch boxes.

Each week, allow your children to participate in their lunch decisions, encouraging change and variety, thus avoiding loss of interest and them giving in to the temptation of unhealthy foods.

Remember, it is more important your children's meals are super-nutritious, not super-big.

No matter the child's age, enclose a little note or photograph of something that will remind them how much they are loved.

Hot Foods

Hot meals comprise approximately 30% of the daily food intake and it is important include them. But try to avoid excessive consumption of hot foods; when eaten in excess, the process of depuration in the body can take hours, causing it to be slow and heavy. A common mistake is to overeat them during the last meal of the day (dinner time). If you can make a hot dish at noontime (lunch), an afternoon of activities will provide for adequate digestion.

If nighttime is the only opportunity to eat hot foods, here are a few suggestions to make the meal healthy and balanced and not detract from the weight loss treatment.

• Eating too much is harmful, but it is worse to go to bed without eating at all (even if done to lose weight).

• The child should have a hot meal that is light but complete. This is a good moment to add some of the foods not included during the day.

• To facilitate digestion, cooking methods should be soft: boiled, oven baked, poached, grilled, etc..

• It is important to eat dinner at a reasonable hour. In general, two to three hours before bedtime is recommended.

- Among the **recommended foods** to be incorporated into a hot meal are:
  - Salads and vegetables.
  - Cereals, rice and pastas, (use whole meal products but always prepare in moderation).
  - Low fat dairy products (milk, yogurt, cheese).
  - If fruit was not eaten during the day, it can be eaten as the evening dessert (and much healthier than cake or chocolate).
  - Moderate amounts of lean meats like veal, chicken or fish.

- To help measure consumer portions, this book provides a list of the serving sizes for different foods.

Get Your Children To Eat More Fish

"I don't like it", is the usual reaction when a child is asked to eat fish. The reason? They think it is boring, difficult to eat, find the taste or odor too strong, etc., but this is no cause to remove it from their diet.

In fact, fish is essential to their diet due to its great nutritional properties (it helps growth, weight maintenance, is good for the heart, and feeds the brain…), making it vital that parents teach their children to eat this type of food. This is not always an easy task, but can be started with grilled fillet or sardines.

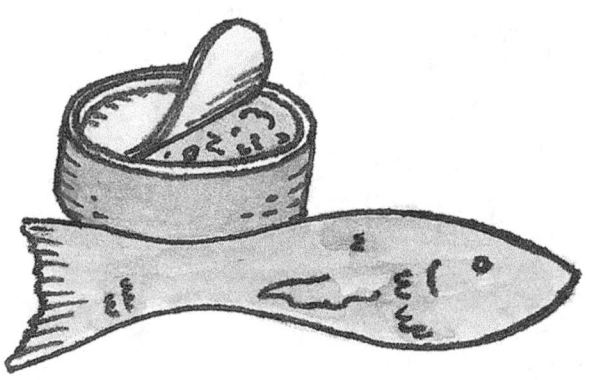

The Regulation and Organization Fund for the Fish and Marine Cultures Market (FROM) offers this advice:

- Children cannot tell the difference between species of fish. As a solution, show them the different variety and flavors of fish they can eat.

- Try to demonstrate that eating fish can also be fun. To achieve this, develop recipes with fish that are more creative, try to add bright colors and new shapes.

- The bones (spines) are the main concern when children eat fish. Therefore, start by using pieces without bones or skin (filet) or fish in a can (preserved). For example, trout, cod, and halibut — fresh or frozen, among the latter, little children seem to like fish sticks.

- Let children collaborate in its preparation to help them to lose their fear of fish and see lunch as a fun and important part of their day.

- Also, "FROM RADIO" (www.fromradio.es) is the first radio station with children talking about fish. It is a fun site for children to discover for themselves how healthy and tasty fish can be as a part of their diet.

Fruit Salads, Crunchy Vegetables, Chicken Fingers And Other Ideas To Accompany School Lunch

- Cut fresh fruit then put in a small plastic container. No need to add sugar or sauce, since fruits contain their own natural juices and sugar.

- Add a cup of yogurt with a small baggie of cereal to mix into the yogurt when ready to eat.

- Dry fruit, raisins and a variety of nuts offer great nutrition and children enjoy eating them.

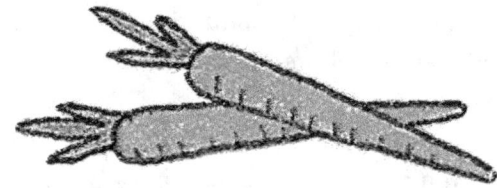

• Cut fresh cucumber (or carrots, peppers, celery) into slices or sticks, and then pack while cold from the refrigerator to make them crunchy.

• Another way to prepare carrots: cut them into sticks, place on tray sprayed with canola oil, bake at 400° for 25 minutes to make crispy, then place in lunch container.

• In the same manner as above prepare:
 – Skinless chicken breast the same: cut into thin slices, add some mustard and honey, and then bake.
 – Fish fingers with mayonnaise or fat free sour cream, and bake for 20 minutes.
 – Pasta in tomato sauce with fresh herbs like oregano, basil and low fat parmesan cheese.

Your children will enjoy their lunch!

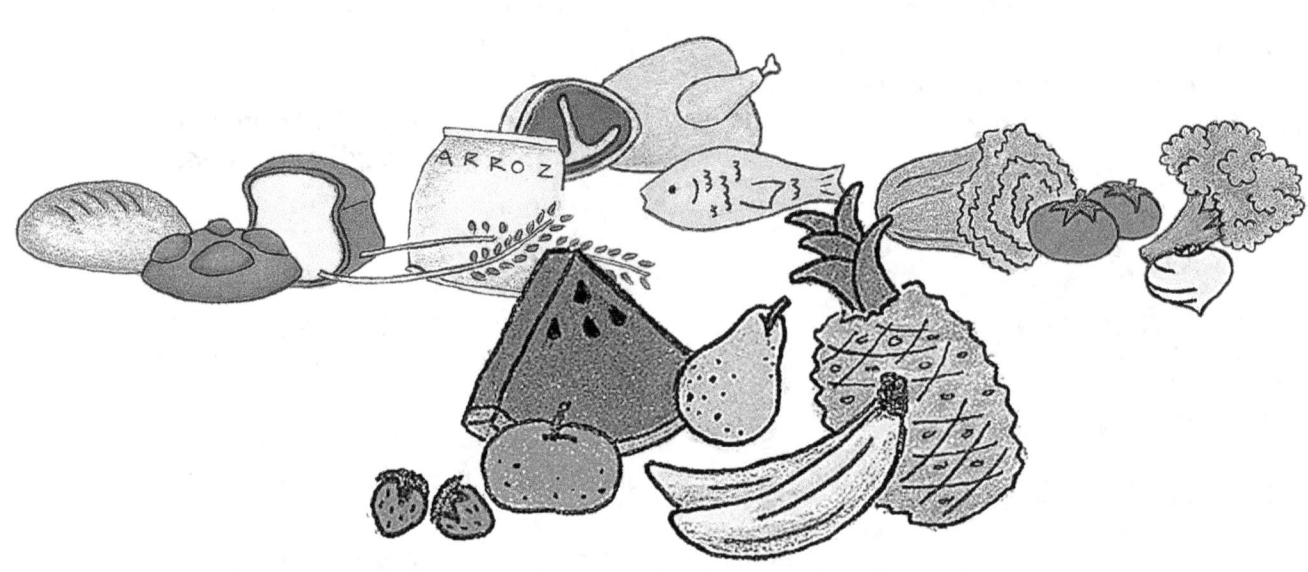

Requirements For School-age Children's Daily Nutrition

Generally, school-age children need 1,000 to 1,400 calories/day and between five to six meals/day to maintain high energy levels.

Vegetables	1 cup
Fruits	1 cup
Grains and cereals	3 ounces
Meats and beans	2 to 3 ounces
Dairy	3 glasses
Oils	2 teaspoons
Fats and sweets	Minimum possible

Elementary School Children

Complex carbohydrates and proteins are particularly important between ages five and eleven years, with normal weight children needing between 1,400 to 2,000 calories/day while obese and inactive children need between 1,000 to 1,500 calories/day:

Vegetables	2 cups
Fruits	1 cup
Grains and cereals	4 ounces
Meats and beans	3 ¼ ounces
Dairy	2 glasses
Oils	2 teaspoons
Fats and sweets	Abstain completely

Middle and High School Children

Generally, obese teenagers should be given between 1,500 to 2,000 calories/day:

Vegetables	3 cups
Fruits	1 cup
Grains and cereals	4 ounces
Meats and beans	3 ¼ ounces
Dairy	2 glasses
Oils	2 teaspoons
Fats and sweets	Abstain completely

Portion Control

Caution should be taken in the management of portions (see page 40):

Meat	3 ounces (equal to size of an open palm)
Pasta or rice	½ cup (size of a tennis ball)
Bread	1 slice
Vegetable	½ cup (equal to a hand full)
Dried fruit	1 ounce (size of an egg)
Nuts	1 ounce (size of a ping-pong ball)

Help Guide For Healthy Food Choices

PERMITTED	PROHIBITED
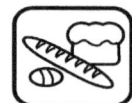	

Group: breads and breakfast cereals

Instead of 1 slice of bread:
½ medium round whole wheat loaf
1 small round whole wheat loaf
½ cup of unsweetened cereal fiber
2 saltine crackers
2 rice crackers or ½ French bread
or ½ cup unsweetened grains (oats, rye, wheat…)

Group: breads and breakfast cereals

All kinds of white bread, with raisins or dried
fruits, fruit fillings or sweet rolls
Muffins, pies, cakes, cookies
Breakfast cereal with sugar
Rice flakes
Oatmeal made with "whole" milk and sugar

Group: cheeses and cold meats

Cheese with 30% or less fat
Cheese spread (low fat)
Cottage cheese (low fat)
Cream cheese (low or nonfat)
Mozzarella (low fat)
Parmesan cheeses
Turkey (low fat)

Group: cheeses and cold meats

Cheese with 40% or more fat
American Cheese (whole milk)
Italian cream cheese 60% fat
Hollandaise cheese 48% fat (i.e., all cream cheese)
All French cheese
Cheese with cumin
Sour cream and parmesan

Group: hot and cold drinks

Freely allowed:
Water, mineral or soda water
Skim or low fat milk, soy milk
Herb tea unsweetened
Coffee with low fat milk,
Hot unsweetened chocolate
Lemonade and fresh fruit juices unsweetened
Salt-free vegetable juices
Salt-free vegetable broth
Yogurt (low or nonfat) unsweetened
Diet soft drinks (maximum 3/week)

Group: hot and cold drinks

Whole milk, or any beverages make with it
Buttermilk with sugar
Regular black tea and coffee
Iced tea or instant tea powder
Naturally sweetened lemonade
Liquid or "whole" yogurt,
Yogurt with fruit or sugar
Vegetable or fruit juices with sugar
Juice packages (if 100% fruit juice dilute ½ water)
Salt vegetable, beef or chicken broth
Soft drinks (soda pop)

Help Guide For Healthy Food Choices

PERMITTED

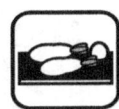

Group: meat, poultry and fish

Beef max. 2x/week: steak, sirloin, ground beef, t-bone, round, loin...
Lean veal, lamb, or goat
Poultry: chicken and turkey (without skin)
Lean fish (fillets): able, captain, grouper, nicuro, red snapper, snook, trout, bocachico...
Seafood: clams, shrimp, crab, lobster, oysters
Tuna, salmon in water

A serving of beef: 100 grams
A serving of poultry: ± 120 grams
A serving of fish: ± 150-200 grams

Prepare lean meats: grilled, baked, boiled, wrapped in aluminum foil
Remove visible fat from meat before preparation

Group: vegetables

Fresh or frozen vegetables, (except "Prohibited")
Only in limited quantities (2 tbsp.)
Peas, corn and mixed vegetables
Eat vegetables and greens daily with meals
Salads are best eaten as a first course to help activate digestive enzymes
Cooked vegetables should be ⅓ of a hot meal

PROHIBITED

Group: meat, poultry and fish

Pork and food containing pork (e.g., bacon, sausage, chops, ribs, ham, hamburgers, Chinese food, canned soups and sauces, ...
Ground beef
Meat cutlets: heart, liver, tongue, menudo, tripe, lung, kidney, brains, udder...
Chicken giblets
Chicken with skin, chicken sausage
Breaded meats or seafood
Fatty (blue) fish: sardines, anchovies, salted fish
Tuna in oil

Meat, poultry or fish grilled or prepared in a lot of fat or fatty sauces

Group: vegetables

Vegetables in heavy sauces or creams (e.g., fatty cheese, cream, sour cream...)
Canned vegetables
Canned tomato juice
Canned vegetable soups
Vegetable soup with potatoes, pasta, banana, cassava, canned corn
Thick soups with flour
Avocado salad with mayonnaise
Roasted banana (banana is NOT a vegetable)

Help Guide For Healthy Food Choices

PERMITTED

PROHIBITED

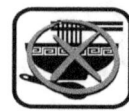

Group: flour, tubers, plantains and legumes

Replace with:

1 tablespoon of pasta (macaroni, spaghetti)

1 potato (max. 3x/week) or 2 small (boiled, steamed or baked)

1 tablespoon of mashed potatoes without milk, butter or margarine

⅓ boiled plantain or 2 slices baked

100 grams of sweet potato or similar radish in similar preparation

300 grams of baked yams

1 cup cooked legumes

2 slices of "vegetarian" pizza with mozzarella

Note: Remember to use only the amounts indicated!

Group: flour, tubers, plantains and legumes

Fried rice

French fries

Instant mashed potatoes

Potato mashed with butter or steamed with sour cream

Macaroni or spaghetti with sauce, fat cheese or butter

Fettucini Alfredo

Pizza with extra cheese or toppings, (pepperoni, salami, or anchovies)

Beans with pork fat or sugar

Refried or canned beans

Group: fruits

Choose from among the following fresh fruits:

1 apple, orange, peach, pear, apricot,

1 large or 2 small tangerine,

2 plums or kiwis, ½ grapefruit,

2 cups strawberries or raspberries,

1 cup grapes, blueberries or cherries,

200 grams of watermelon, melon or papaya,

100grams of pineapple,

1 glass of guava or cranberry juice,

1 glass of sugar-free juice package,

Coconut water without inside pulp

Instead of 1 fruit — drink 1 glass/day of fresh fruit juice (homemade and unsweetened)

Avoid powder and premade juices — if no other option: mix ½ unsweetened juice + ½ water.

Group: fruits

Fruits you should not eat: sapodilla, coconut, dried fruits, dates, raisins, plums and figs, dehydrated fruits (apples, pears, peaches...)

All types of nectars

Fruits canned or jar preserved with molasses or syrup

Fruit flavored syrups

Fruit juices with sugar packet

Instant fruit juice powder

Fruit ices and popsicles with sugar

Fruit "Permitted" within limitations:

Mango (1x/week)

Prunes (max 3 to 4 units)

Help Guide For Healthy Food Choices

PERMITTED

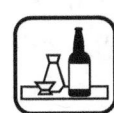

Group: spices and seasonings
Fresh herbs and spices: garlic, onion, tomato, pepper, celery, red pepper...

Do not combine a variety of condiments that contain salt: flavor cubes + soy sauce + garlic salt

Use only one seasoning that contains salt.

Sauces with salt: black, soy and Tabasco®

Dried spices without salt: curry, pepper, paprika, nutmeg, turmeric, ginger, ginseng...

PROHIBITED

Group: spices and seasonings
Any tomato sauces, ketchup and dips
Any packaged or canned soups and sauces
Mayonnaise (100 kcal per tablespoon)
Oil based sauces or gravies

Group: desserts and sweets
Pudding, custard, gelatin, pies, cakes, cookies, chips...
Hard and soft candies, sweet and sours, mints, milk chocolate, caramels...

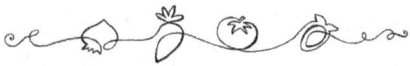

97

Practical Ideas For Healthy Cooking

• Whenever oil is needed, replace it with low sodium chicken broth. If oil is absolutely required, use canola oil in small quantities. For baking sweets, replace oil with applesauce or pureed raisins.

• Instead of frying, bake using canola oil spray or an oil soaked napkin to lightly cover a tray, then place food on the tray and spray lightly again. Food will be golden brown and crispy.

• Instead of cream, use low fat evaporated milk mixed with low fat 1% milk, or use nonfat sour cream or nonfat yogurt.

• Use nonfat or low fat mayonnaise.

• If a recipe requires cheese or chocolate, use a small amount of low or nonfat, for flavor only.

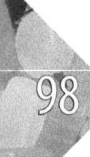

98

• Use small quantities of low sodium sea salt, or replace it with low sodium soy sauce.

• Instead of regular eggs use egg whites or an egg substitute.

• Use sauces or dressings that are low fat or nonfat, or preferably natural fruit juice.

• Use pastas and cereals preferably from whole grains, especially oats or corn.

• Look for diet recipes that are low in calories and follow their instructions to the letter.

• To thicken food, use cooked potato or wheat flour in small quantities, or avoid when possible.

• Reduce or eliminate sugar in recipes or replace with molasses, maple syrup (without sugar), a little honey, or a sugar substitute.

• Give color and variety to your meals with: green veggies like spinach, broccoli or green beans; red veggies like beets or peppers; yellow veggies like carrots, pumpkin or zucchini; and white veggies like cauliflower or parsnips.

• Give flavor to your meals by seasoning with fresh herbs and avoid heavy sauces/gravies. For soups, use leeks, onions, turnips, celery or cole.

• If possible, shop at farmers markets and fresh food marts which sell vegetables and "organic products" that are grown free of pesticides.

• Replace meat during the week with legumes in moderate quantities. They are very rich in vitamins A & C, and protein with no cholesterol.

• Tofu, made from soybeans, is healthy replacement for meat in most recipes. It is a great companion for vegetables and most other foods.

• Avoid recipes high in saturated fat or cholesterol. Whenever possible, decrease the consumption of beef, pork, lamb and eggs and replace with soy milk, soybeans or tofu. Replace meat sausages with nonfat turkey or vegetarian.

• It is very important to read the "Nutrition Facts" product labels to ensure they contain the proper amount of calories and nutritional value.

• Lastly, make mealtime the most important time of day and establish your own rules: wash hands, use table manners, and most important, eat slowly in a relaxed environment while having pleasant conversations with family members, (minus television or other background noise).

NOTE:
If you have any questions please contact: **recetas@obesidadtratamiento.com** and we will gladly respond as soon as possible.

6. Recipes
For The Whole Family

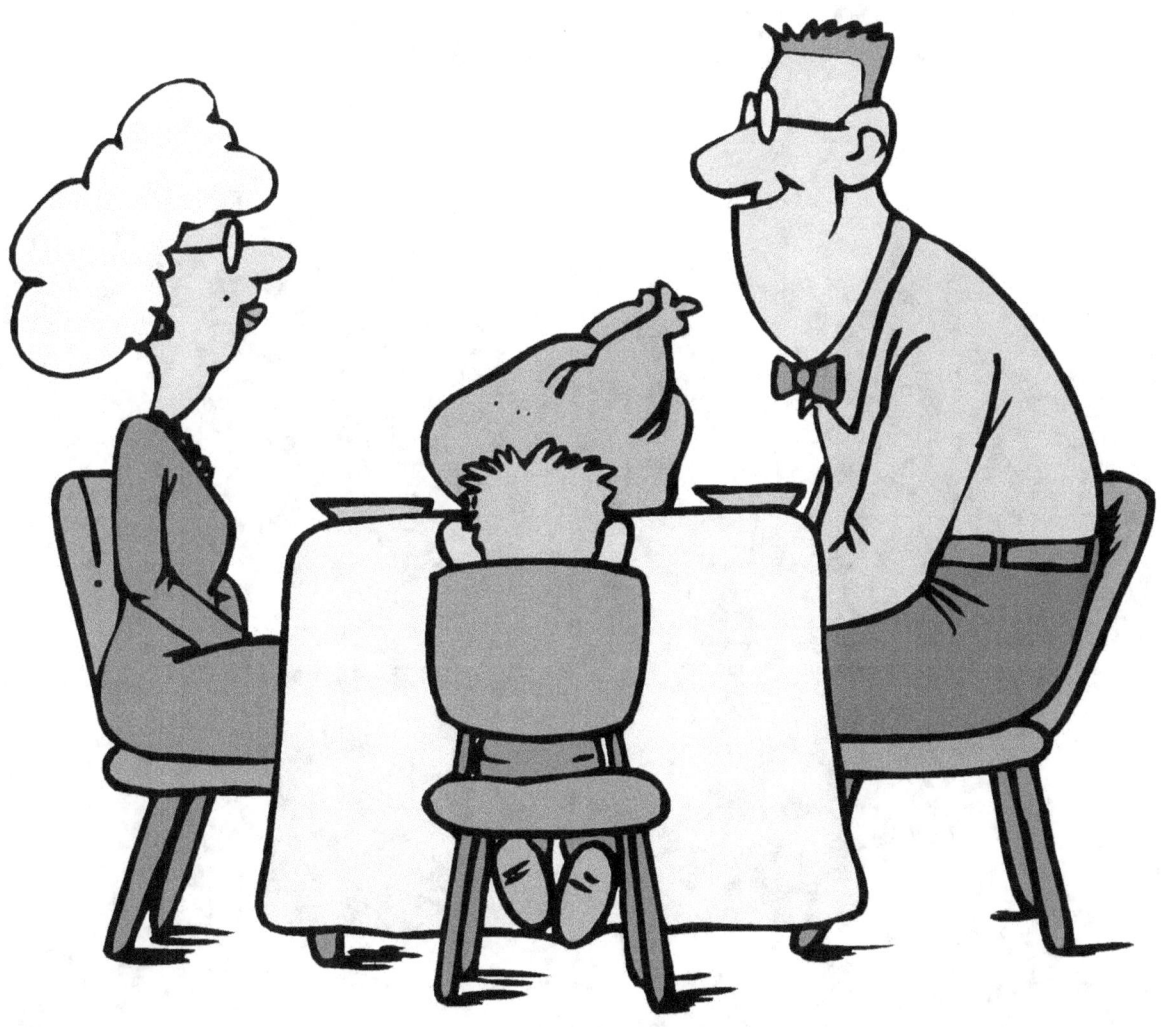

Best School Lunches

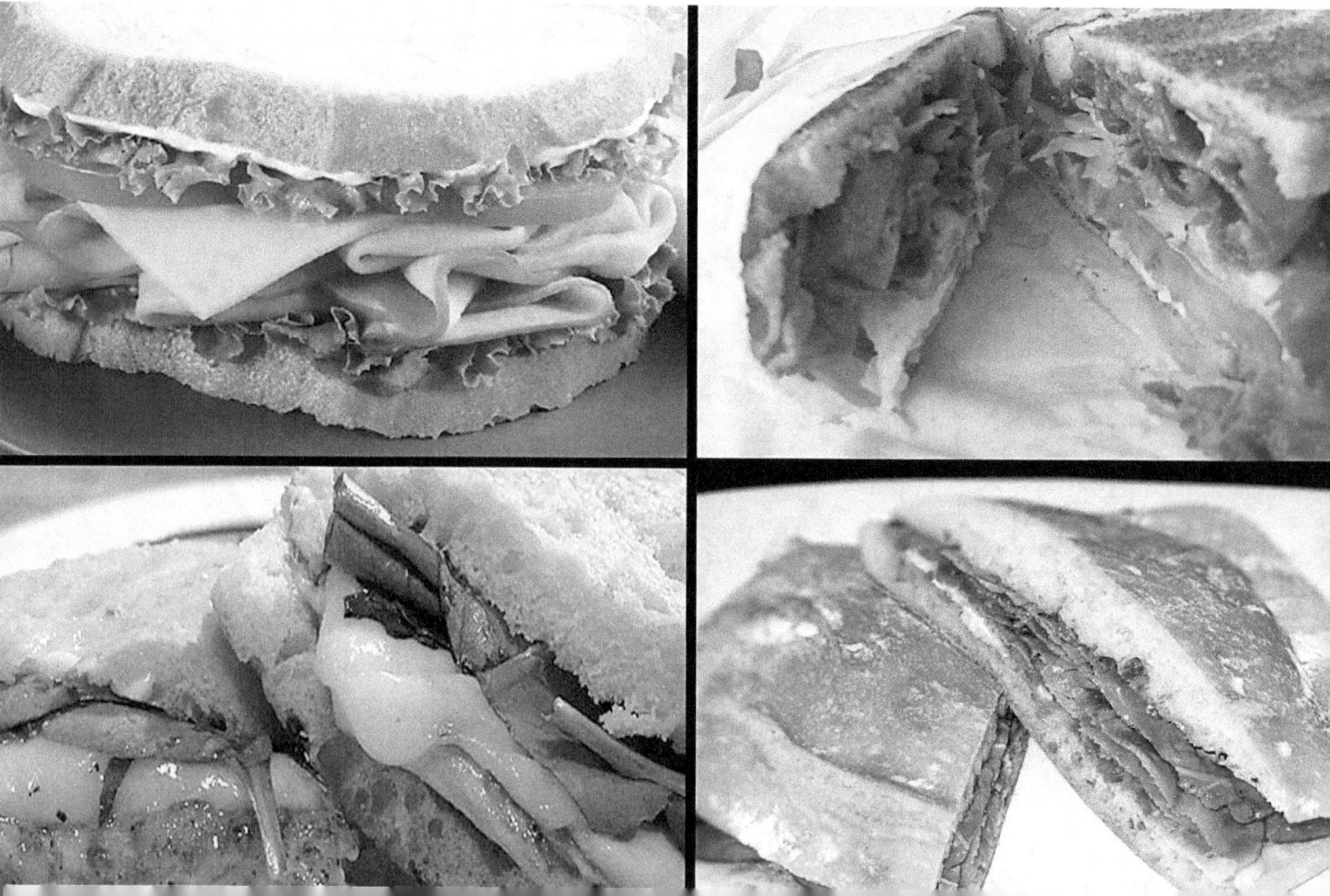

1. Vegetarian Burrito

Preparation Time: 10 minutes
6 servings

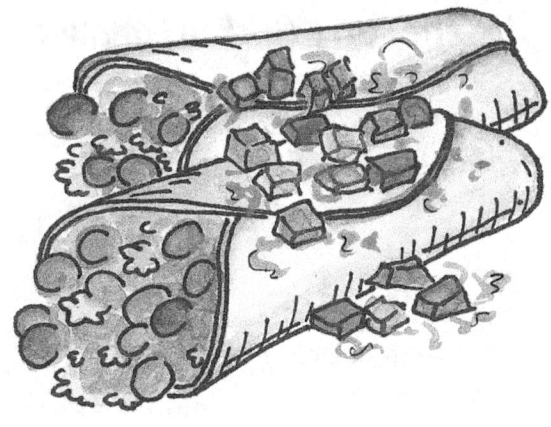

Ingredients

1 red pepper, seeded and chopped
1 yellow pepper, seeded and chopped
1 onion, peeled and sliced
1 can (8 oz.) black beans, drained and rinsed in water
½ avocado, peeled and cut into squares
½ cup chopped cilantro
1 lime, squeezed for juice
1 tsp. chili powder (optional)
½ cup nonfat sour cream
6 tortillas, 8" wheat
8 tbsp. "pico de gallo" salsa made with skinned tomatoes, onions, cilantro, garlic and spices
Canola oil spray

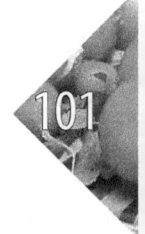

Preparation

In a pan, previously sprayed with canola oil, saute the peppers and onion 5 minutes over medium heat. Add beans, mix well and cook 5 minutes more.

In a separate medium bowl, combine the avocado, lime juice, cilantro and chili powder.

Divide mixture into two and leave one half aside. In the other half add the sour cream and mix well.

Warm tortillas on the stove or in the microwave. Spread on each warm tortillas the avocado mixture and a quarter of the bean mixture, then add 2 teaspoons of "pico de gallo".

Fold each tortilla up and down over the filling and roll the rest to form a burrito.

This is a complete source of nutrition and fiber.

Latin food is tasty and healthy.

Nutrition Facts	
Serving Size 1/6 of recipe 216g (215 g)	
Servings per container 6	
Amount Per Serving	
Calories 343	Calories from Fat 49
	% Daily Value*
Total Fat 6g	9%
Saturated Fat 1g	4%
Trans Fat 0g	
Cholesterol 2mg	1%
Sodium 365mg	15%
Total Carbohydrate 61g	20%
Dietary Fiber 8g	32%
Sugars 3g	
Protein 15g	

2. Rotisserie Curry Chicken Sandwich

Preparation Time: 15 minutes
2 servings

Ingredients

1 ¾ shredded rotisserie chicken
2 tbsp. chopped celery
2 tbsp. plain yogurt
2 tbsp. nonfat sour cream
1 tbsp. lemon juice
½ tbsp. curry powder
⅛ tbsp. cumin
Salt and pepper to taste
1 pita bread
4 leaves red lettuce

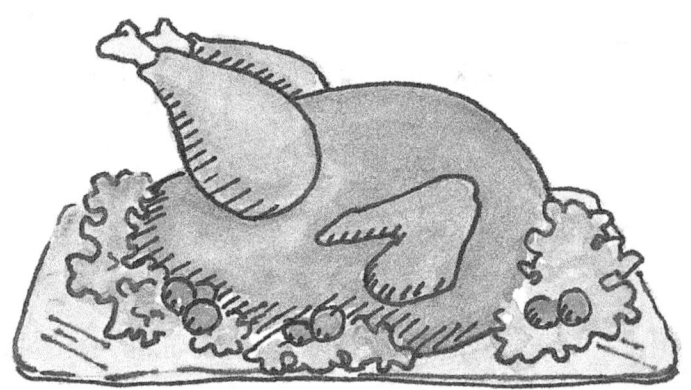

Preparation

In a medium bowl, mix chicken and celery.

Separately, mix together the yogurt, sour cream, lemon juice, curry powder and cumin. Add the chicken and celery. Mix well and add salt and pepper to taste.

Cut pita bread in half to form 2 pockets and put them to roast slightly.

Fill each warmed pocket with an equal servings of chicken mixture then serve on 2 lettuce leaves.

Nutrition Facts	
Serving Size 1/2 of recipe 235g (234 g)	
Servings per container 2	
Amount Per Serving	
Calories 351	Calories from Fat 97
	% Daily Value*
Total Fat 11g	17%
Saturated Fat 3g	15%
Trans Fat 0g	
Cholesterol 116mg	39%
Sodium 295mg	12%
Total Carbohydrate 21g	7%
Dietary Fiber 3g	11%
Sugars 3g	
Protein 42g	

3. Sweet Chicken Wraps

Preparation Time: 5 minutes
4 servings

Ingredients

1 lb. cooked chicken breast, sliced thin
1 green pepper, chopped
4 green olives, chopped
1 red pepper, chopped
1 tomato, diced
¼ cup nonfat ranch salad dressing
4 medium-size flour tortillas

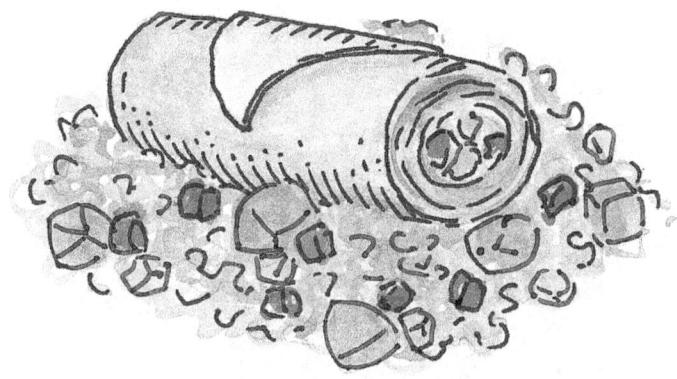

Preparation

In a medium bowl, place the first 5 ingredients and the ranch dressing, then mix together well.

Put a quantity of the mixture in the center of each tortilla then wrap well.

Use lettuce leaves, wax paper or foil to transport in school lunch box or bag.

Children will love them combined with a juice, yogurt or fruit.

Nutrition Facts		
Serving Size 1/4 of recipe 258g (258 g)		
Servings per container 4		
Amount Per Serving		
Calories 366	Calories from Fat 80	
		% Daily Value*
Total Fat 9g		14%
Saturated Fat 2g		11%
Trans Fat 0g		
Cholesterol 96mg		32%
Sodium 469mg		20%
Total Carbohydrate 30g		10%
Dietary Fiber 3g		12%
Sugars 4g		
Protein 39g		

4. Turkey Ham Submarine Sandwich

Preparation Time: 15 minutes
6 servings

Ingredients

1 tbsp. fruit vinegar
2 tsp. dried oregano
2 tbsp. chicken broth
1 French bread (baguette)
1 head iceberg lettuce shredded
1 large tomato, cut into thin round slices
6 slices of turkey ham (92% fat)
6 thin slices of nonfat cheddar cheese
3 red bell peppers (baked, skinless), cut lengthwise into strips
2 eggs hard-boiled, sliced
Salt and pepper to taste

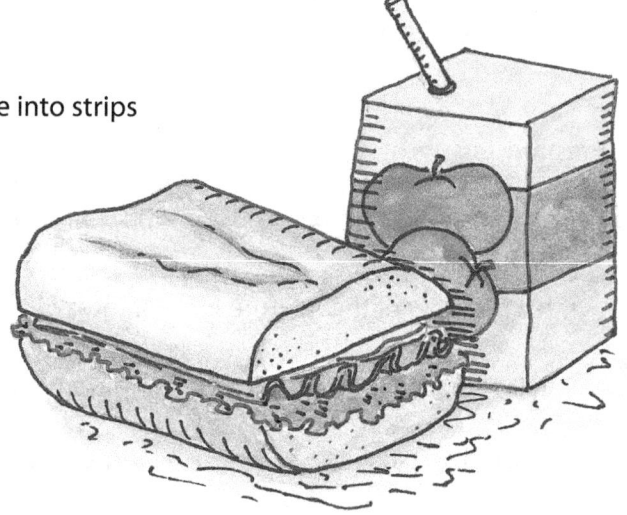

Preparation

In a small bowl, place the vinegar, oregano
and chicken broth.

Cut the bread open on one side for filling,
then sprinkle one side with half the vinegar mixture.

On the vinegar side, place shredded lettuce,
tomato, slices of turkey ham, cheese, red peppers, and finish with the sliced boiled eggs. Sprinkle with
remaining vinegar then firmly press closed the two sides of the sandwich.

Cut the sandwich into 6 portions and serve.

This is another delicious lunch accompanied by a juice, yogurt or fruit.

Nutrition Facts	
Serving Size 1/6 of recipe 338g (337 g)	
Servings per container 6	
Amount Per Serving	
Calories 351	Calories from Fat 76
	% Daily Value*
Total Fat 8g	13%
Saturated Fat 4g	21%
Trans Fat 0g	
Cholesterol 69mg	23%
Sodium 984mg	41%
Total Carbohydrate 47g	16%
Dietary Fiber 4g	18%
Sugars 8g	
Protein 23g	

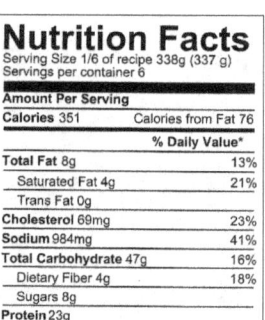

5. Grilled Vegetable Sandwich

Preparation Time: 35 minutes
6 servings

Ingredients

2 medium zucchini
1 eggplant, skinned
1 sweet onion, peeled
2 cloves garlic, minced
½ cup chopped fresh basil
½ cup canola oil
10 sun-dried tomatoes (packed in oil), chopped
2 anchovies (packed in oil), chopped
½ lb. of nonfat mozzarella
1 French bread (baguette)
Salt and pepper to taste

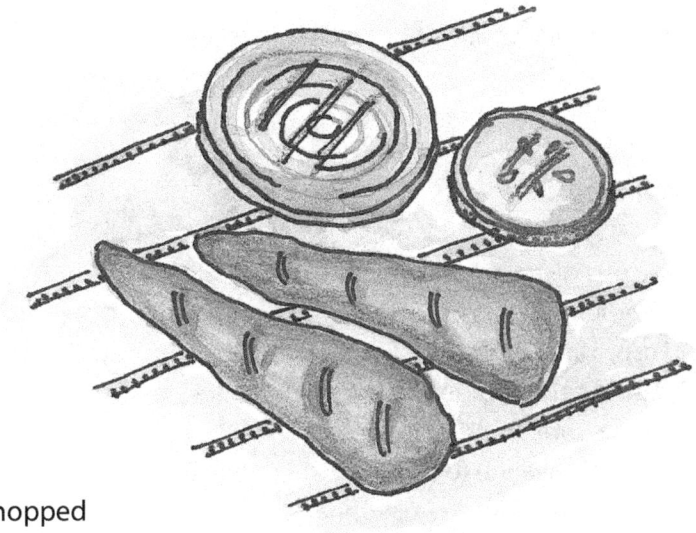

Preparation

Preheat Grill. Cut zucchini lengthwise into thin slices and place in large bowl. Cut eggplant and onion in half lengthwise then crosswise into thin slices and add to bowl. Then add garlic and half the basil, and drizzle with 4 tablespoons of oil. Season with salt and pepper to taste. Stir well.

Move vegetables to a baking tin then grill them, turning each until lightly browned. Allow to cool.

Combine tomatoes with anchovies and remaining basil in a blender. Add 3 tablespoons of oil then blend until chunky, adding more oil to make a spreadable paste.

Cut bread open lengthwise and hollow out the center leaving a retaining wall of bread. Spread paste on both sides, then carefully lay the grilled vegetables on top.
Finish with mozzarella cheese placed over the vegetables.

Carefully close sandwich then, using a spatula, press any protruding cheese or vegetables back into the sandwich. Wrap in waxed paper then top the sandwich with cast-iron skillet or other heavy weight. Let stand for a half hour to compact then cut into thick slices to serve.

Wash this healthy lunch down with a delicious fruit juice or 1% milk.

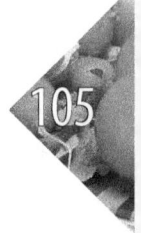

Nutrition Facts		
Serving Size 1/6 of recipe 317g (317 g)		
Servings per container 6		
Amount Per Serving		
Calories 437	Calories from Fat 186	
		% Daily Value*
Total Fat 21g		32%
Saturated Fat 2g		11%
Trans Fat 0g		
Cholesterol 5mg		2%
Sodium 992mg		41%
Total Carbohydrate 47g		16%
Dietary Fiber 5g		22%
Sugars 11g		
Protein 17g		

6. Braised Ham Sandwich

Preparation Time: 5 minutes
2 servings

Ingredients

1 ½ cups diced naturally-cured ham
½ medium apple, diced
1 tbsp. minced sweet red onion
1 tbsp. finely chopped celery
1 tbsp. chopped green pepper
1 dash of cayenne (optional)
2 - 3 tbsp. nonfat tofu mayonnaise
4 slices wheat bread
Salt to taste

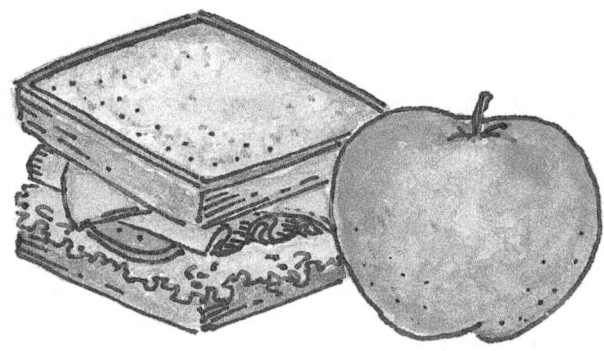

Preparation

In a medium bowl, mix the first 6 ingredients until well combined, then add mayonnaise until uniformly moistened.

Spread 2 bread slices with remaining mayonnaise, then with ham mixture. Close sandwiches with the other bread slices, then cut both in half and serve.

Nutrition Facts	
Serving Size 1/2 of recipe 228g (228 g)	
Servings per container 2	
Amount Per Serving	
Calories 348	Calories from Fat 106
	% Daily Value*
Total Fat 12g	18%
Saturated Fat 3g	13%
Trans Fat 0g	
Cholesterol 32mg	11%
Sodium 1572mg	66%
Total Carbohydrate 31g	10%
Dietary Fiber 3g	11%
Sugars 7g	
Protein 29g	

7. Tuna Salad Sandwich

Preparation Time: 10 minutes
2 servings

Ingredients

1 can (6 oz.) albacore tuna (without water)
2 tbsp. finely chopped jicama
2 tbsp. grated carrot
2 tbsp. minced green onion
2 tbsp. lemon juice
3 tbsp. tofu mayonnaise
Salt and pepper to taste
4 slices wheat bread

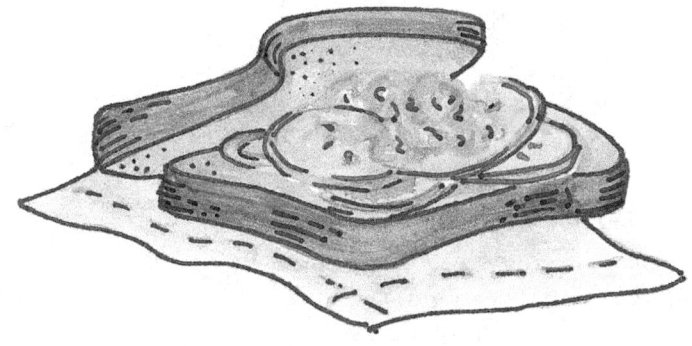

Preparation

In a medium bowl, mix the first 6 Ingredients until well combined.

Add 2 tablespoons of tofu mayonnaise, salt and pepper to taste, then mix again.

Spread remaining mayonnaise on 2 bread slices then with tuna mixture. Close sandwiches with other bread slices, then cut both in half and serve.

Nutrition Facts		
Serving Size 1/2 of recipe 196g (196 g)		
Servings per container 2		
Amount Per Serving		
Calories 323	Calories from Fat 88	
		% Daily Value*
Total Fat 10g		15%
Saturated Fat 1g		6%
Trans Fat 0g		
Cholesterol 26mg		9%
Sodium 488mg		20%
Total Carbohydrate 29g		10%
Dietary Fiber 3g		11%
Sugars 4g		
Protein 29g		

8. Mediterranean Turkey Sandwich

Preparation Time: 30 minutes
5 servings

Ingredients

½ lb. turkey ham, sliced thin
1 green pepper, sliced thin
1 onion, sliced thin
¼ cup water
¼ tsp. each: garlic powder, oregano powder, and pepper
1 cup nonfat yogurt
1 ½ tsp. lemon juice
Salt and pepper to taste
10 batavia lettuce leaves, washed and dried
1 French bread (baguette),
   cut open lengthwise
Canola oil spray

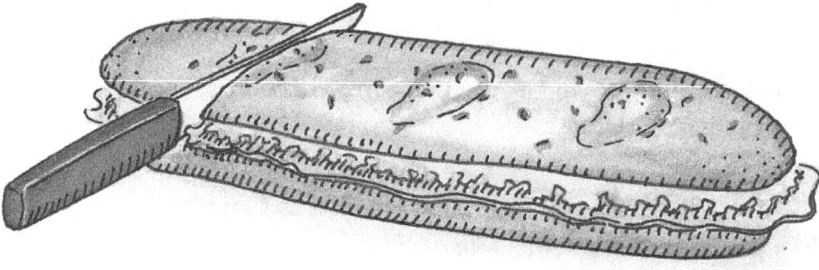

Preparation

Spray pan with canola oil and place over medium heat for about 30 seconds. Add turkey ham, bell pepper and onion, then cook and stir for 5 minutes or until turkey is lightly browned. Add water, garlic powder, oregano and pepper, then cook 5 minutes or until water is absorbed.

In a small bowl, mix the yogurt with lemon juice then salt and pepper to taste. Spread on both sides of bread, then place the lettuce on top and evenly fill it with turkey ham mixture.

Close the sandwich, then cut into 5 portions and serve.

Delicious for lunch.

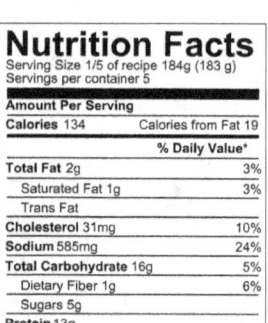

Nutrition Facts	
Serving Size 1/5 of recipe 184g (183 g)	
Servings per container 5	
Amount Per Serving	
Calories 134	Calories from Fat 19
	% Daily Value*
Total Fat 2g	3%
Saturated Fat 1g	3%
Trans Fat	
Cholesterol 31mg	10%
Sodium 585mg	24%
Total Carbohydrate 16g	5%
Dietary Fiber 1g	6%
Sugars 5g	
Protein 13g	

9. Egg and Vegetable Stuffed Pita

Preparation Time: 5 minutes
4 servings

Ingredients

3 large eggs
½ cup shredded nonfat cheddar cheese
½ cup chopped green and red peppers
4 small mushrooms, chopped
4 small flour pitas with pockets
1 small tomato, chopped
Salt and pepper to taste
Canola oil spray

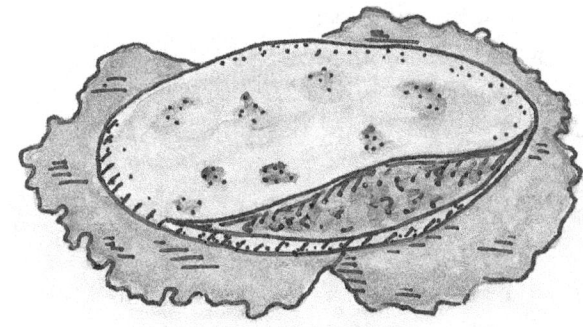

Preparation

In a regular bowl, whisk the eggs with salt and pepper then set aside.

Spray a large pan with oil then heat. Add eggs and cook until golden on one side. Flip eggs over with rubber spatula then add remaining ingredients on top and cook until eggs look dry.

Remove from heat, place in dish and cross-cut into 4 portions, then cut each of 4 in half to make 8 portions.

Cut 4 pitas in half, then lightly toast. Open each pita half and fill with 1 egg portion to make 8 pockets.

Serve 2 warm pitas per serving with a side of fruit.

Nutrition Facts	
Serving Size 1/4 of recipe 178g (178 g)	
Servings per container 4	
Amount Per Serving	
Calories 245	Calories from Fat 61
	% Daily Value*
Total Fat 7g	11%
Saturated Fat 2g	10%
Trans Fat 0g	
Cholesterol 267mg	89%
Sodium 436mg	18%
Total Carbohydrate 28g	9%
Dietary Fiber 2g	8%
Sugars 2g	
Protein 17g	

10. Peanut Butter Sandwich with Ham and Strawberries

Preparation Time: 5 minutes
2 servings

Ingredients

2 tbsp. nonfat peanut butter
4 slices wheat or banana bread
4 slices turkey ham
2 tbsp. nonfat sour cream
4 strawberries, cut into round slices
2 tsp. molasses

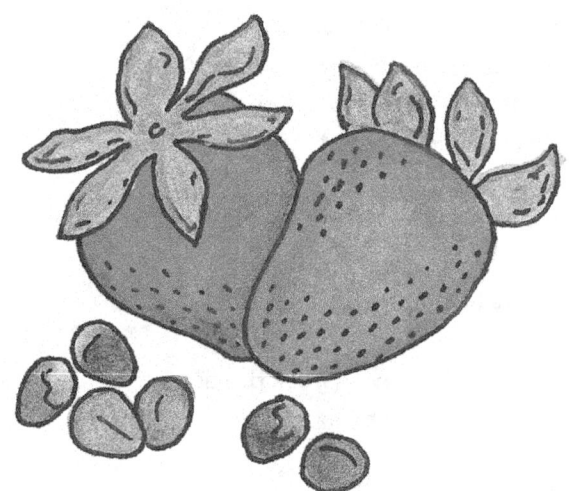

Preparation

Spread peanut butter on 2 slices of bread, then place 2 slices of turkey ham on each.

Spread other 2 slices of bread with sour cream and set aside.

In a small bowl, mix strawberries with molasses, then spread over the turkey ham slices.

Cover with the sour cream coated bread slices, then cut each sandwich in halves or in fours.

Combines nicely with a side of fruit juice.

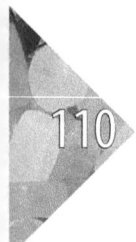
Nutrition Facts	
Serving Size 1/2 of recipe 164g (164 g)	
Servings per container 2	
Amount Per Serving	
Calories 294	Calories from Fat 63
	% Daily Value*
Total Fat 7g	11%
Saturated Fat 2g	8%
Trans Fat	
Cholesterol 37mg	12%
Sodium 830mg	35%
Total Carbohydrate 40g	13%
Dietary Fiber 3g	11%
Sugars 12g	
Protein 18g	

11. Delicious Tofu (Soy) Burgers

Preparation Time: 15 minutes
6 servings

Ingredients

1 lb. hard tofu
1 cup breadcrumbs
1 egg, beaten
1 tbsp. tomato sauce.
1 tbsp. Worcestershire sauce
1 small onion
1 tsp. mustard
1 tsp. salt
¼ tsp. pepper
Canola oil spray
12 slices wheat bread

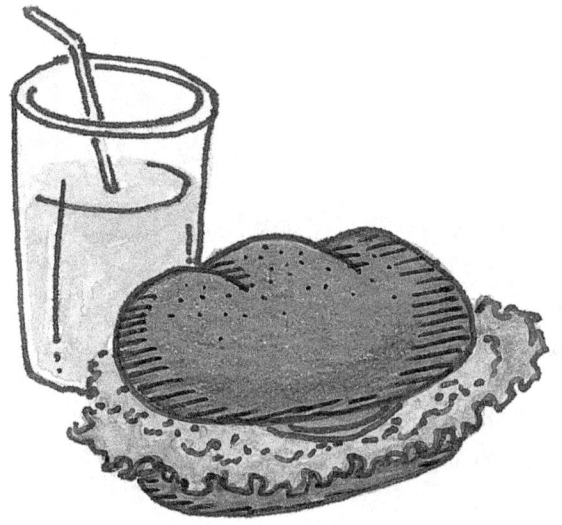

Preparation

In a large bowl, crumble tofu and separate.

In a separate bowl, whisk the egg then mix together with breadcrumbs until well combined. Add egg mixture with remaining ingredients to the tofu and mix well.

Wet hands and using 4 tbsp. of mixture form thin, round patties the size of a regular hamburger.

Preheat oven to 350F and spray baking sheet with canola oil. Place burgers on sheet and cook each side for 10 minutes.

Serve on toasted bread with lettuce, sliced tomato and pickles or any other vegetables of your choice.

Burgers may be saved in the refrigerator then later reheated in the microwave for 30 seconds.

This is a high protein, low calorie, meat substitute lunch.

Nutrition Facts	
Serving Size 1/6 of recipe 125g (125 g)	
Servings per container 6	
Amount Per Serving	
Calories 207	Calories from Fat 88
	% Daily Value*
Total Fat 10g	16%
Saturated Fat 2g	8%
Trans Fat 0g	
Cholesterol 35mg	12%
Sodium 617mg	26%
Total Carbohydrate 20g	7%
Dietary Fiber 2g	6%
Sugars 2g	
Protein 10g	

12. Mexican Chicken Tacos with Avocado and Cheese

Preparation Time: 10 minutes
10 servings

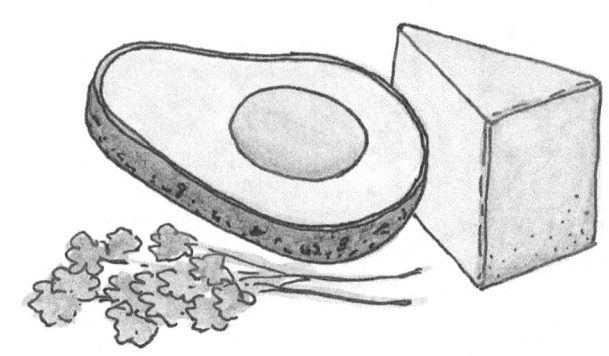

Ingredients

1 ripe avocado, sliced
1 lemon, squeezed for juice
½ tsp. salt
2 tbsp. canola oil
2 cups cooked chicken, chopped into small pieces
1 jar (4 oz.) green chiles, drained and chopped
1 small white onion, chopped
10 taco shells
½ cup sliced pimento stuffed green olives
2 cups nonfat Monterey Jack cheese, grated
1 cup shredded lettuce
½ cup nonfat sour cream
Taco sauce

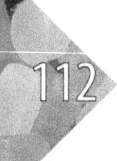
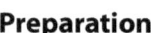

Preparation

Sprinkle avocado with lemon juice and salt to taste.

In a medium pan, heat the oil then cook the chicken and stir in chiles, onion and salt.

Warm taco shells in oven, then fill each with chicken mixture, olives, cheese, lettuce and avocado.

Serve with taco sauce and sour cream with pickles on the side.

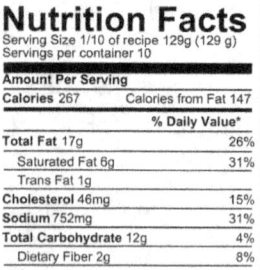

Nutrition Facts	
Serving Size 1/10 of recipe 129g (129 g)	
Servings per container 10	
Amount Per Serving	
Calories 267	Calories from Fat 147
	% Daily Value*
Total Fat 17g	26%
Saturated Fat 6g	31%
Trans Fat 1g	
Cholesterol 46mg	15%
Sodium 752mg	31%
Total Carbohydrate 12g	4%
Dietary Fiber 2g	8%
Sugars 1g	
Protein 18g	

Easy Salads

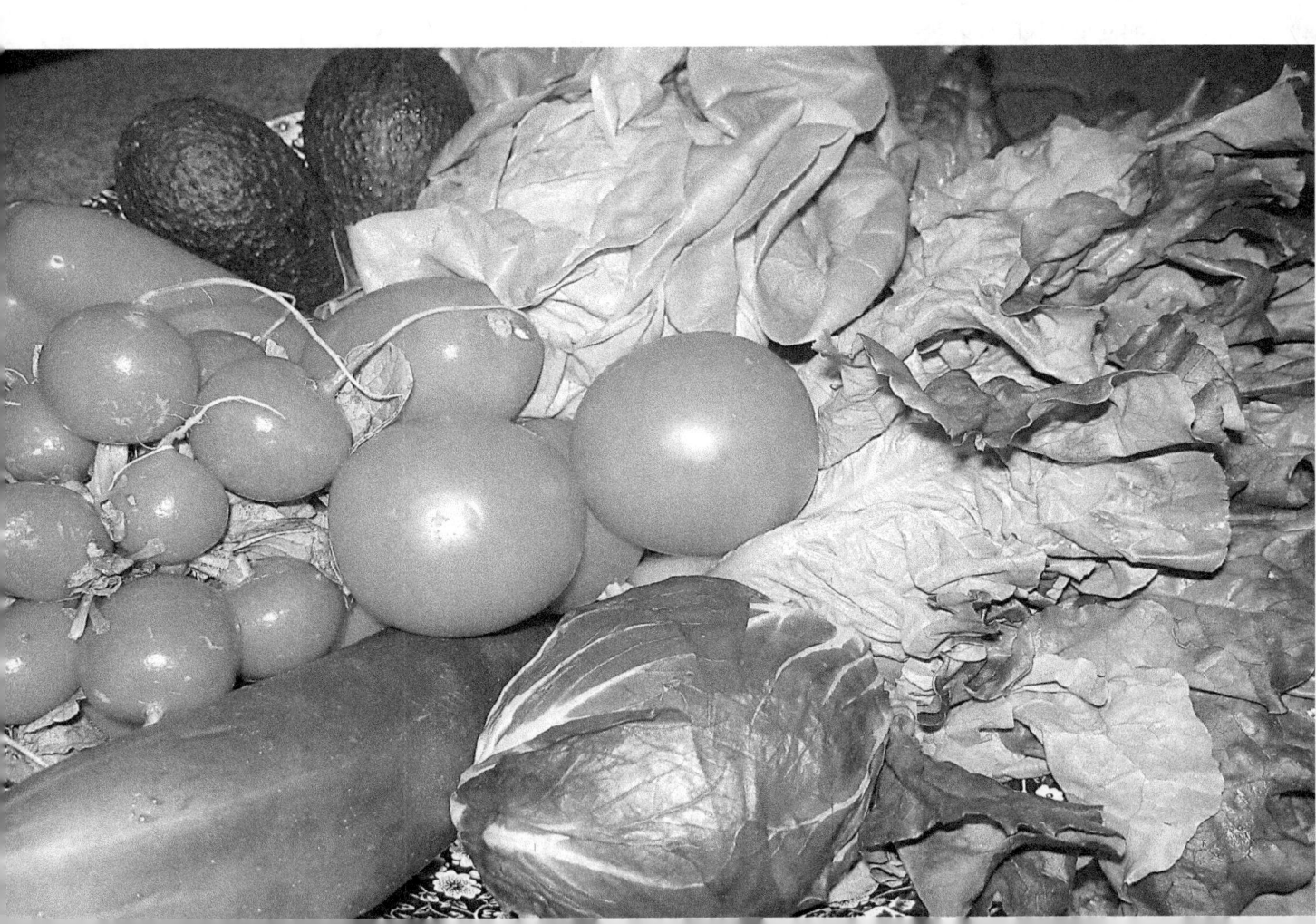

1. Spinach Salad with Cottage Cheese and Strawberry Dressing

Preparation Time: 10 minutes
6 servings

Ingredients

1 ½ cup strawberries, sliced
3 tbsp. rice vinegar
1 tbsp. olive oil
1 tsp. ground tarragon
1 tbsp. finely chopped onion
1 tsp. lemon juice
1 clove garlic, crushed
¼ cup water
6 cups spinach leaves well-washed
6 red onion rounds, sliced very thin
4 kiwi fruit, peeled and sliced crosswise
¼ lb. nonfat cottage cheese
Salt and pepper to taste

Preparation

In a blender, puree 1 cup of strawberries and water, then mix in vinegar, olive oil, tarragon, onion, garlic, and lemon juice. Salt and pepper to taste.

On each of 6 serving dishes, place 1 cup of spinach with 1 red onion round slices, add kiwi, strawberry and cottage cheese slices. Sprinkle salad with strawberry dressing.

An exquisite side dish served with any fish.

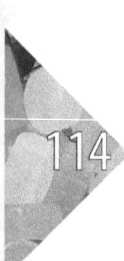

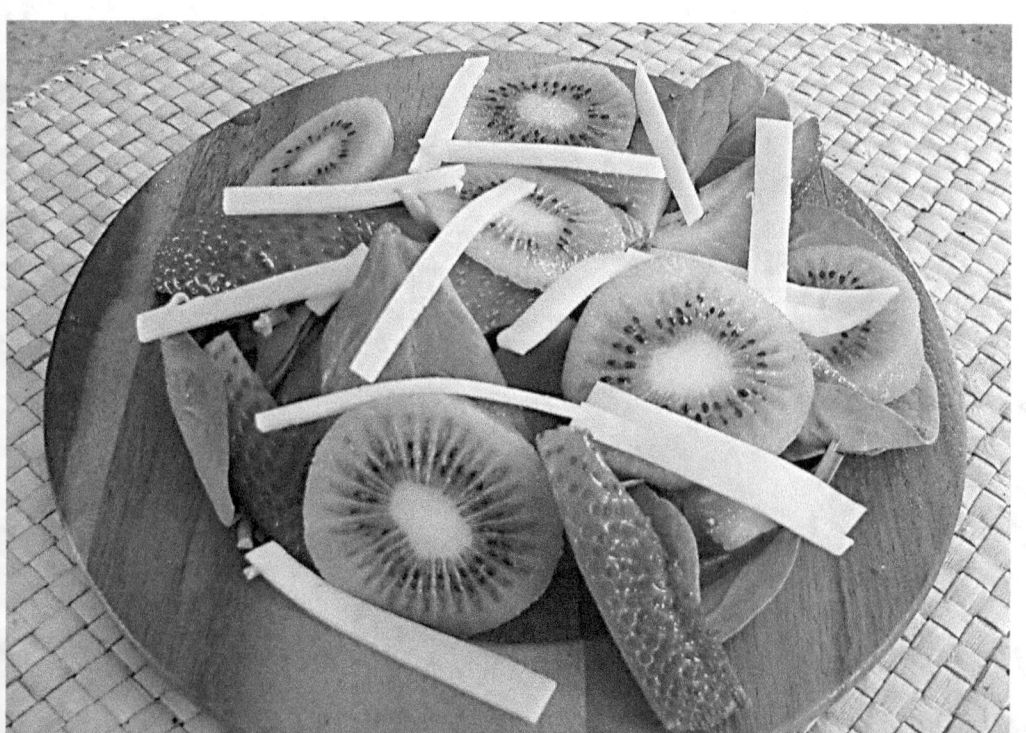

Nutrition Facts	
Serving Size 1/6 of recipe 131g (130 g)	
Servings per container 6	
Amount Per Serving	
Calories 66	Calories from Fat 11
	% Daily Value*
Total Fat 1g	2%
Saturated Fat 0g	1%
Trans Fat 0g	
Cholesterol 1mg	0%
Sodium 69mg	3%
Total Carbohydrate 12g	4%
Dietary Fiber 3g	12%
Sugars 6g	
Protein 4g	

2. Delicious "Eggless" Salad

Preparation Time: 5 minutes
2 servings

Ingredients

1 ½ cups tofu, drained and cut into 1" cubes
2 tbsp. finely chopped celery
1 heaping tsp. finely minced scallion or chives
1 tbsp. black olives, drained and minced
2 tsp. Dijon mustard
3 tbsp. nonfat or tofu mayonnaise
1 pinch turmeric
4 slices bread
Salt to taste

Preparation

In medium bowl, place first 4 ingredients and stir with fork until well combined; allow diced tofu cubes to break into uneven pieces similar to the appearance of egg whites.

Add remaining ingredients and gently fold into tofu mixture until evenly distributed and uniformly moistened.

Serve over bread slices previously spread with tofu mayonnaise.

Nutrition Facts		
Serving Size Entire Recipe 367g (367 g)		
Amount Per Serving		
Calories 373	Calories from Fat 245	
		% Daily Value*
Total Fat 28g		43%
Saturated Fat 4g		20%
Trans Fat 0g		
Cholesterol 4mg		1%
Sodium 636mg		27%
Total Carbohydrate 10g		3%
Dietary Fiber 3g		13%
Sugars 5g		
Protein 24g		

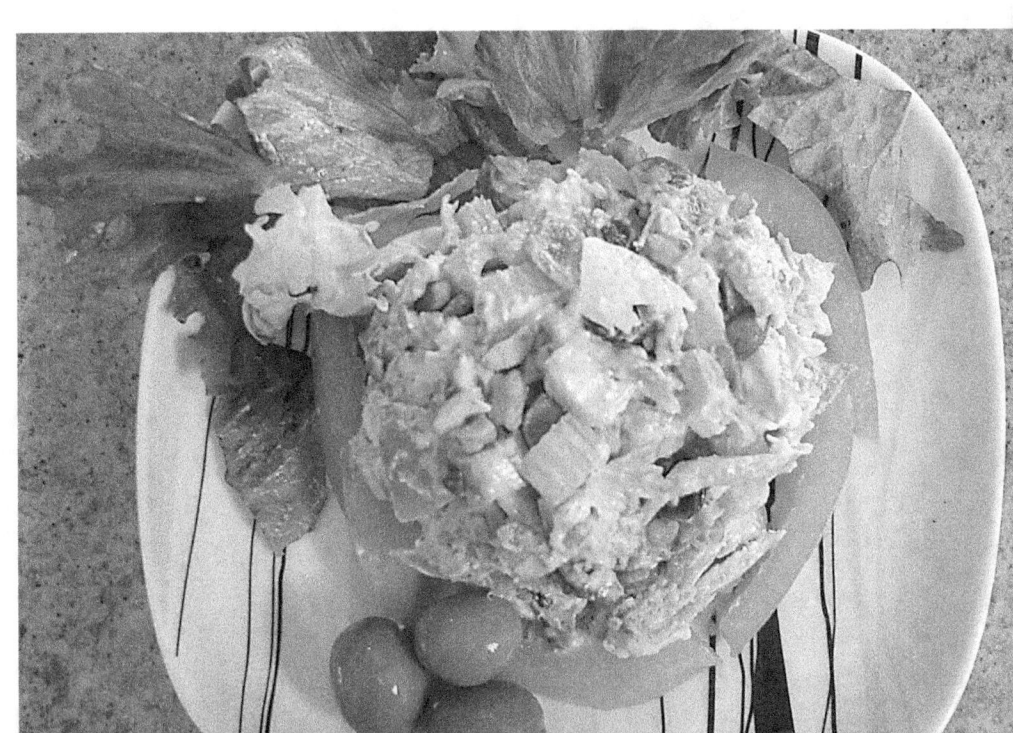

3. French Green Salad

Preparation Time: 5 minutes
6 servings

Ingredients

- ⅓ cup Canola oil
- 2 tbsp. wine vinegar
- ¼ tsp. salt
- ¼ tsp. ground mustard
- ⅛ tsp. pepper
- 10 cups mixed lettuce: arugula, radicchio, escarole, and endive

Preparation

In a tightly covered jar, shake well first 5 ingredients then store in refrigerator.

Wash and dry lettuce well, then put in large bowl and mix together. Reshake salad dressing before pouring over lettuce.

Add thin almond slices for even more flavor.

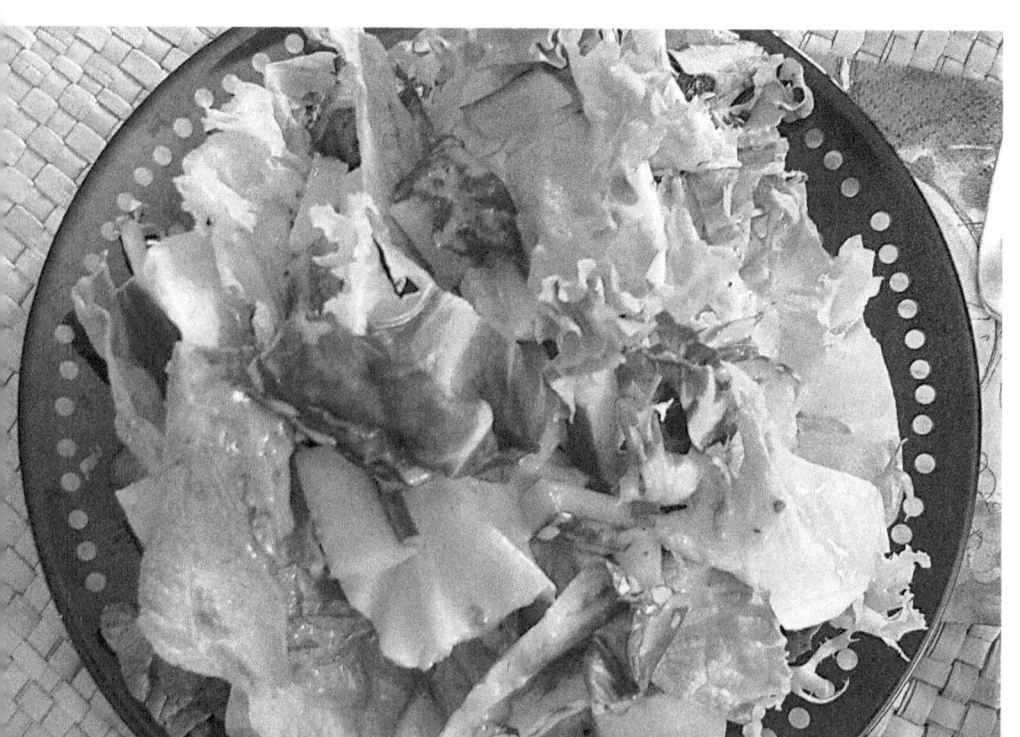

Nutrition Facts		
Serving Size 1/6 of recipe 75g (74 g)		
Servings per container 6		
Amount Per Serving		
Calories 117	Calories from Fat 107	
		% Daily Value*
Total Fat 12g		19%
Saturated Fat 1g		5%
Trans Fat 0g		
Cholesterol 0mg		0%
Sodium 120mg		5%
Total Carbohydrate 2g		1%
Dietary Fiber 1g		4%
Sugars 0g		
Protein 1g		

4. Cooked Vegetable Salad

Preparation Time: 15 minutes
8 servings

Ingredients

2 medium beetroot leaves, cooked and diced
2 medium carrots, cooked and diced
2 medium potatoes, peeled, cooked and diced
1 Dill (or fennel), diced
1 red apple, diced
1 white onion, diced
1 cup nonfat sour cream
2 tbsp. white vinegar
Salt and pepper to taste

Preparation

Peel and dice cooked beets, carrots and potatoes, dill, apple and onion then combine in large bowl.

Stir in sour cream, which will turn pink from the beets, and mix well. Season with vinegar, salt and pepper.

Put everything in a salad bowl, add sour cream and mix well. Season with vinegar, salt and pepper to taste.

Salad pairs well with any beef or chicken dish.

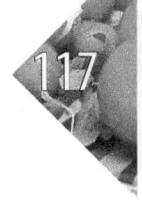

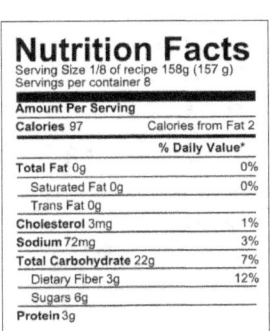

Nutrition Facts
Serving Size 1/8 of recipe 158g (157 g)
Servings per container 8

Amount Per Serving	
Calories 97	Calories from Fat 2
	% Daily Value*
Total Fat 0g	0%
Saturated Fat 0g	0%
Trans Fat 0g	
Cholesterol 3mg	1%
Sodium 72mg	3%
Total Carbohydrate 22g	7%
Dietary Fiber 3g	12%
Sugars 6g	
Protein 3g	

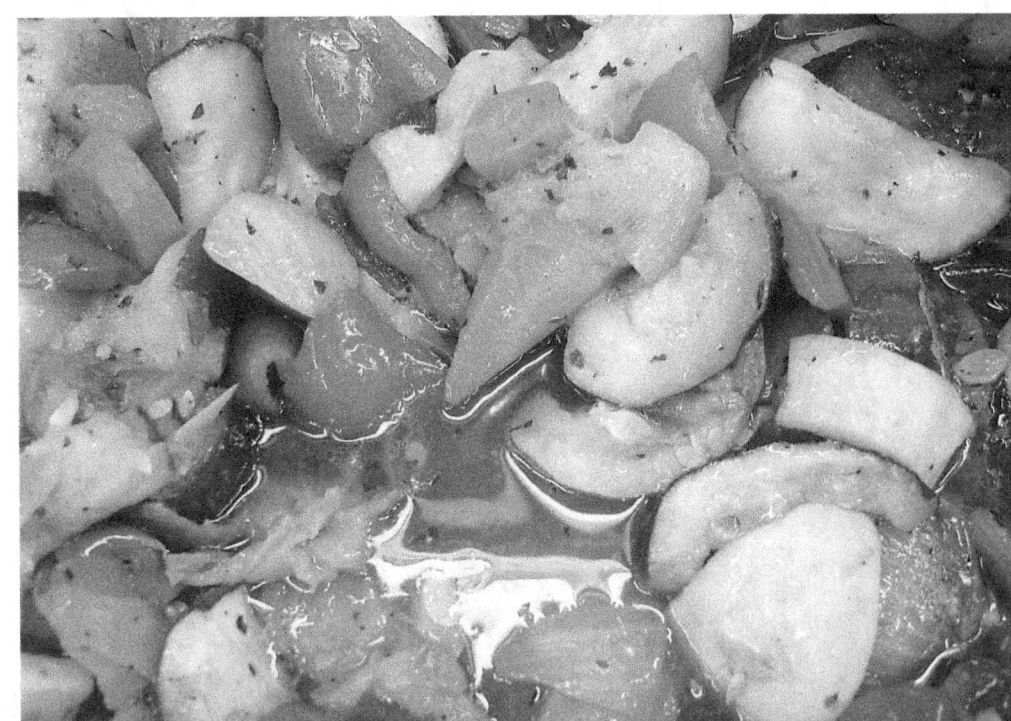

5. Chinese Chicken Salad

Preparation Time: 15 minutes
4 servings

Ingredients

1 tbsp. orange marmalade
3 tbsp. rice vinegar
1 tbsp. sesame oil
3 - 4 tbsp. nonfat mayonnaise
1 ¼ cup chopped celery
¼ cup walnut pieces
1 tbsp. sweet red onion, finely chopped
1 cup shredded carrots
1 tsp. ground ginger
Salt to taste
4 Romaine lettuce leaves
1 ½ cups cooked chicken breast, diced
¼ cup chopped fresh cilantro
¼ cup chopped green onions

Preparation

In a large bowl, combine marmalade, vinegar, oil, and mayonnaise, mix and add celery, walnuts, red onion, carrots, ginger, salt and lettuce, then mix well again.

Add chicken, cilantro and green onions then toss salad and serve.

This is a wonderful dish for lunch.

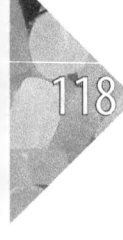

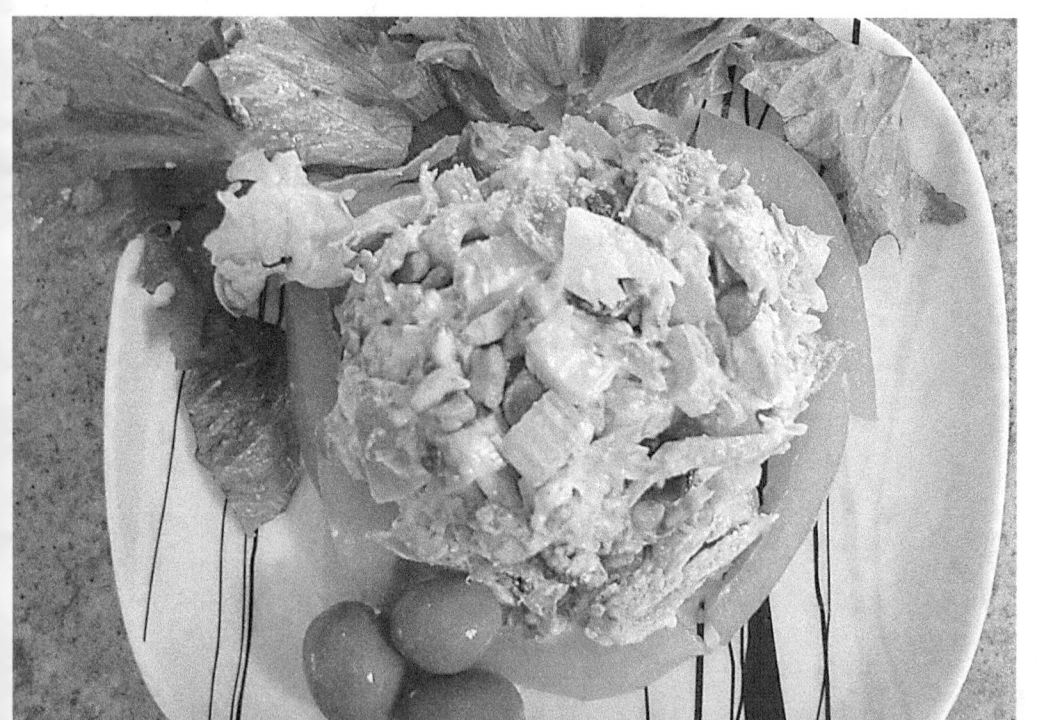

Nutrition Facts	
Serving Size 1/4 of recipe 96g (96 g)	
Servings per container 4	
Amount Per Serving	
Calories 214	Calories from Fat 118
	% Daily Value*
Total Fat 14g	21%
Saturated Fat 2g	10%
Trans Fat 0g	
Cholesterol 44mg	15%
Sodium 134mg	6%
Total Carbohydrate 6g	2%
Dietary Fiber 1g	3%
Sugars 4g	
Protein 18g	

6. Cucumber, Carrot and Sesame Seed Salad

Preparation Time: 15 minutes
6 servings

Ingredients

3 large cucumbers, peeled and seeded,
  cut lengthwise into thin strips
6 medium carrots, grated
2 ½ tsp. sesame oil
2 tsp. grated orange rind
⅛ tsp. cayenne pepper
½ cup seasoned rice vinegar
3 tbsp. chopped green onion
Salt to taste

Preparation

In a large bowl, mix well the cucumber and carrot.

In a small bowl, mix the vinegar with 2 teaspoons of sesame oil, orange zest and cayenne pepper, then add to vegetables and mix well again. Cover large bowl mixture and refrigerate for 6 hours.

After, remove from refrigerator and drain juice then add remaining sesame oil, salt, and fresh green onions. Stir again and serve well-chilled.

Also delicious when served with fish or chicken dishes.

Nutrition Facts	
Serving Size 1/6 of recipe 227g (226 g)	
Servings per container 6	
Amount Per Serving	
Calories 64	Calories from Fat 20
	% Daily Value*
Total Fat 2g	3%
Saturated Fat 0g	2%
Trans Fat 0g	
Cholesterol 0mg	0%
Sodium 46mg	2%
Total Carbohydrate 9g	3%
Dietary Fiber 3g	11%
Sugars 5g	
Protein 1g	

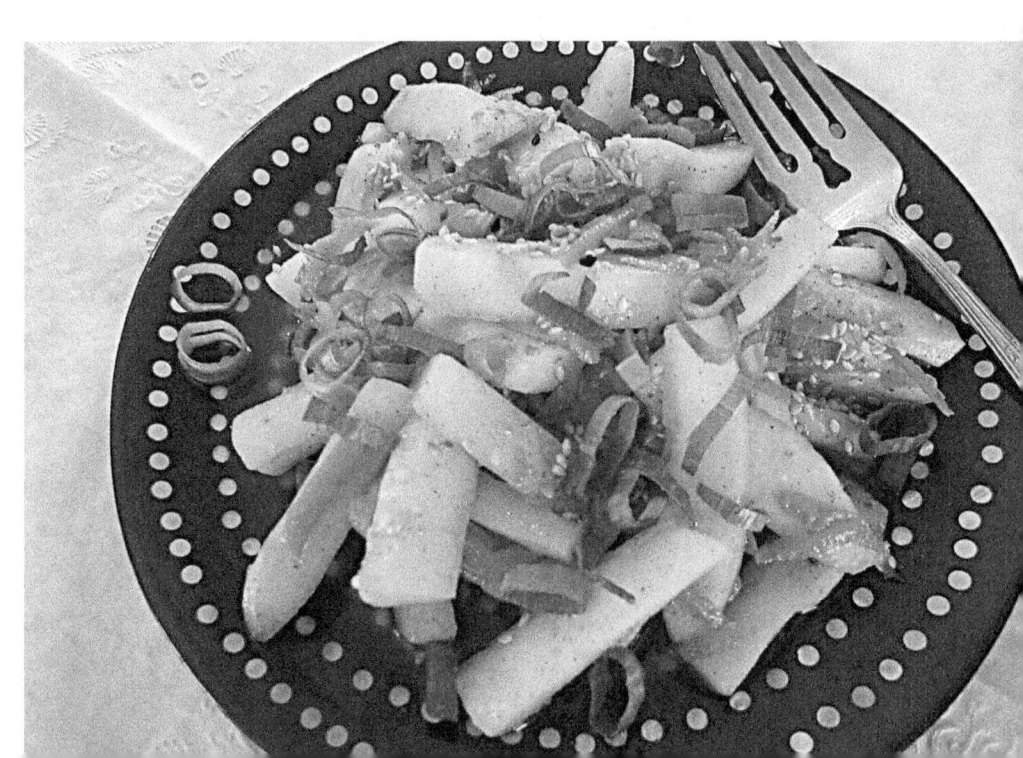

7. Greek Salad

Preparation Time: 10 minutes
8 servings

Ingredients

2 large Romaine lettuce, chopped to bite size
10 red radish lettuce
1 medium cucumber, seeded and diced
6 green onions, cut into ½" pieces
1 cup diced plum tomatoes
½ cup chopped red onion
⅓ cup olive oil
⅓ cup red wine vinegar
1 tsp. salt
1 tsp. oregano
12 green Greek olives
12 black Greek olives
¼ cup finely chopped fresh parsley
¼ cup crumbled nonfat feta cheese
1 can (2 oz.) anchovies with capers, drained

Preparation

In a plastic bag, combine lettuce, radish, cucumbers, tomatoes and onions, then shake to mix and store in refrigerator for about 2 hours.

In a tightly capped jar, combine oil, vinegar, salt and oregano and store in the refrigerator.

Just before serving, shake the vinaigrette well and add with Greek olives to the vegetable bag. Close the bag and shake until ingredients are well mixed.

Pour the salad onto a platter and top with feta cheese, anchovies and parsley.

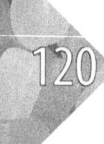

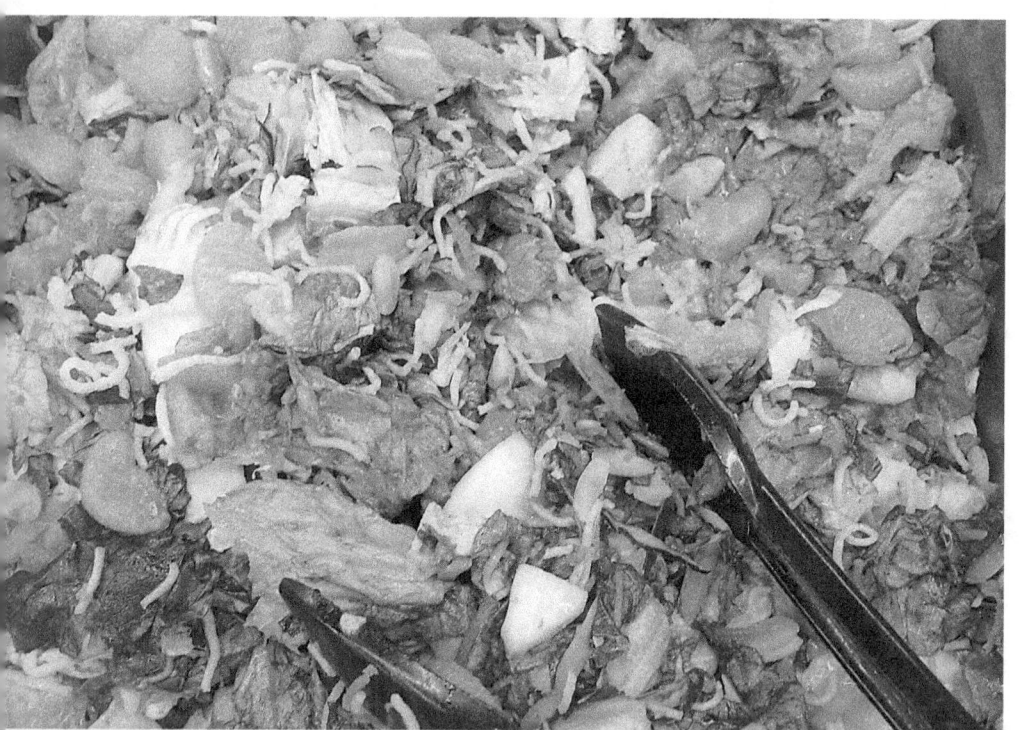

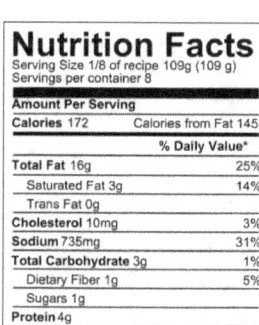

Nutrition Facts

Serving Size 1/8 of recipe 109g (109 g)
Servings per container 8

Amount Per Serving	
Calories 172	Calories from Fat 145

	% Daily Value*
Total Fat 16g	25%
Saturated Fat 3g	14%
Trans Fat 0g	
Cholesterol 10mg	3%
Sodium 735mg	31%
Total Carbohydrate 3g	1%
Dietary Fiber 1g	5%
Sugars 1g	
Protein 4g	

8. Green Plantain Salad

Preparation Time: 10 minutes
8 servings

Ingredients

3 green plantain, peeled
2 cups water
1 tsp. salt
2 medium carrots, grated
1 small cucumber, diced
1 medium tomato, chopped
1 avocado, diced
1 celery stalk, diced

Vinaigrette

½ cup olive oil
1 clove garlic, crushed
½ tsp. mustard
2 tablespoons wine vinegar
Salt and pepper to taste

Preparation

Put the plantains in a pot of salted water and, at medium temperature, bring to boil for 10 minutes or until soft. Drain and cool.

Cut the plantain into ½" cubes and place in bowl, then mix in the remaining ingredients. Add the dressing, mix well and serve.

A perfect salad to accompany any meat, fish or chicken dish.

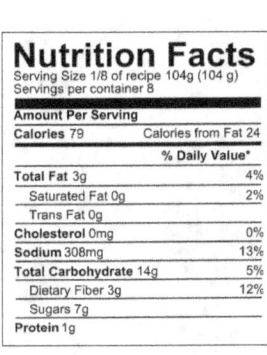

Nutrition Facts	
Serving Size 1/8 of recipe 104g (104 g)	
Servings per container 8	
Amount Per Serving	
Calories 79	Calories from Fat 24
	% Daily Value*
Total Fat 3g	4%
Saturated Fat 0g	2%
Trans Fat 0g	
Cholesterol 0mg	0%
Sodium 308mg	13%
Total Carbohydrate 14g	5%
Dietary Fiber 3g	12%
Sugars 7g	
Protein 1g	

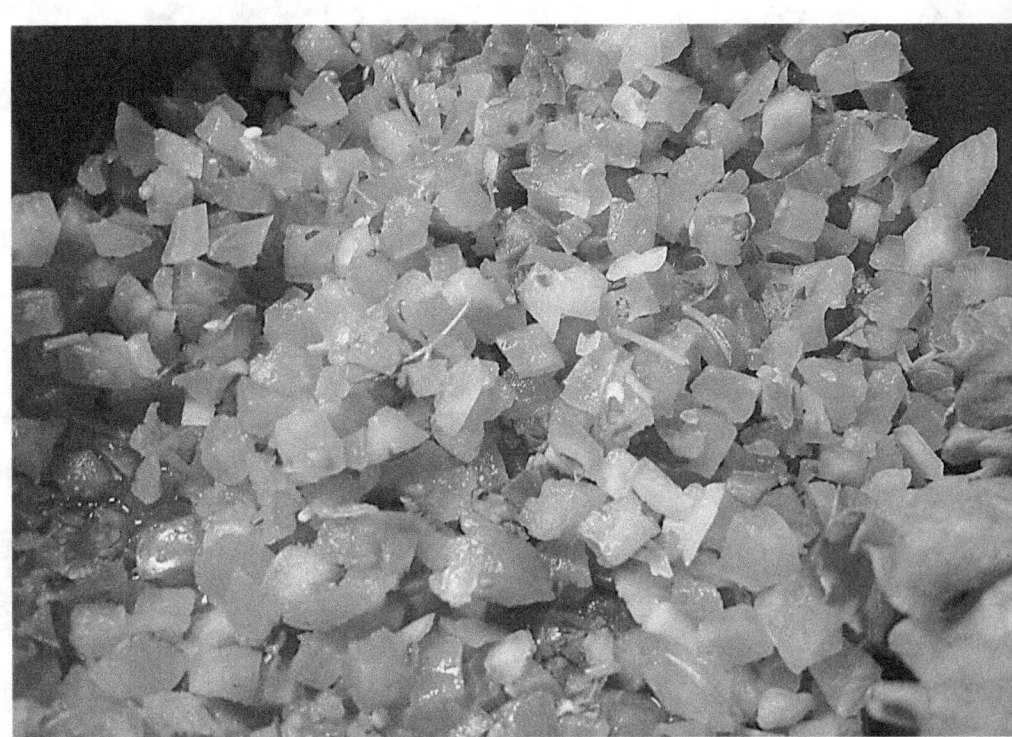

The Latest Soups

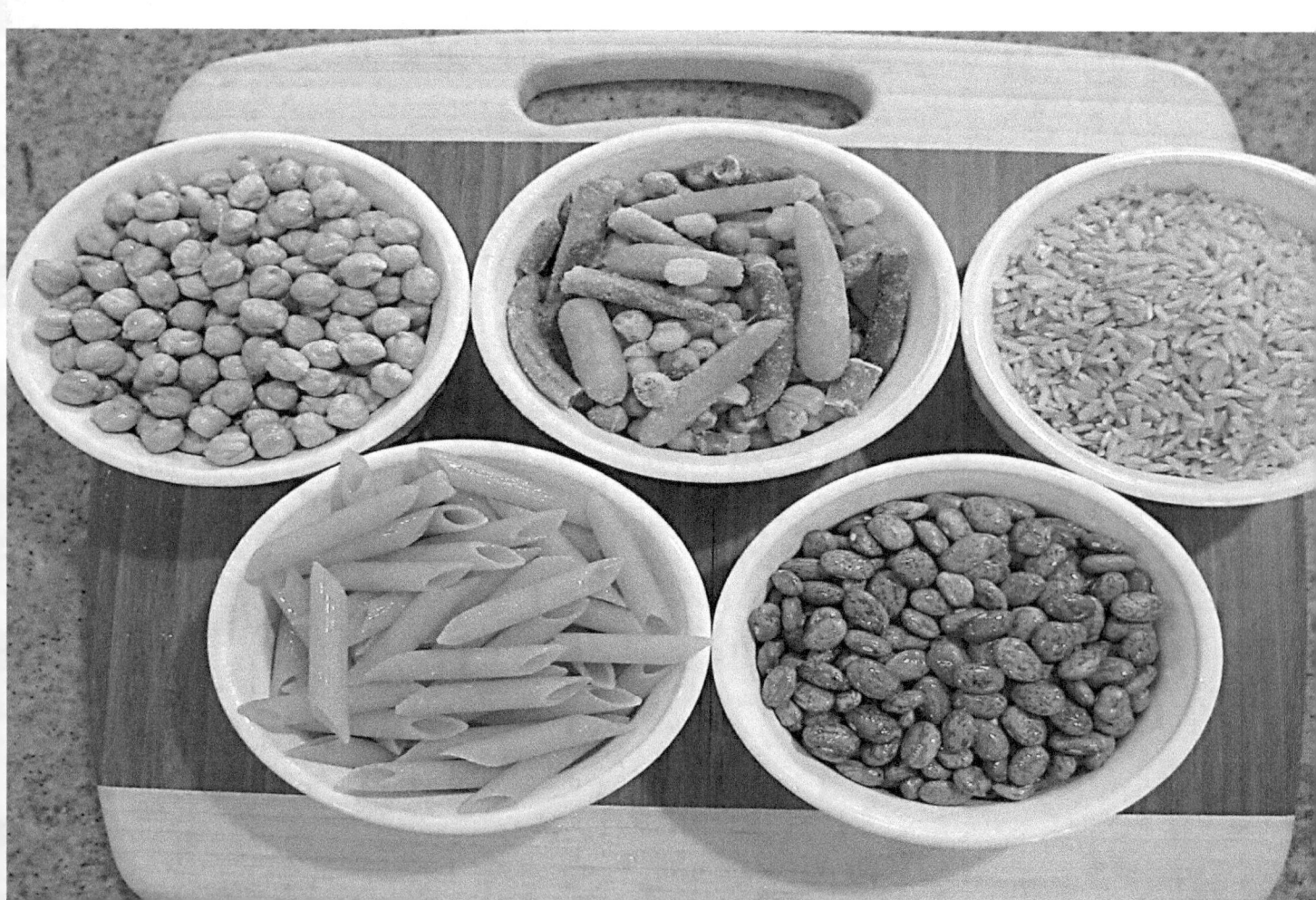

1. Colombian Barley Soup with Radishes and Turnips

Preparation Time: 45 minutes
6 servings

Ingredients

½ cup chopped celery
½ cup chopped carrot
1 onion, chopped
2 cloves garlic, minced
2 large radishes, peeled and diced
2 large turnips, peeled and diced
1 potato, peeled and diced
8 cups chicken or beef broth
2 tbsp. soy sauce
⅓ cup pearl barley, (soak for one day prior)
1 handful chopped cilantro
Canola oil spray
Salt and pepper to taste

Preparation

In a large pot, spray oil then cook until hot.

Add celery and carrots, stirring occasionally for 2 minutes, then add onion and garlic, cook for 3 minutes more. Reduce heat to medium and add radishes, turnips, potatoes, broth, soy sauce and barley. Simmer for 45 minutes. If necessary, add more water.

Season with salt, pepper, and chopped cilantro to taste then serve.

Add a warm piece of French bread on the side.

Nutrition Facts	
Serving Size 1/6 of recipe 451g (451 g)	
Servings per container 6	

Amount Per Serving	
Calories 109	Calories from Fat 5
	% Daily Value*
Total Fat 1g	1%
Saturated Fat 0g	1%
Trans Fat 0g	
Cholesterol 0mg	0%
Sodium 867mg	36%
Total Carbohydrate 21g	7%
Dietary Fiber 5g	19%
Sugars 4g	
Protein 6g	

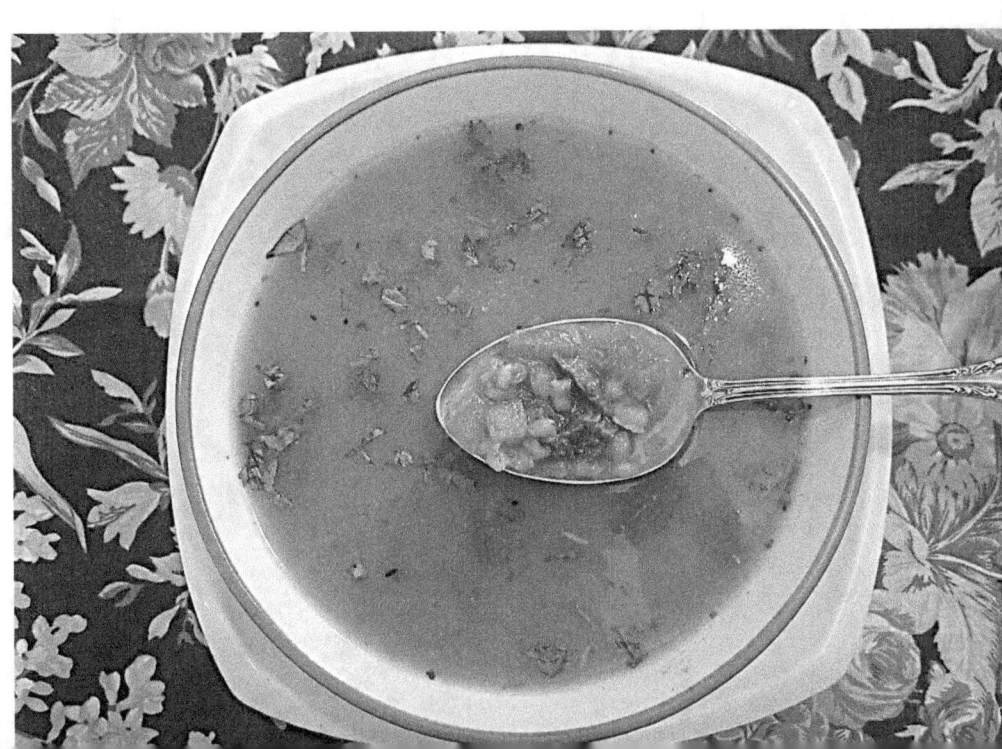

2. Argentinian Bean Soup

Preparation Time: 70 minutes
6 servings

Ingredients

3 Spanish sausage, skinned and chopped
8 cups chicken broth
1 white onion, finely chopped
2 celery stalks, finely chopped
2 carrots, sliced round
2 ½ cup white beans, medium cooked
¼ cup tomato paste
2 cups tomato juice
2 cloves garlic, minced
1 tbsp. chili powder
1 tbsp. salt
½ tsp. each: black pepper, paprika, oregano, thyme and pepper

Preparation

In a saucepan, cook sausages until browned then peel skin and remove fat from pan.

Add broth, onion, celery and carrots then simmer until tender.

Add beans, tomato paste and spices then simmer for 40 minutes more.

Serve hot with toasted olive bread.

Beans are a great source of vitamins A & C, and are very rich in protein with no cholesterol.

124

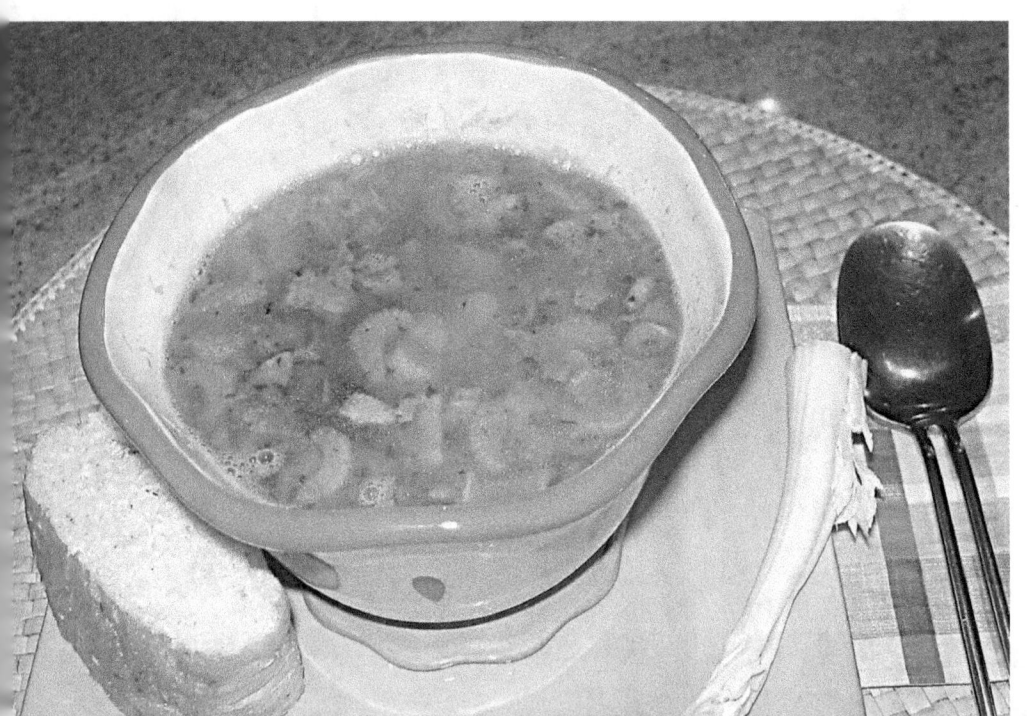

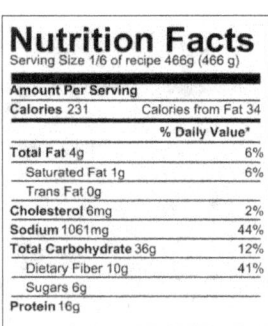

Nutrition Facts
Serving Size 1/6 of recipe 466g (466 g)

Amount Per Serving

Calories 231	Calories from Fat 34
	% Daily Value*
Total Fat 4g	6%
Saturated Fat 1g	6%
Trans Fat 0g	
Cholesterol 6mg	2%
Sodium 1061mg	44%
Total Carbohydrate 36g	12%
Dietary Fiber 10g	41%
Sugars 6g	
Protein 16g	

3. Caribbean Fish Soup with Swiss Chard

Preparation Time: 60 minutes
6 servings

Ingredients

Canola oil spray
1 small onion, chopped
3 cloves garlic, crushed
1 celery stalk with leaves, chopped
1 bay leaf, cut into ½ inch cubes
8 cups chicken broth
4 tomatoes, peeled and diced
2 white potatoes, peeled and chopped
1 tbsp. paprika
1 bunch fresh Swiss chard, washed and
   finely chopped
1 lb. swordfish, sliced into chunks
1 lb. white fish, sliced into chunks
Salt and pepper to taste
1 bunch fresh basil, chopped

Preparation

In a large pot, spray oil then add onion, garlic and celery, and let cook for 2 minutes. Add bay leaf and broth, bring to boil, then reduce heat to medium and simmer 30 minutes.

Add tomatoes, potatoes, paprika and cook for 15 minutes more.

Add the chard and cook for 10 minutes.

Lastly, add the swordfish and white fish and simmer everything for 8 minutes more. Add salt and pepper to taste.

Sprinkle each bowl of soup with basil and serve with toasted French bread.

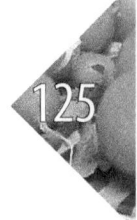

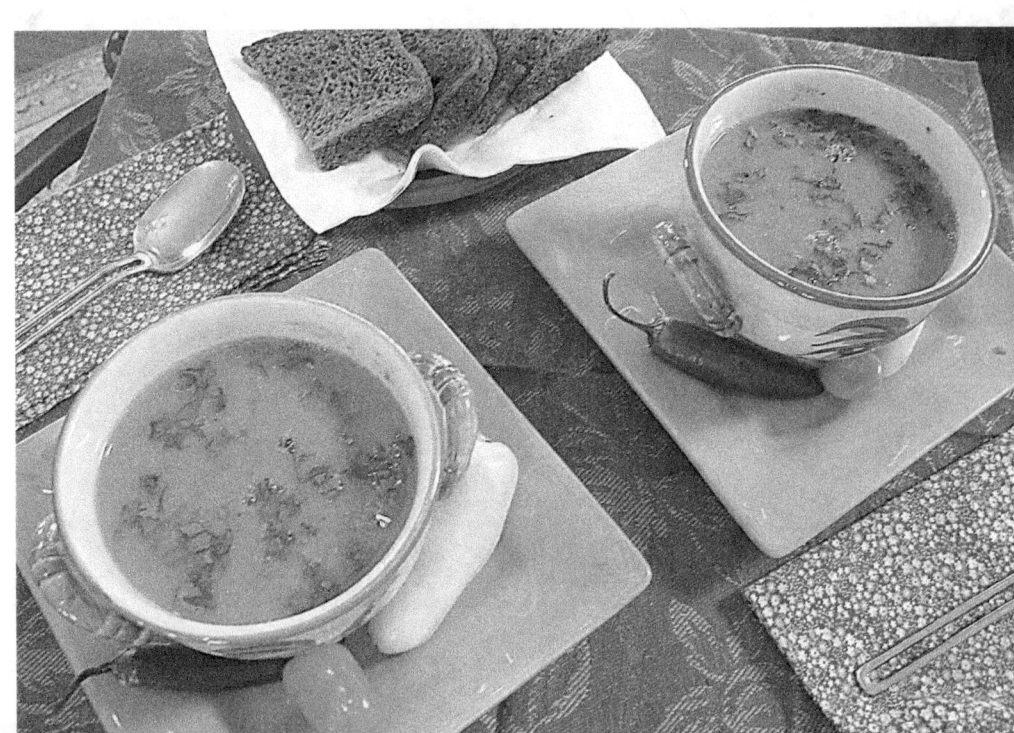

Nutrition Facts	
Serving Size 1/6 of recipe 636g (636 g)	
Servings per container 6	

Amount Per Serving	
Calories 260	Calories from Fat 42
	% Daily Value*
Total Fat 5g	7%
Saturated Fat 1g	6%
Trans Fat	
Cholesterol 79mg	26%
Sodium 618mg	26%
Total Carbohydrate 21g	7%
Dietary Fiber 5g	21%
Sugars 5g	
Protein 34g	

4. Italian Minestrone Soup

Preparation Time: 1 ½ hours
4 servings

Ingredients

1 cup water
4 cups chicken broth
½ cup white beans, half cooked
2 tomatoes, chopped
2 medium carrots, sliced round
1 celery stalk, chopped
1 medium onion, chopped
2 cloves garlic, minced
½ cup fussily pasta
1 tbsp. chopped parsley
1 tsp. salt
½ tsp. basil leaves
⅛ tsp. pepper
1 bay leaf
12 green beans, cut into 1" pieces
2 courgettes (or zucchini), cut into 1" pieces
Parmesan Cheese, grated

Preparation

In medium saucepan, bring to boil the chicken broth, cooked beans, tomatoes, carrots, celery, onion, garlic, pasta, parsley, salt, basil, pepper and bay leaf.

Once boiling, reduce heat to medium, cover pot and simmer for 15 minutes.

Then add the beans and courgettes (or zucchini) and simmer another 15 minutes.

Once all the vegetables are cooked, turn off heat and remove bay leaf. Sprinkle each bowl of soup with grated parmesan cheese.

126

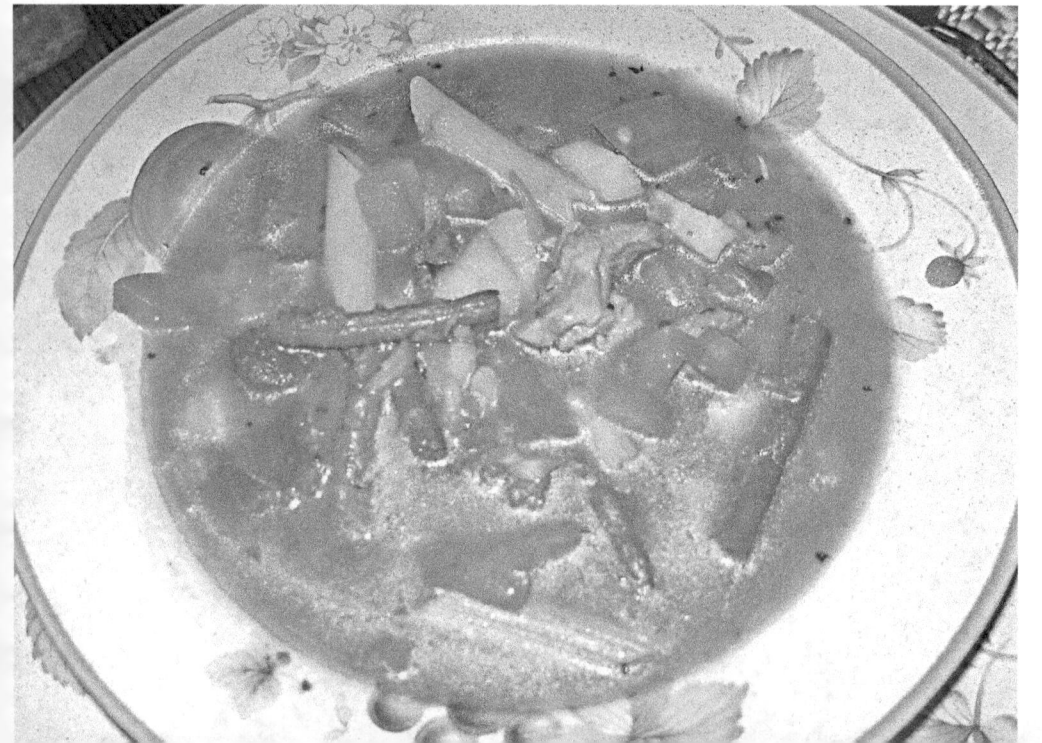

Nutrition Facts	
Serving Size Entire Recipe 343g (343 g)	
Amount Per Serving	
Calories 93	Calories from Fat 6
	% Daily Value*
Total Fat 1g	1%
Saturated Fat 0g	1%
Trans Fat 0g	
Cholesterol 0mg	0%
Sodium 769mg	32%
Total Carbohydrate 18g	6%
Dietary Fiber 3g	14%
Sugars 4g	
Protein 6g	

5. Colombian Carrot and Cilantro Soup

Preparation Time: 15 minutes
6 servings

Ingredients

- 6 large carrots, peeled and cut into thick rounds
- 2 potatoes, peeled and diced
- 7 cups chicken broth
- 2 tbsp. canola oil
- ¼ cup white onion, chopped
- 2 cloves garlic, crushed
- 1 tsp. salt
- ¼ tsp white pepper
- ⅛ tsp. cayenne pepper
- 2 tbsp. chopped cilantro
- 2 cups nonfat sour cream

Preparation

In a medium pot, bring to boil 3 carrots, potatoes and 3 cups of chicken broth until tender, then puree them in a blender.

In a saucepan, saute the oil, onion and garlic until light brown. Add remaining chicken broth and carrots and puree then simmer on medium heat for 3 minutes.

Add spices and cook for another 5 minutes.

To serve, sprinkle each bowl with cilantro and 1 teaspoon of sour cream.

It can also be served with a rich salad of lettuce and tomatoes.

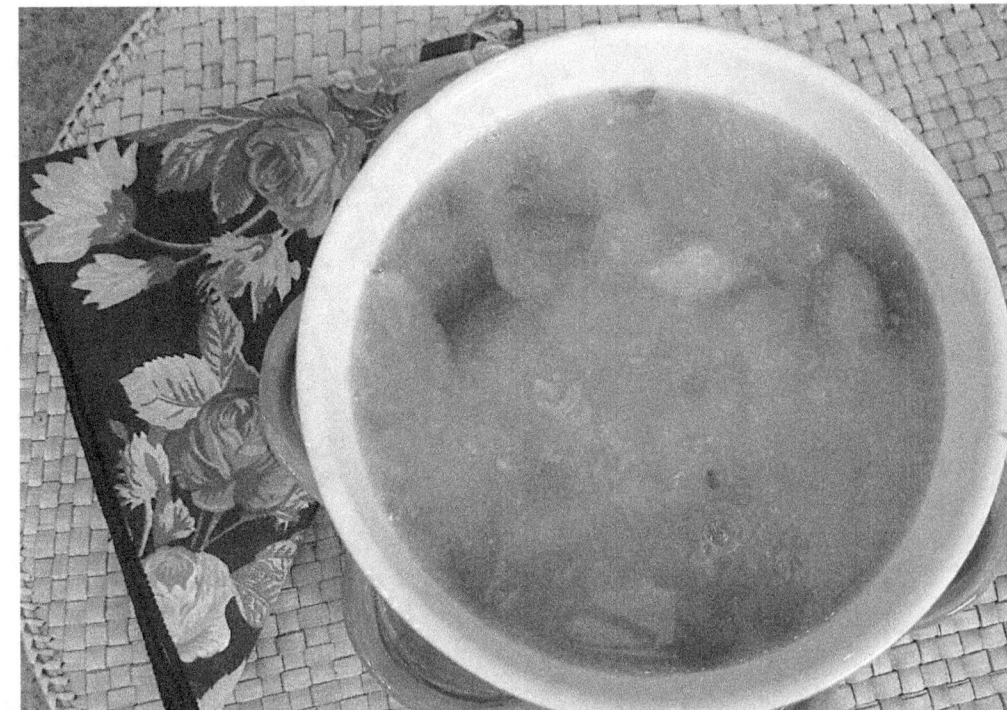

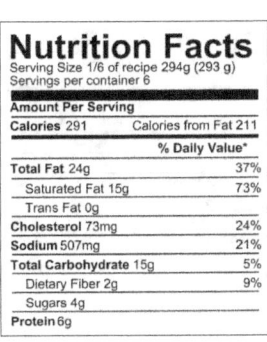

Nutrition Facts

Serving Size 1/6 of recipe 294g (293 g)
Servings per container 6

Amount Per Serving	
Calories 291	Calories from Fat 211
	% Daily Value*
Total Fat 24g	37%
Saturated Fat 15g	73%
Trans Fat 0g	
Cholesterol 73mg	24%
Sodium 507mg	21%
Total Carbohydrate 15g	5%
Dietary Fiber 2g	9%
Sugars 4g	
Protein 6g	

6. *Italian Pasta Fagioli Soup*

Preparation Time: 30 minutes
5 servings

Ingredients

8 oz. navy beans (about 1 ¼ cups), soak in
    water overnight to soften
6 cups chicken broth
1 large onion, chopped
1 large tomato, chopped
2 medium celery stalks, chopped
2 cloves garlic, minced
½ tsp. salt
¼ tsp. pepper
½ lb. smoked ham, chopped
2 tsp. instant beef bouillon
½ cup small pasta, uncooked
Parmesan cheese, grated

Preparation

In a big pot, put pre-soaked beans, broth,
onion, tomato, celery, garlic, salt, pepper,
smoked ham and beef bouillon. Let simmer
1 hour or until beans are tender.

Add the pasta and simmer 10 minutes more.

Sprinkle each bowl of soup with grated
parmesan cheese.

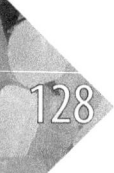

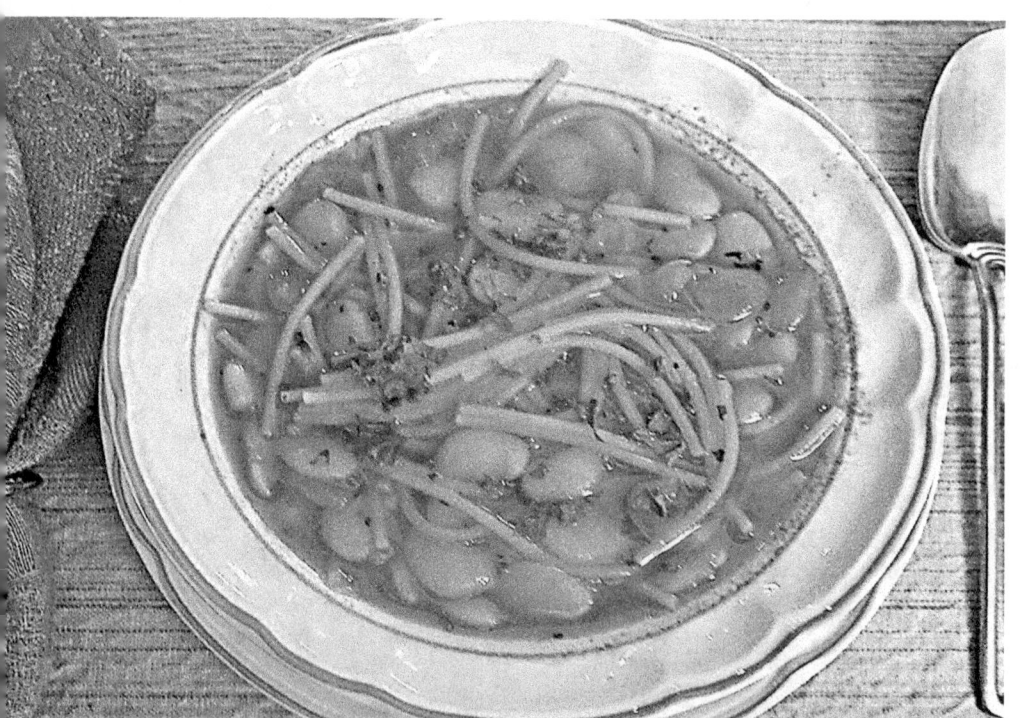

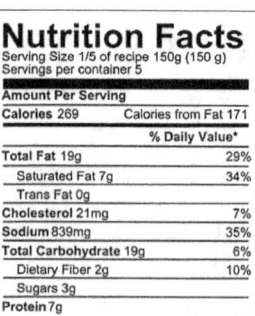

Nutrition Facts	
Serving Size 1/5 of recipe 150g (150 g)	
Servings per container 5	
Amount Per Serving	
Calories 269	Calories from Fat 171
	% Daily Value*
Total Fat 19g	29%
Saturated Fat 7g	34%
Trans Fat 0g	
Cholesterol 21mg	7%
Sodium 839mg	35%
Total Carbohydrate 19g	6%
Dietary Fiber 2g	10%
Sugars 3g	
Protein 7g	

7. Original Spanish Gazpacho

Preparation Time: 20 minutes
6 servings

Ingredients

2 cups sweet tomato sauce
4 large ripe tomatoes, chopped
2 medium cucumbers, chopped
1 medium green pepper, chopped
1 medium white onion, finely chopped
2 tbsp. cilantro, finely chopped
2 tsp. garlic, finely chopped
2 cups of water
2 tbsp. olive oil
⅓ cup red wine vinegar
2 tbsp. fresh basil, finely chopped
2 tbsp. ground dry oregano
2 tsp. salt
1 tsp. ground cumin
⅛ tsp. freshly ground pepper

Preparation

Wash the vegetables well.

In a bowl, cut and mix all the ingredients.

Take 1 cup of mix and blend on high speed.

Combine blended mix back into bowl, cover and store in refrigerator for 2 hours.

Serve cold with a piece of warm fresh bread.

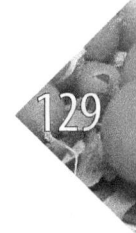

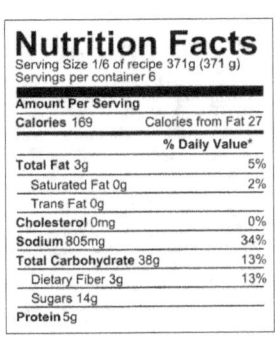

Nutrition Facts	
Serving Size 1/6 of recipe 371g (371 g)	
Servings per container 6	

Amount Per Serving	
Calories 169	Calories from Fat 27

	% Daily Value*
Total Fat 3g	5%
Saturated Fat 0g	2%
Trans Fat 0g	
Cholesterol 0mg	0%
Sodium 805mg	34%
Total Carbohydrate 38g	13%
Dietary Fiber 3g	13%
Sugars 14g	
Protein 5g	

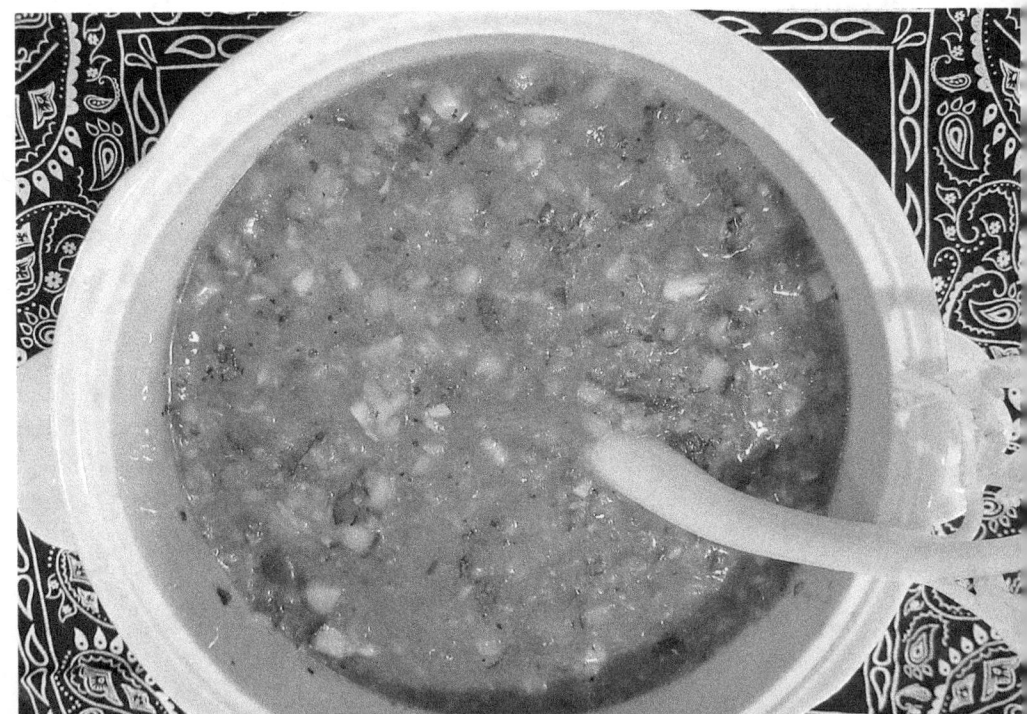

8. Mexican Vegetable Soup

Preparation Time: 45 minutes
6 servings

Ingredients

1 tbsp. olive oil
1 white onion, finely chopped
2 celery stalks, finely chopped
2 carrots, finely chopped
6 cups chicken broth
2 potatoes, peeled and cooked then mashed
2 cups red cabbage, sliced rounds
2 cups tomatoes, peeled and seeded then chopped.
¼ tsp. each: oregano, thyme, basil, garlic powder, onion powder
1 tsp. salt
½ tsp. black pepper

Preparation

In a large pot, heat oil then add onion, celery, carrots, and broth, then cook for 5 minutes.

Mash the potatoes then add to soup with red cabbage and simmer for 30 minutes.

Add tomatoes and seasonings, then continue cooking over low heat for 10 minutes more.

Serve hot with wheat tortillas.

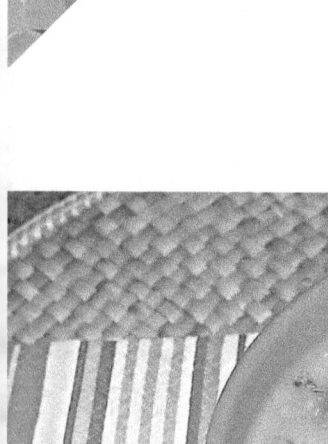

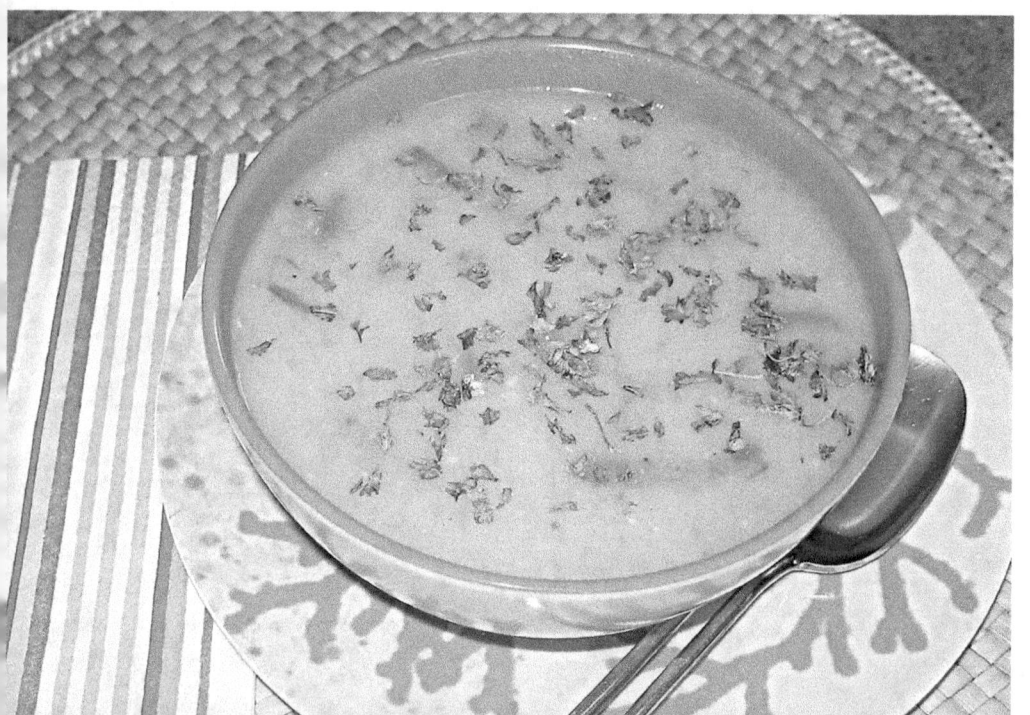

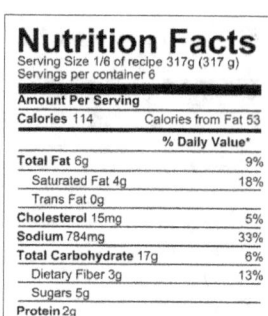

Nutrition Facts
Serving Size 1/6 of recipe 317g (317 g)
Servings per container 6

Amount Per Serving	
Calories 114	Calories from Fat 53

	% Daily Value*
Total Fat 6g	9%
Saturated Fat 4g	18%
Trans Fat 0g	
Cholesterol 15mg	5%
Sodium 784mg	33%
Total Carbohydrate 17g	6%
Dietary Fiber 3g	13%
Sugars 5g	
Protein 2g	

Favorite Chicken Recipes

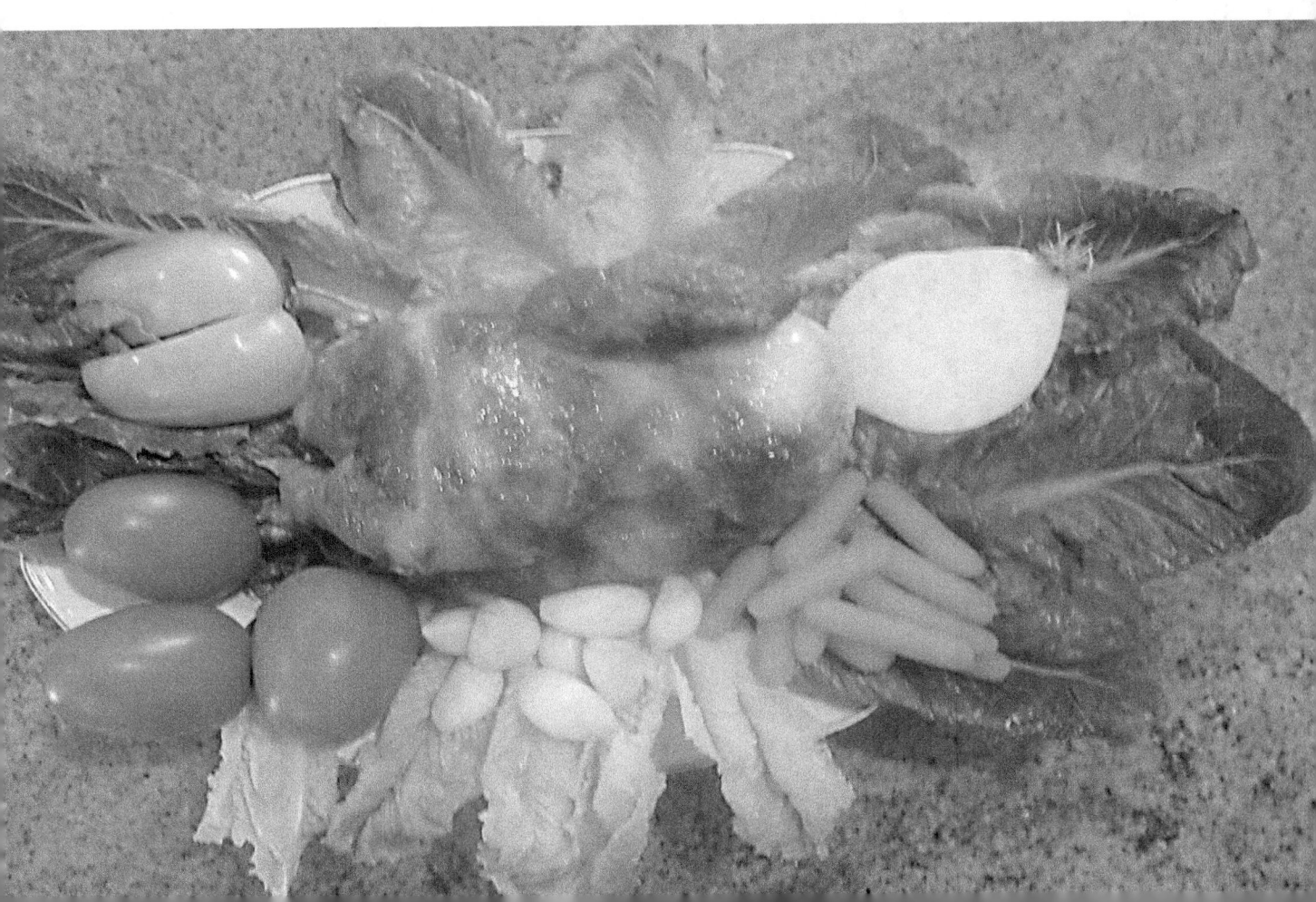

1. California Chicken

Preparation Time: 35 minutes
6 servings

Ingredients

6 skinless chicken drumsticks
Canola oil spray
½ cup milk
1 cup nonfat sour cream
2 green peppers, chopped
2 dried California chilies, cut with scissor along
  edges and discard seeds
Salt and pepper to taste
¼ cup chicken broth
3 tbsp. sesame seeds, toasted
6 corn tortillas, warm to serve

Preparation

Lightly season drumsticks with salt and pepper. Spray bottom of a Dutch oven with oil, then put in drumsticks to brown on all sides.

In a separate pan, mix milk, ½ cup sour cream, chilies, green peppers and a pinch of salt and pepper. Simmer on stove for 15 minutes, then puree in blender to make sauce.

Place the sauce and chicken broth in with the drumsticks, then cook for 15 minutes over low heat, turning drumsticks until evenly cooked. Add remaining sour cream and bring to boil.

Serve hot drumsticks on a tray with sesame seeds drizzled over hind legs and warm tortillas on the side.

This is a delightful dish!

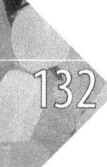

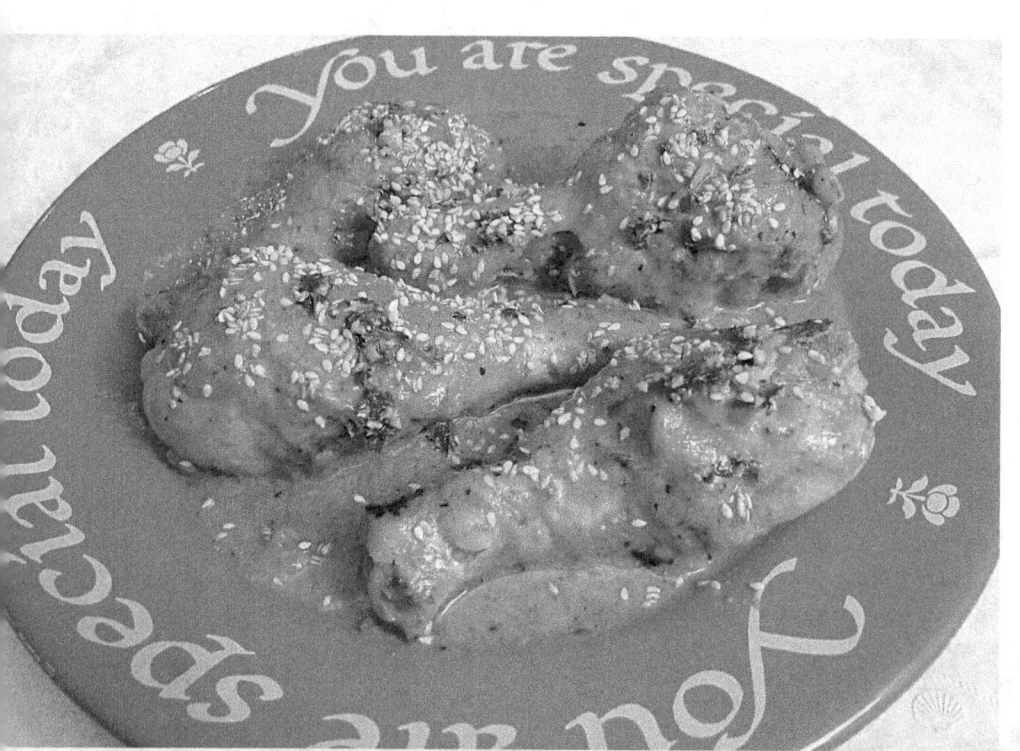

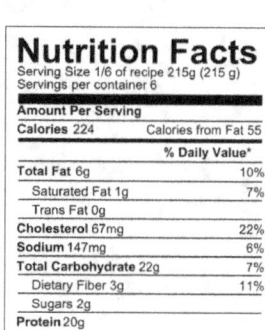

Nutrition Facts	
Serving Size 1/6 of recipe 215g (215 g)	
Servings per container 6	
Amount Per Serving	
Calories 224	Calories from Fat 55
	% Daily Value*
Total Fat 6g	10%
Saturated Fat 1g	7%
Trans Fat 0g	
Cholesterol 67mg	22%
Sodium 147mg	6%
Total Carbohydrate 22g	7%
Dietary Fiber 3g	11%
Sugars 2g	
Protein 20g	

2. Lemon and Ginger Roast Chicken

Preparation Time: 30 minutes
6 servings

Ingredients

1 whole (4 lb.) chicken
2 large lemons
2 tbsp. ground ginger
2 tbsp. yellow mustard powder
Salt and pepper to taste

* Optional:
  3 onions, crosscut
  4 medium red potatoes, crosscut

Preparation

Preheat oven to 425°. Wash chicken and pat dry. Squeeze lemons over chicken, including inside cavity.

Mix ginger and mustard powder with salt and pepper to taste. Smear and rub chicken with mixture, inside and out for added flavor.

Place chicken in baking pan, (if desired, add onions and red potatoes). Bake for 1 hour, until the chicken juice looks cooked. (Not bleeding, indicating that it is well cooked)

Better to serve without skin, to avoid fat.

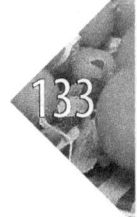

Nutrition Facts	
Serving Size 1/6 of recipe 173g (172 g)	
Servings per container 6	
Amount Per Serving	
Calories 186	Calories from Fat 44
	% Daily Value*
Total Fat 5g	8%
Saturated Fat 1g	5%
Trans Fat	
Cholesterol 91mg	30%
Sodium 106mg	4%
Total Carbohydrate 5g	2%
Dietary Fiber 2g	6%
Sugars 1g	
Protein 30g	

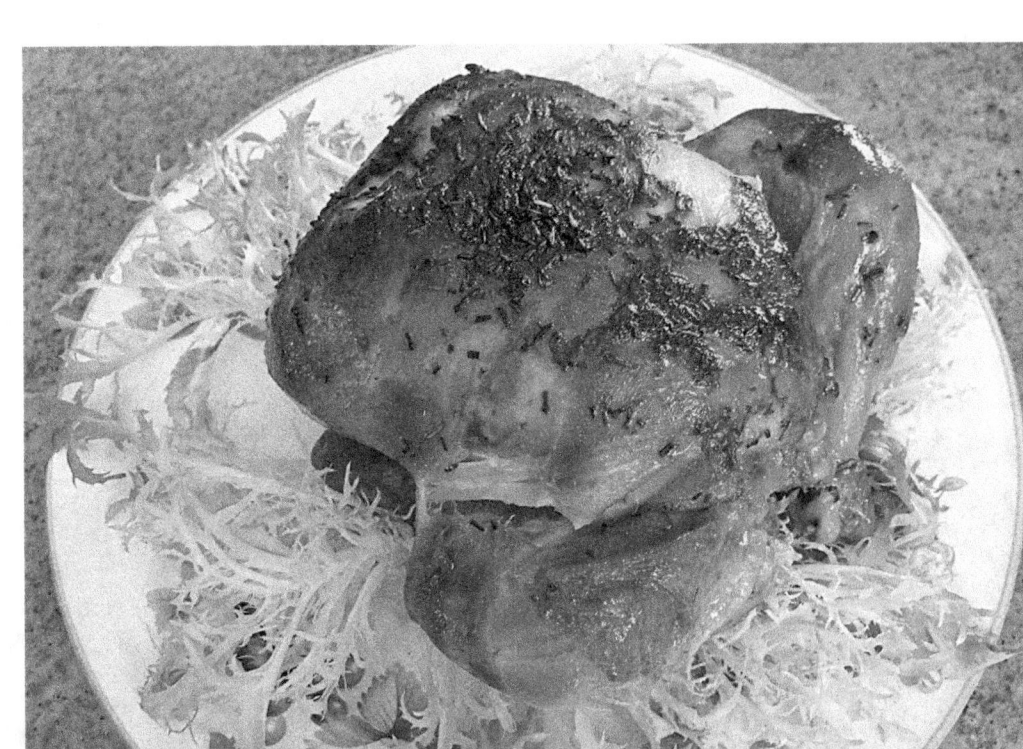

3. Puerto Rican Rice and Chicken Stew

Preparation Time: 30 minutes
10 servings

Ingredients

3 lb. chicken, diced
2 tsp. salt
1 tsp. ground basil
½ tsp. ground cumin
¼ tsp. pepper
2 cups water
1 can (16 oz.) stewed tomato
1 onion, chopped
1 clove garlic, crushed
1 cup uncooked white rice
1 cup green peas
1 green pepper, diced
½ cup beef, diced and cooked tender
⅓ cup green olives, pitted and halved
1 tbsp. capers
Parmesan cheese, grated

Preparation

In a medium 12" skillet with lid, sprinkle the chicken pieces with salt, oregano, cumin and pepper. Add water, tomato sauce, onion and garlic. Bring to a boil, then cover and reduce heat to medium for 30 minutes.

Then add rice, cover again and simmer 20 minutes more. When chicken is tender, add the fresh peas, paprika, cooked beef, olives, and capers. Sprinkle a tablespoon of water, then cook another 5 minutes.

Sprinkle each dish with grated parmesan cheese and serve.

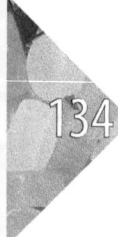

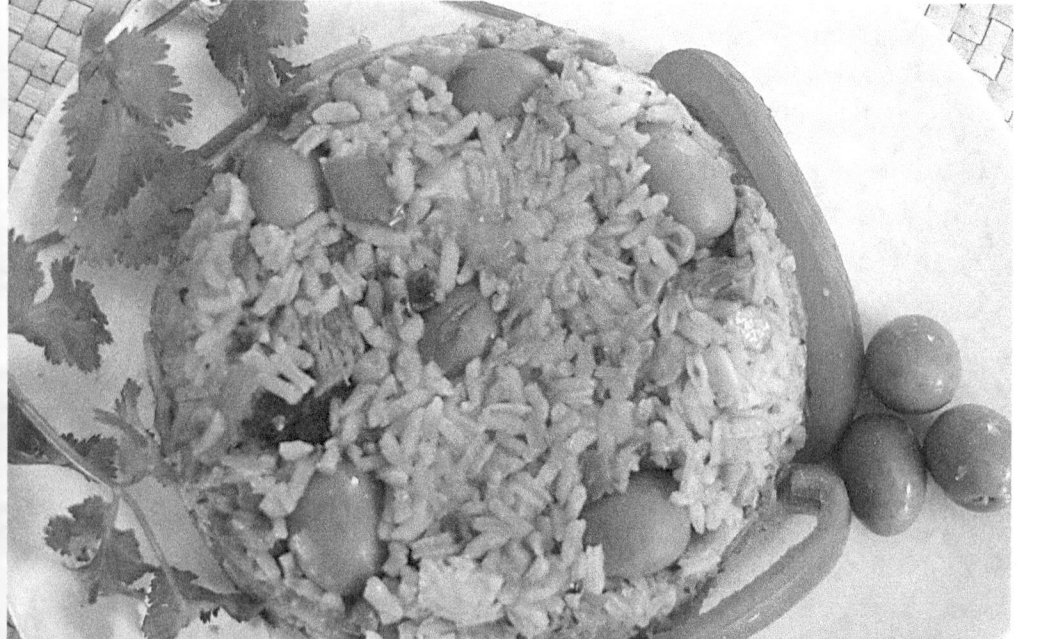

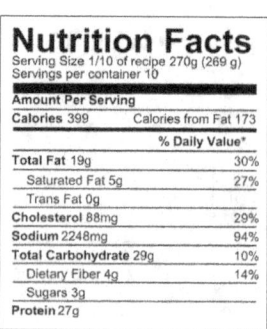

Nutrition Facts
Serving Size 1/10 of recipe 270g (269 g)
Servings per container 10

Amount Per Serving

Calories 399	Calories from Fat 173

	% Daily Value*
Total Fat 19g	30%
Saturated Fat 5g	27%
Trans Fat 0g	
Cholesterol 88mg	29%
Sodium 2248mg	94%
Total Carbohydrate 29g	10%
Dietary Fiber 4g	14%
Sugars 3g	
Protein 27g	

4. Italian Stuffed Chicken Leg with Capellini

Preparation Time: 25 minutes
8 servings

Ingredients

½ cup of mixed cilantro and basil
½ cup parmesan cheese, grated
8 legs of chicken
3 large red peppers
½ lb. capellini pasta
1 tbsp. olive oil
1 cup rice vinegar mixed with
½ cup capers, drained
2 tbsp. finely grated lemon peel
4 tbsp. molasses or diet maple syrup
Cilantro leaves
Salt and pepper to taste

Preparation

Combine cilantro and basil with grated cheese and mix in blender until minced. Cut slit in skin of each leg, slide fingers in to separate skin from meat, then tuck and spread mixture evenly inside. Set aside.

Bake red peppers in foil for 20 minutes, then cover until cool. Remove skin and seeds, then cut into thin strips.

Rub legs with molasses or diet maple syrup. Bake chicken at 375° until cooked and brown.

Meanwhile, cook pasta as directed until tender then drain. In a large pan, bring to boil oil, vinegar, capers, grated lemon then add pasta.

Serve dish with chicken on top of pasta, then sprinkle with peppers, cilantro, parmesan cheese, salt and pepper to taste.

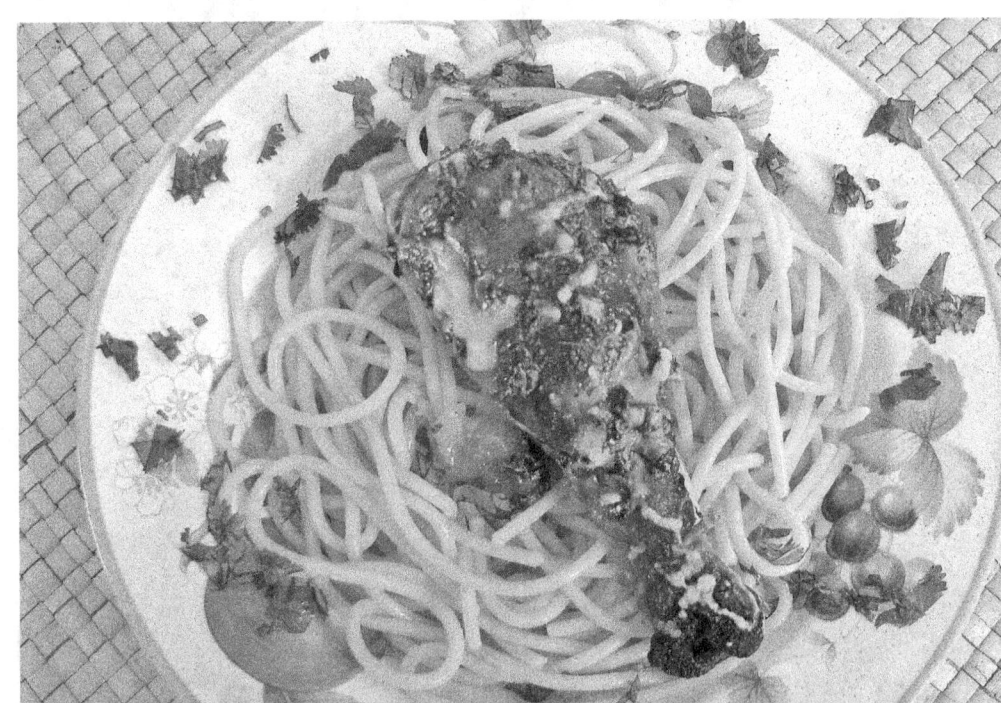

Nutrition Facts	
Serving Size 1/8 of recipe 197g (197 g)	
Servings per container 8	
Amount Per Serving	
Calories 326	Calories from Fat 128
	% Daily Value*
Total Fat 14g	22%
Saturated Fat 3g	17%
Trans Fat 0g	
Cholesterol 52mg	17%
Sodium 568mg	24%
Total Carbohydrate 33g	11%
Dietary Fiber 5g	20%
Sugars 7g	
Protein 17g	

5. Chicken Casserole with Macaroni (Pasticcio)

Preparation Time: 30 minutes
8 servings

Ingredients

1 lb. macaroni or ziti pasta
Canola oil spray
1 lb. chicken breast, cooked and diced
2 cloves garlic, crushed
1 cup 1% milk
2 tbsp. breadcrumbs
½ cup nonfat parmesan cheese
2 cups chicken broth
Salt and pepper to taste
1 cup fresh parsley and basil, finely chopped
1 tomato, finely chopped

Preparation

Preheat oven to 375°. In a large pot, cook pasta according to package directions, then drain.

Meanwhile, spray a large pan with oil and add cooked chicken, garlic, milk, breadcrumbs and parmesan cheese, mix well, then bake in oven for 10 minutes, stirring frequently.

Mix in cooked pasta and chicken broth, season with salt and pepper to taste, then bake for another 10 minutes.

Serve with fresh parsley, basil and chopped tomatoes drizzled on top.

This is a high energy food.

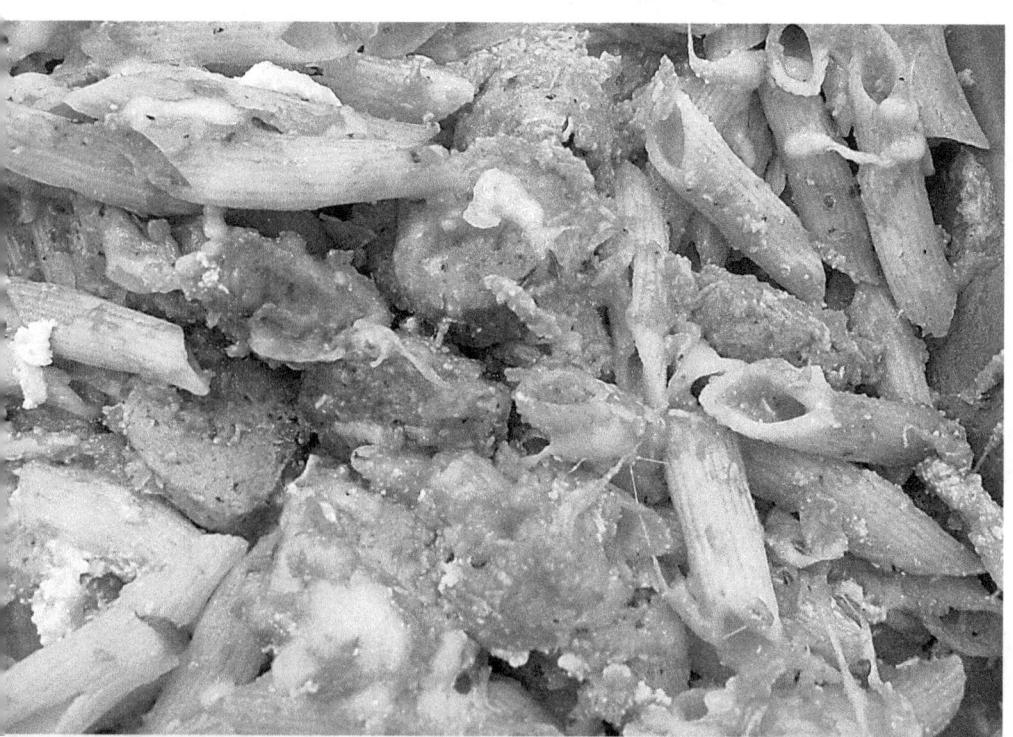

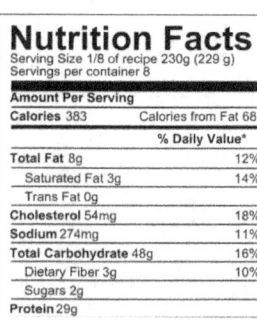

Nutrition Facts		
Serving Size 1/8 of recipe 230g (229 g)		
Servings per container 8		
Amount Per Serving		
Calories 383	Calories from Fat 68	
		% Daily Value*
Total Fat 8g		12%
Saturated Fat 3g		14%
Trans Fat 0g		
Cholesterol 54mg		18%
Sodium 274mg		11%
Total Carbohydrate 48g		16%
Dietary Fiber 3g		10%
Sugars 2g		
Protein 29g		

6. Brazilian Chicken with Garlic and Thyme

Preparation Time: 30 minutes
6 servings

Ingredients

6 boneless chicken breasts (6 oz.), skinned
3 tbsp. olive oil
6 cloves garlic, minced
1 tsp. ginger, grated
1 tbsp. fresh thyme, chopped
1 jalapeno pepper, chopped
¼ cup fine breadcrumbs

Preparation

Preheat oven to 350°.

Wash chicken breasts and place in baking pan.

In a small bowl, combine oil, garlic, ginger, thyme, pepper and breadcrumbs.

Rub mixture over each breast then bake for 20 minutes or until golden brown.

Serve with fresh vegetables and homemade salad of lettuce and tomatoes.

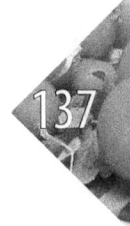

Nutrition Facts		
Serving Size 1/6 of recipe 191g (190 g)		
Servings per container 6		
Amount Per Serving		
Calories 383	Calories from Fat 195	
		% Daily Value*
Total Fat 22g		34%
Saturated Fat 8g		41%
Trans Fat 0g		
Cholesterol 123mg		41%
Sodium 173mg		7%
Total Carbohydrate 8g		3%
Dietary Fiber 1g		3%
Sugars 1g		
Protein 37g		

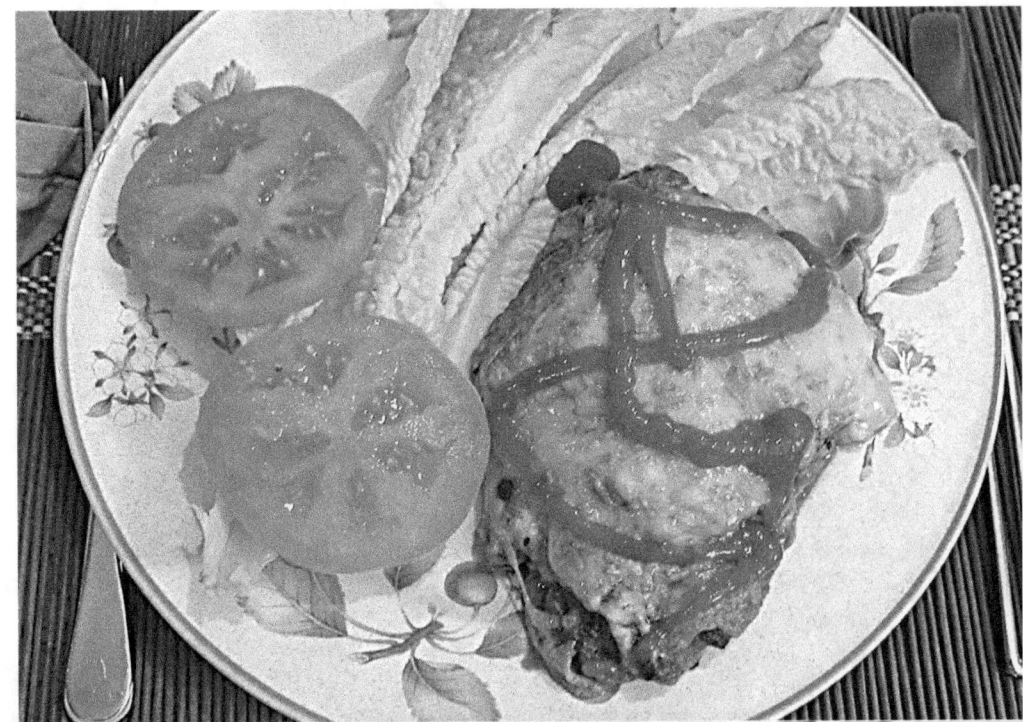

7. Caribbean Chicken with Mango Salsa

Preparation Time: 45 minutes
4 servings

Ingredients

¼ cup molasses (or honey)
¼ cup lemon juice
2 tsp. grated lemon rind
1 ripe mango, peeled and diced
1 small onion, peeled and cut in fourths
2 jalapenos peppers, halved and seeded
2 tsp. paprika
1 ½ tsp. garlic salt
½ tsp. ground cinnamon
½ tsp. freshly ground black pepper
½ tsp. allspice
4 boneless chicken breasts, skinned and halved
Canola oil spray

Preparation

Preheat oven to 375°. Spray medium baking pan with oil.

In a small bowl, combine molasses, lemon juice and grated lemon then whisk well. Remove ¼ cup of mixture, pour in blender and set aside. Add mango to remaining mixture, stir well then store in refrigerator.

In blender, add onions, jalapenos, paprika, garlic, salt, cinnamon, ground pepper and allspice, then mix until finely chopped. Spread mixture evenly over both sides of chicken breast, then place in baking pan and cook for 25 minutes or until cooked through.

Serve chicken with refrigerated mango mixture on top. Delicious with white rice.

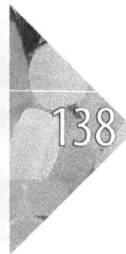

138

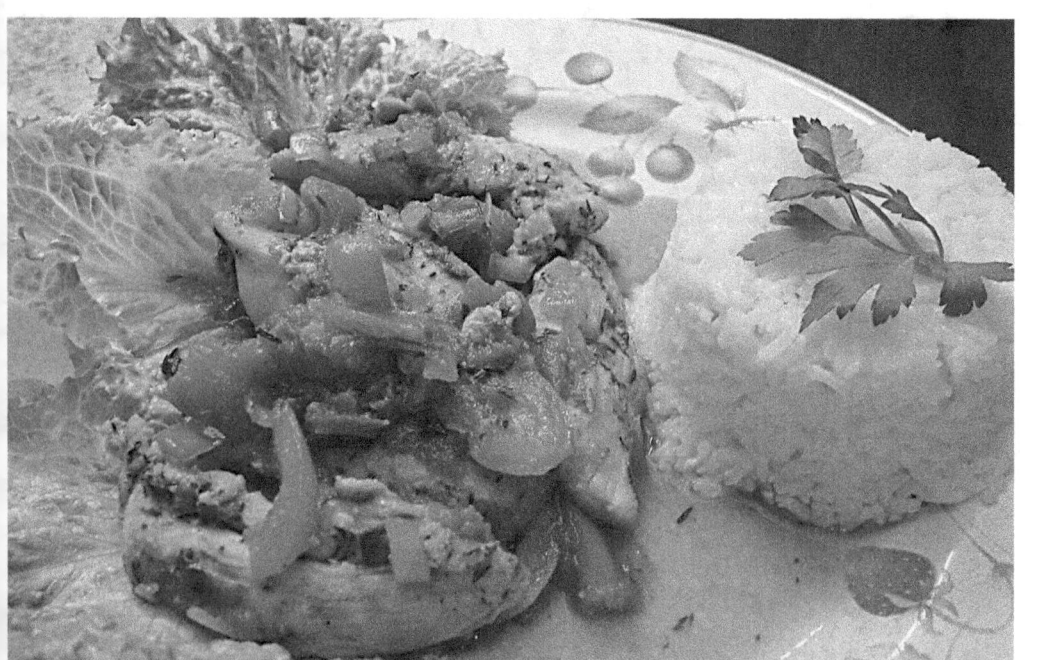

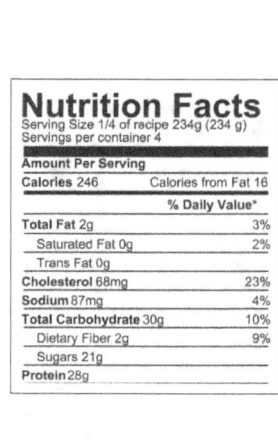

Nutrition Facts
Serving Size 1/4 of recipe 234g (234 g)
Servings per container 4

Amount Per Serving

Calories 246	Calories from Fat 16
	% Daily Value*
Total Fat 2g	3%
Saturated Fat 0g	2%
Trans Fat 0g	
Cholesterol 68mg	23%
Sodium 87mg	4%
Total Carbohydrate 30g	10%
Dietary Fiber 2g	9%
Sugars 21g	
Protein 28g	

8. Spiced Chicken with Orange Sauce

Preparation Time: 30 minutes
6 servings

Ingredients

6 boneless chicken thighs, skinned
Canola oil spray
1 tsp. paprika
1 tsp. salt
⅛ tsp. pepper
1 large onion, chopped fine
1 cup orange juice (concentrate)
¼ cup honey
2 tbsp. lemon juice
½ tsp. ground ginger
¼ tsp. ground nutmeg
¼ cup black olives, pitted and sliced
3 tbsp. fine wheat breadcrumbs
Chopped cilantro

Preparation

Preheat oven to 375º.

Spray baking pan with oil, place chicken and sprinkle with paprika, salt, pepper and onions then bake for 15 minutes.

In a medium bowl, whisk orange juice, honey, lemon juice, ginger and nutmeg then pour over chicken, sprinkle with olives and bake for another 15minutes.

In a medium saucepan, pour the baking pan juice and heat to boiling, then add breadcrumbs and cook 2 minutes.

Pour sauce over chicken and garnish with chopped cilantro. Serve with a side of brown rice.

139

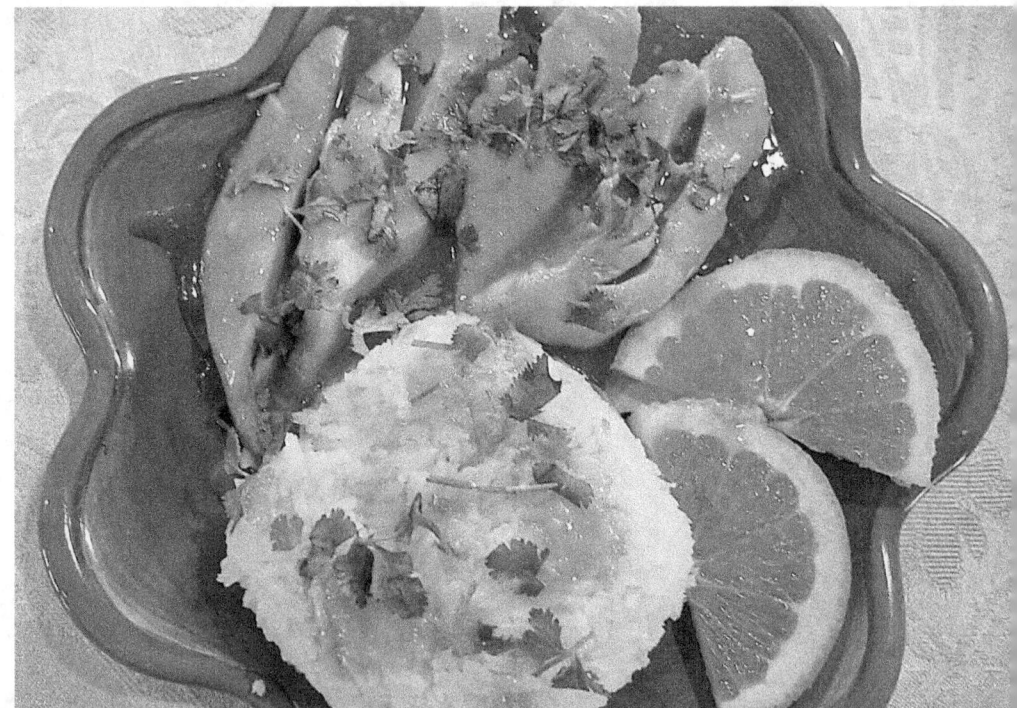

Nutrition Facts	
Serving Size 1/6 of recipe 325g (324 g)	
Servings per container 6	
Amount Per Serving	
Calories 366	Calories from Fat 53
	% Daily Value*
Total Fat 6g	9%
Saturated Fat 1g	7%
Trans Fat 0g	
Cholesterol 104mg	35%
Sodium 485mg	20%
Total Carbohydrate 39g	13%
Dietary Fiber 14g	56%
Sugars 10g	
Protein 39g	

The Latest Beef And Lamb Recipes

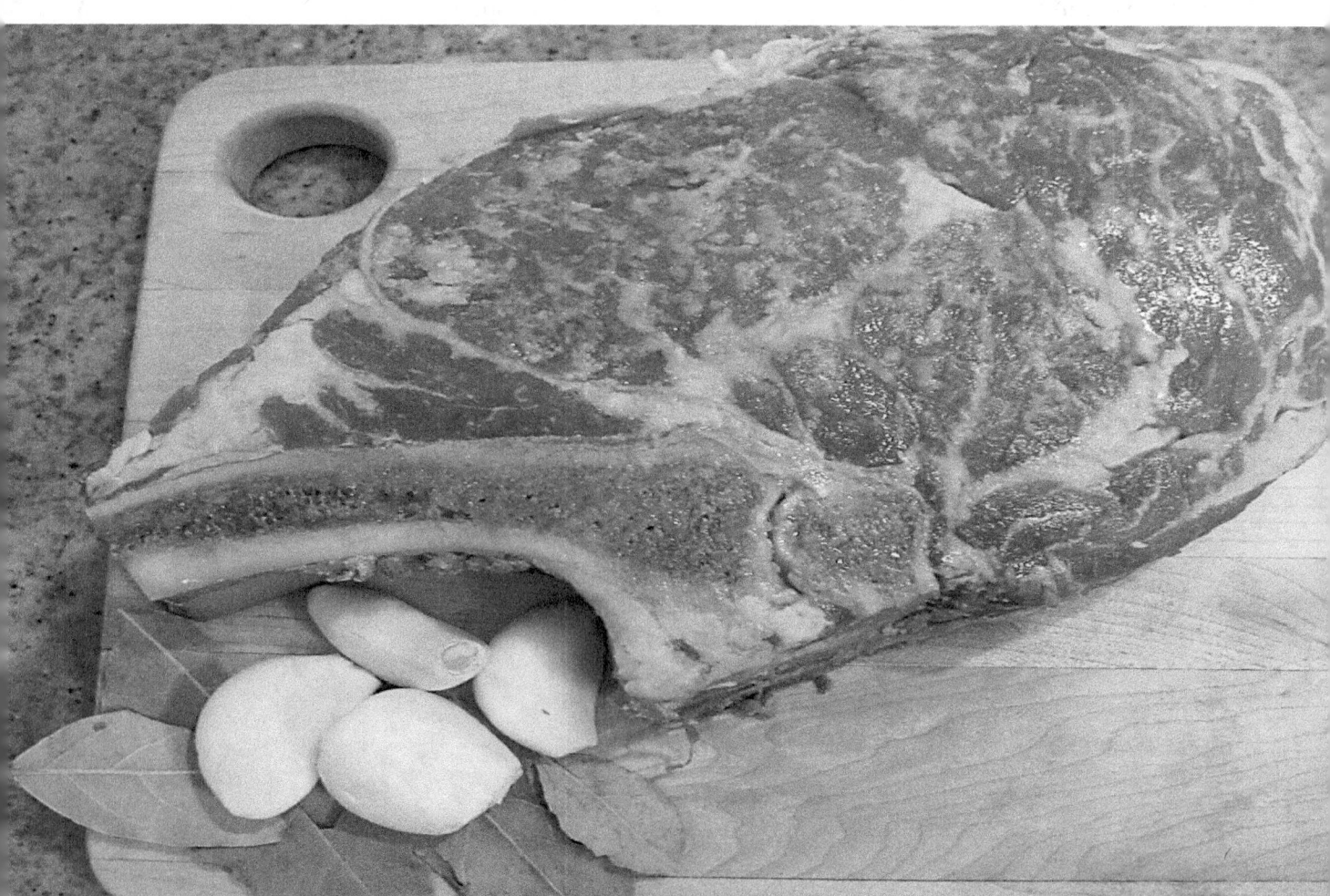

1. Spanish Shredded Beef (Ropa Vieja)

Preparation Time: 40 minutes
6 servings

Ingredients

- 1 ½ lb. boneless beef chuck, tip or round
- ½ cup water
- 2 tsp. salt
- ¼ tsp. pepper
- 1 bay leaf
- 1 tbsp. Canola oil
- 2 white onion, chopped
- 2 cloves garlic, minced
- 1 can (4 oz.) green chiles, drained, seeded and chopped
- 3 medium tomatoes, chopped
- 2 green peppers, ½" diced
- 1 tbsp. white vinegar
- ⅛ tsp. ground cinnamon
- ⅛ tsp. ground cloves
- 1 can (16 oz.) black beans

Preparation

Trim fat from meat, then cut into 1 ½ inch pieces. In a Dutch oven, place beef, water, salt, pepper and bay leaf. Cover pot and simmer 1 ½ hours or until beef is tender. Remove beef from broth and pull apart into shreds.

In a saucepan, saute oil, onions and garlic until tender.

In beef broth, add shredded beef, sauted onion mix, green chiles, tomatoes, green peppers, white vinegar, cinnamon and cloves. Heat to boiling, then simmer uncovered for 30 minutes.

Serve with a side of black beans on each plate. This is a Latin American specialty.

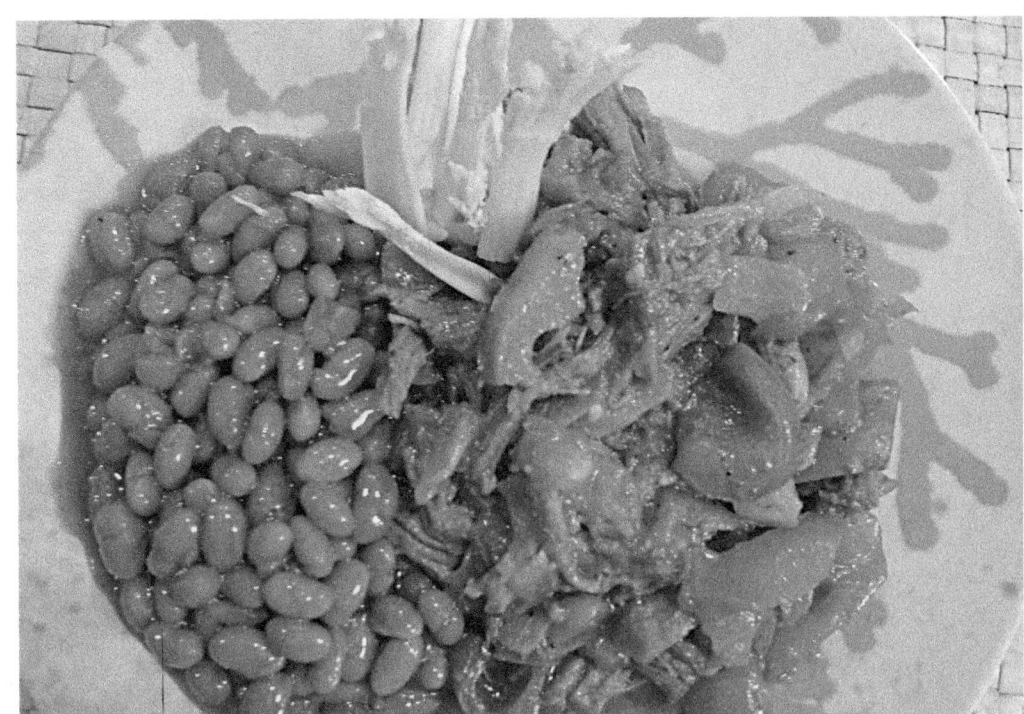

Nutrition Facts	
Serving Size 1/6 of recipe 259g (259 g)	
Amount Per Serving	
Calories 401	Calories from Fat 197
	% Daily Value*
Total Fat 22g	34%
Saturated Fat 9g	43%
Trans Fat 0g	
Cholesterol 106mg	35%
Sodium 907mg	38%
Total Carbohydrate 14g	5%
Dietary Fiber 4g	17%
Sugars 3g	
Protein 36g	

2. Stuffed Irish Lamb

Preparation Time: 80 minutes
6 servings

Ingredients

2 lb. boneless lamb, neck or shoulder
3 medium potatoes, peeled and ½" diced
3 carrots, peeled and sliced thin rounds
3 onions, peeled and sliced thin rounds
2 tsp. salt
¼ tsp. pepper
1 can beer
1 cup water
¼ parsley, chopped

Preparation

Trim fat from lamb, then cut into 1 inch cubes.

In a Dutch oven, create layer with half of each: lamb, potatoes, carrots and onions. Sprinkle with half of salt and pepper. Repeat with new layer using other half of ingredients, then add beer and water.

Heat to boiling, then cover and simmer 1 ½ hours or until lamb is tender. Skim fat from broth and sprinkle with parsley.

Serve in bowls with a side of red cabbage.

Note

To remove fat easily, prepare it the day before, cover and refrigerate. Once cold remove the fat before reheating.

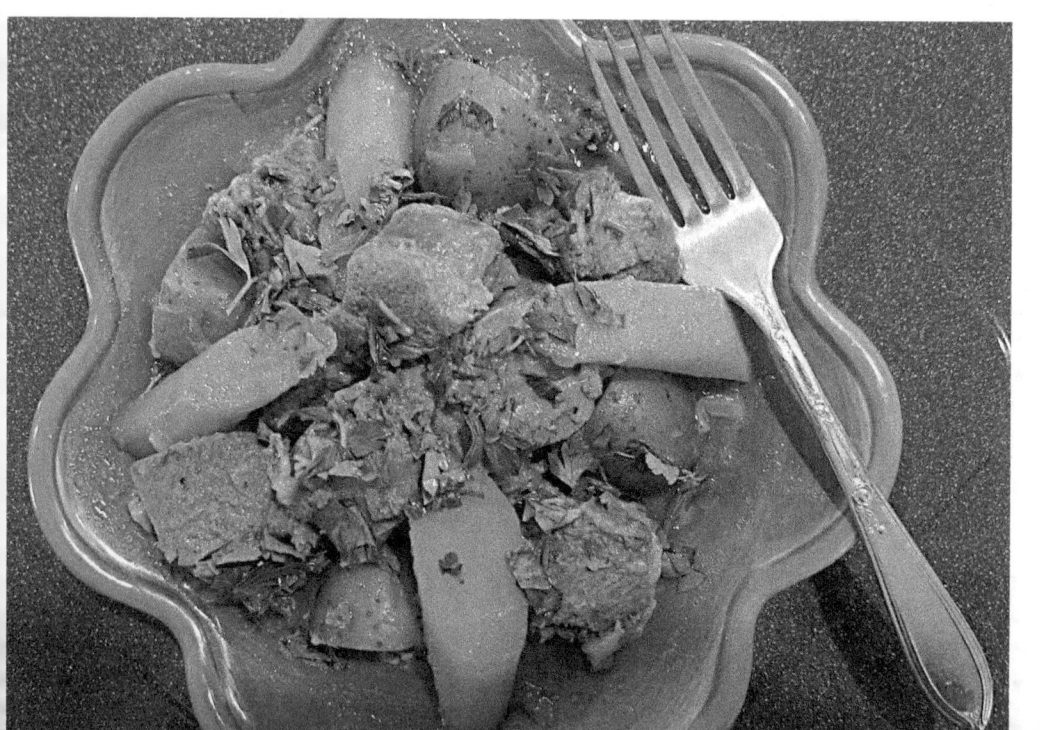

Nutrition Facts	
Serving Size 1/8 of recipe 305g (305 g)	
Servings per container 6	
Amount Per Serving	
Calories 321	Calories from Fat 131
	% Daily Value*
Total Fat 15g	22%
Saturated Fat 7g	34%
Trans Fat 0g	
Cholesterol 76mg	25%
Sodium 715mg	30%
Total Carbohydrate 21g	7%
Dietary Fiber 3g	13%
Sugars 3g	
Protein 24g	

3. Brazilian Black Bean Stew (Feijoada)

Preparation Time: 60 minutes
14 servings

Ingredients

1 smoked beef tongue (2 lb.)
8 cups cold water
3 cups black beans, pre-soaked day prior
½ lb. dried beef, chopped bite size
3 turkey smoked sausage, skinned and
    chopped and flattened with fork
1 large orange, sliced thin
2 cups cooked white rice

Salsa

4 jalapeno peppers, finely chopped
2 large tomatoes, chopped
1 white onion, chopped
2 cloves garlic, minced
¼ tsp. salt
⅛ tsp. ground red pepper
(1 cup mashed black beans)

Preparation

Cook tongue in salted water 2 hours or until tender, then remove skin and fat, and cut into ¼ inch pieces

Separately, boil black beans in water, then cook gently for 1 hour or until tender. Let cool, then crush 1 cup and set aside for salsa.

Combine tongue with remaining beans, beef and sausage, then mix well. Add water to cover ingredients and cook for 30 minutes.

Combine salsa ingredients then add to stew, with a little water if necessary. Simmer together for another 30 minutes.

Serve stew on a bed of white rice and garnish with orange slices.

Nutrition Facts	
Serving Size 1/14 of recipe 210g (210 g)	
Servings per container 14	
Amount Per Serving	
Calories 421	Calories from Fat 153
	% Daily Value*
Total Fat 17g	26%
Saturated Fat 6g	29%
Trans Fat 1g	
Cholesterol 112mg	37%
Sodium 641mg	27%
Total Carbohydrate 36g	12%
Dietary Fiber 7g	29%
Sugars 4g	
Protein 31g	

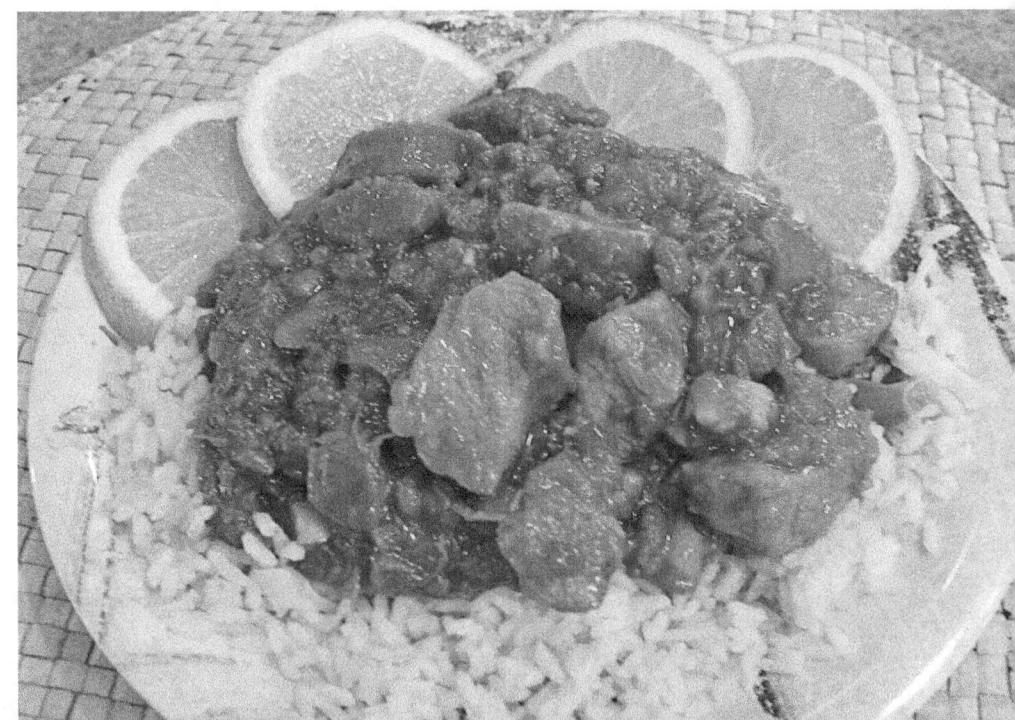

4. Hawaiian Veal Chops

Preparation Time: 30 minutes
6 servings

Ingredients

6 veal chops, (1 ½ - 2 lb.)
Salt and pepper to taste
¼ cup milk
1 egg
½ cup breadcrumbs
2 tbsp. canola oil
4 kiwi, peeled and chopped
2 tangerines, peeled and sectioned
½ cup jicama, peeled and chopped
¼ cup chopped arugula leaves
½ cup finely chopped red pepper
1 jalapeno pepper, chopped
1 tbsp. lime juice

Preparation

Tenderize veal with mallet, then sprinkle both sides with salt and pepper to taste. Mix egg and milk together, then dip veal in mixture, coating both sides.

In a plastic bag, place breadcrumbs and veal, then shake well.

Heat oil in large skillet, then fry veal until golden brown on both sides.

In a large bowl, mix kiwi, tangerine, jicama, arugula, red pepper, jalapeno, and lime juice, then marinate for 30 minutes.

Serve veal hot and cover with sauce.

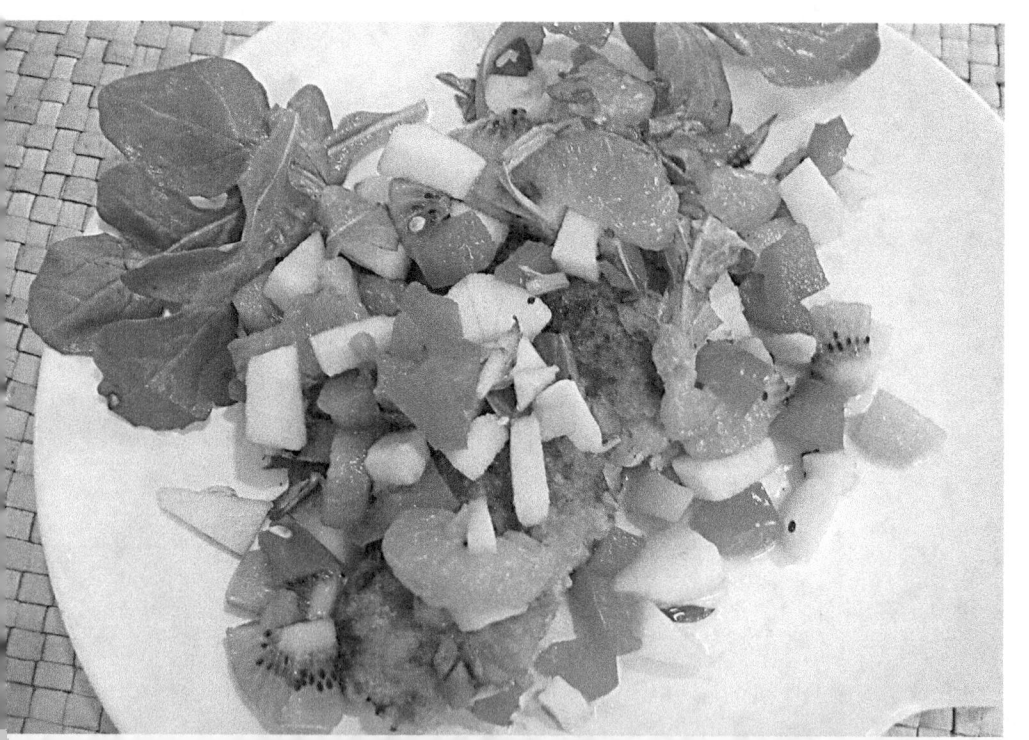

Nutrition Facts
Serving Size 1/6 of recipe 213g (213 g)
Servings per container 6

Amount Per Serving		
Calories 411	Calories from Fat 136	
		% Daily Value*
Total Fat 15g		23%
Saturated Fat 5g		25%
Trans Fat 0g		
Cholesterol 166mg		55%
Sodium 272mg		11%
Total Carbohydrate 27g		9%
Dietary Fiber 2g		10%
Sugars 4g		
Protein 39g		

5. African Beef and Rice (Moui Nagden)

Preparation Time: 1 ¼ hours
6 servings

Ingredients

1 lb. beef round steak, ½" thick,
    cut into 1" pieces
1 tbsp. canola oil
1 white onion, chopped
1 bay leaf
1 tsp. salt
¼ tsp. ground red pepper
1 cup water
1 can (16oz.) red kidney beans, drained
1 cup uncooked white rice
2 green peppers cut into ½" pieces
1 ½ tsp. salt
½ tsp. curry powder
¼ tsp. pepper

Preparation

Preheat oven to 350°.

Heat oil in a 10-inch skillet, stir in beef and cook 15 minutes, or until brown on all sides. Add onion, bay leaf, salt and red pepper, heat to boiling, then cover and simmer for 30 minutes.

Drain beef, reserving broth. Add enough water to broth to measure 2 cups. Mix beef, broth and remaining ingredients and pour into ungreased 2-quart casserole dish.

Cover and bake 30 minutes, or until all liquid is absorbed.

Serve with sliced tomatoes

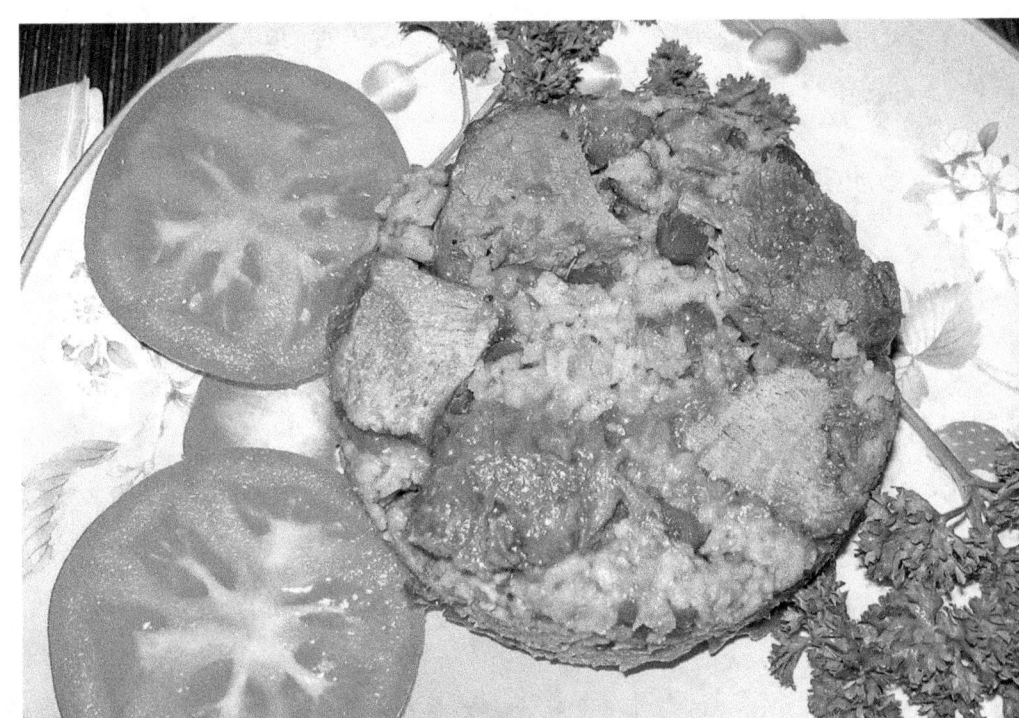

Nutrition Facts	
Serving Size Entire Recipe 243g (242 g)	
Amount Per Serving	
Calories 383	Calories from Fat 87
	% Daily Value*
Total Fat 10g	15%
Saturated Fat 3g	16%
Trans Fat 1g	
Cholesterol 74mg	25%
Sodium 654mg	27%
Total Carbohydrate 42g	14%
Dietary Fiber 6g	24%
Sugars 3g	
Protein 32g	

6. Spanish Stewpot (Puchero)

Preparation Time: 80 minutes
8 servings

Ingredients

1 ½ lb. sirloin steak
8 cups water
1 medium onion, chopped
2 cloves garlic, minced
1 bay leaf
2 ½ tsp. salt
¼ tsp. pepper
1 lb. sausage, cut into ½" slices
3 medium carrots, sliced round
3 celery stalks, slice round
½ lb. cooked chickpeas
1 head white cabbage, cut lengthwise into
   8 slices

Preparation

Trim fat from steak, then cook in water with onion, garlic, bay leaf, salt and pepper until meat is tender. Cut steak into lengthwise pieces.

In a large pan, cook sausages without water, stirring frequently until golden. Then add the steak and broth with carrots, celery, chickpeas, cabbage, and enough water to cover ingredients like a soup.

Cover pot and simmer 20 minutes more. Then remove all ingredients from broth and divide onto serving plates. Serve the broth in separate soup cups.

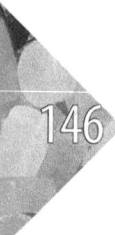

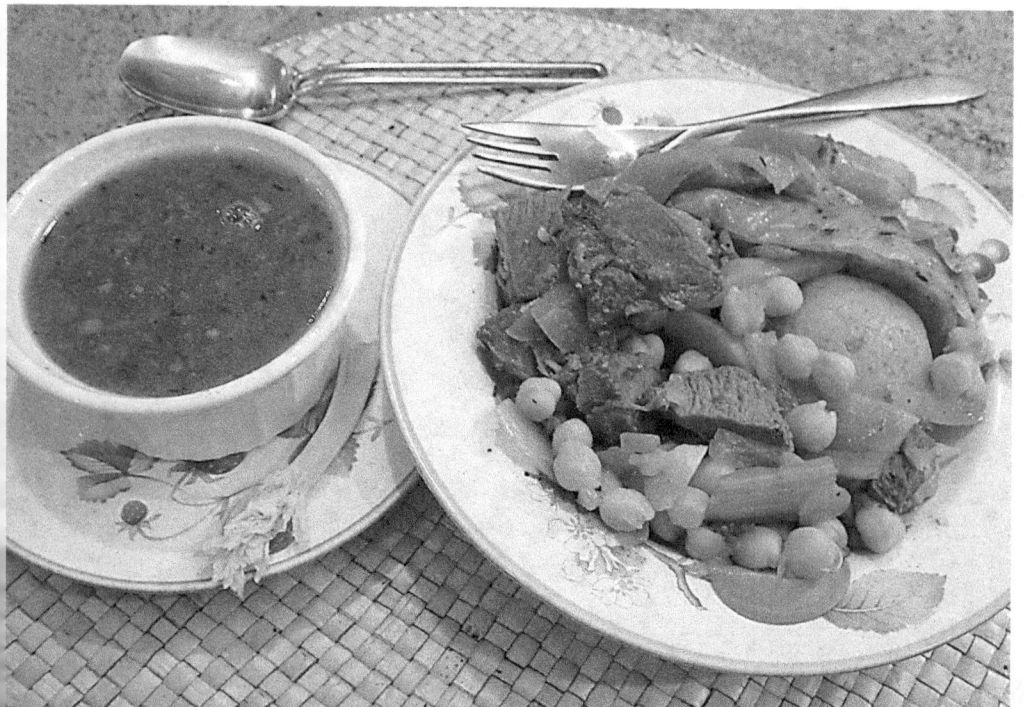

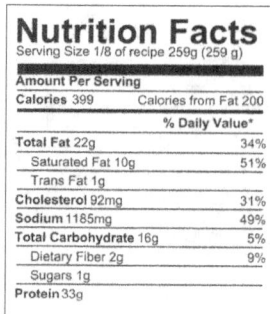

Nutrition Facts	
Serving Size 1/8 of recipe 259g (259 g)	
Amount Per Serving	
Calories 399	Calories from Fat 200
	% Daily Value*
Total Fat 22g	34%
Saturated Fat 10g	51%
Trans Fat 1g	
Cholesterol 92mg	31%
Sodium 1185mg	49%
Total Carbohydrate 16g	5%
Dietary Fiber 2g	9%
Sugars 1g	
Protein 33g	

7. Russian Beef Stroganov

Preparation Time: 30 minutes
6 servings

Ingredients

4 tbsp. low fat margarine
8 oz. mushrooms, sliced
2 medium onions, sliced
1 clove of garlic, crushed
1 lb. boneless sirloin or top sirloin, ½" thick,
    cut across grain into 1 ½" strips
½ cup water
1 tsp. beef bouillon
Salt and pepper to taste
1 cup low fat sour cream
½ tsp. mustard sauce
3 cups cooked white rice
Snipped parsley

Preparation

In skillet, melt 2 tablespoons margarine, then add mushrooms, onions and garlic. Cover and simmer, stirring until onions are tender. Remove vegetables and any liquid from skillet.

In same skillet over medium heat, cook steak in 2 tablespoons of margarine for 10 minutes or until brown. Add water, bouillon, salt and pepper to taste. Heat to boiling, reduce heat, cover and simmer until beef is done to desired wellness. Add cooked vegetable mixture and heat to boil, reduce heat, then stir in sour cream and mustard.

Serve with white rice and garnish with parsley.

Nutrition Facts	
Serving Size 1/6 of recipe 258g (258 g)	
Servings per container 6	
Amount Per Serving	
Calories 288	Calories from Fat 107
	% Daily Value*
Total Fat 12g	18%
Saturated Fat 4g	22%
Trans Fat 0g	
Cholesterol 54mg	18%
Sodium 199mg	8%
Total Carbohydrate 25g	8%
Dietary Fiber 2g	8%
Sugars 2g	
Protein 20g	

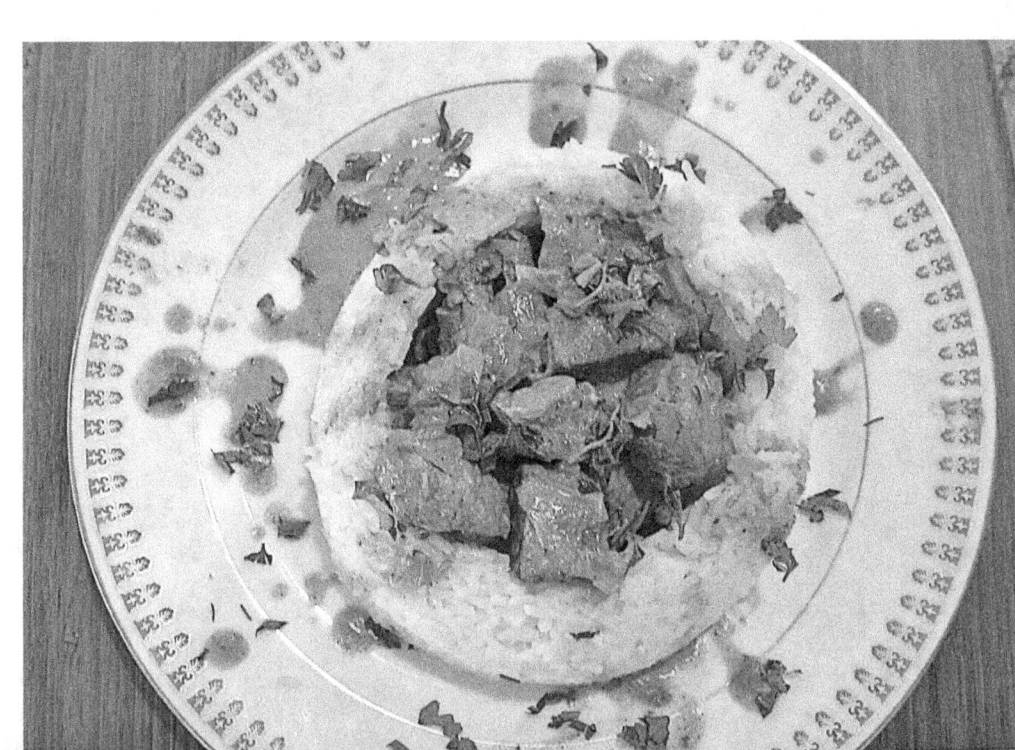

8. *Italian Meat and Spinach Lasagna*

Preparation Time: 45 minutes
8 servings

Ingredients

¾ lb. 90% lean ground beef
Canola oil spray
1 medium onion, chopped
1 clove garlic, minced
3 cups tomato sauce
2 tbsp. chopped parsley
1 tsp. brown sugar
½ tsp. each: salt, basil, oregano
¾ tsp. pepper
1 egg, beaten
1 cup cooked spinach, drained with salt
1 package (8oz.) lasagna pasta
1 carton (15 oz.) nonfat ricotta cheese
1 cup nonfat cheddar cheese, shredded
½ cup parmesan cheese

Preparation

Spray skillet with oil, lightly brown beef, onion and garlic, then add tomato sauce, parsley, sugar, salt, basil, oregano and pepper. Cover and simmer for 20 minutes .

In a small bowl, mix egg and spinach. Cook pasta according to package directions and drain.

In baking pan, cover bottom with 1 cup sauce. Add layer of pasta, then another layer of sauce, then a layer with half ricotta, then half cheddar. Add layer of pasta then remaining sauce and cheeses. Top with pasta layer, then spread egg and spinach layer. Sprinkle top with parmesan.

Preheat oven to 350º, bake uncovered for 45 minutes until golden, let stand 15 minutes.

Serve with a small salad or vegetables.

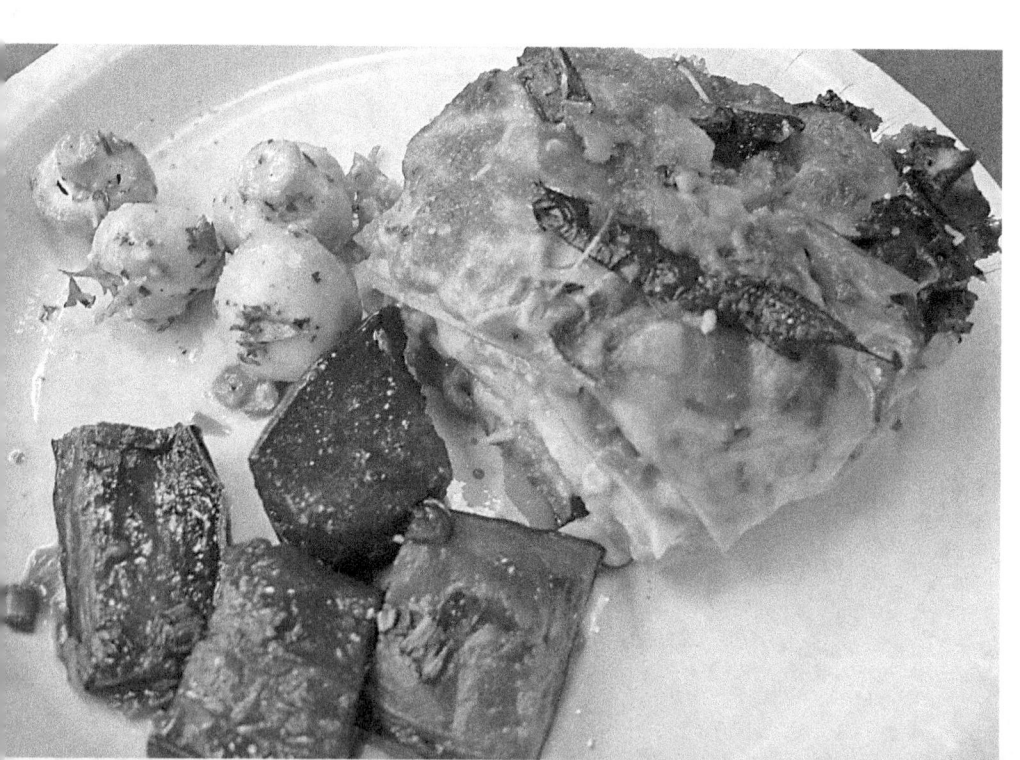

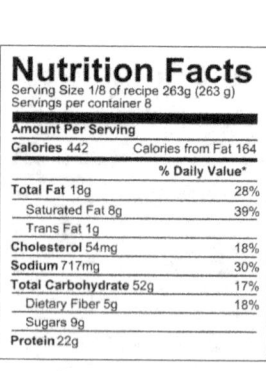

Nutrition Facts	
Serving Size 1/8 of recipe 263g (263 g)	
Servings per container 8	
Amount Per Serving	
Calories 442	Calories from Fat 164
	% Daily Value*
Total Fat 18g	28%
Saturated Fat 8g	39%
Trans Fat 1g	
Cholesterol 54mg	18%
Sodium 717mg	30%
Total Carbohydrate 52g	17%
Dietary Fiber 5g	18%
Sugars 9g	
Protein 22g	

Tasty Turkey Recipes

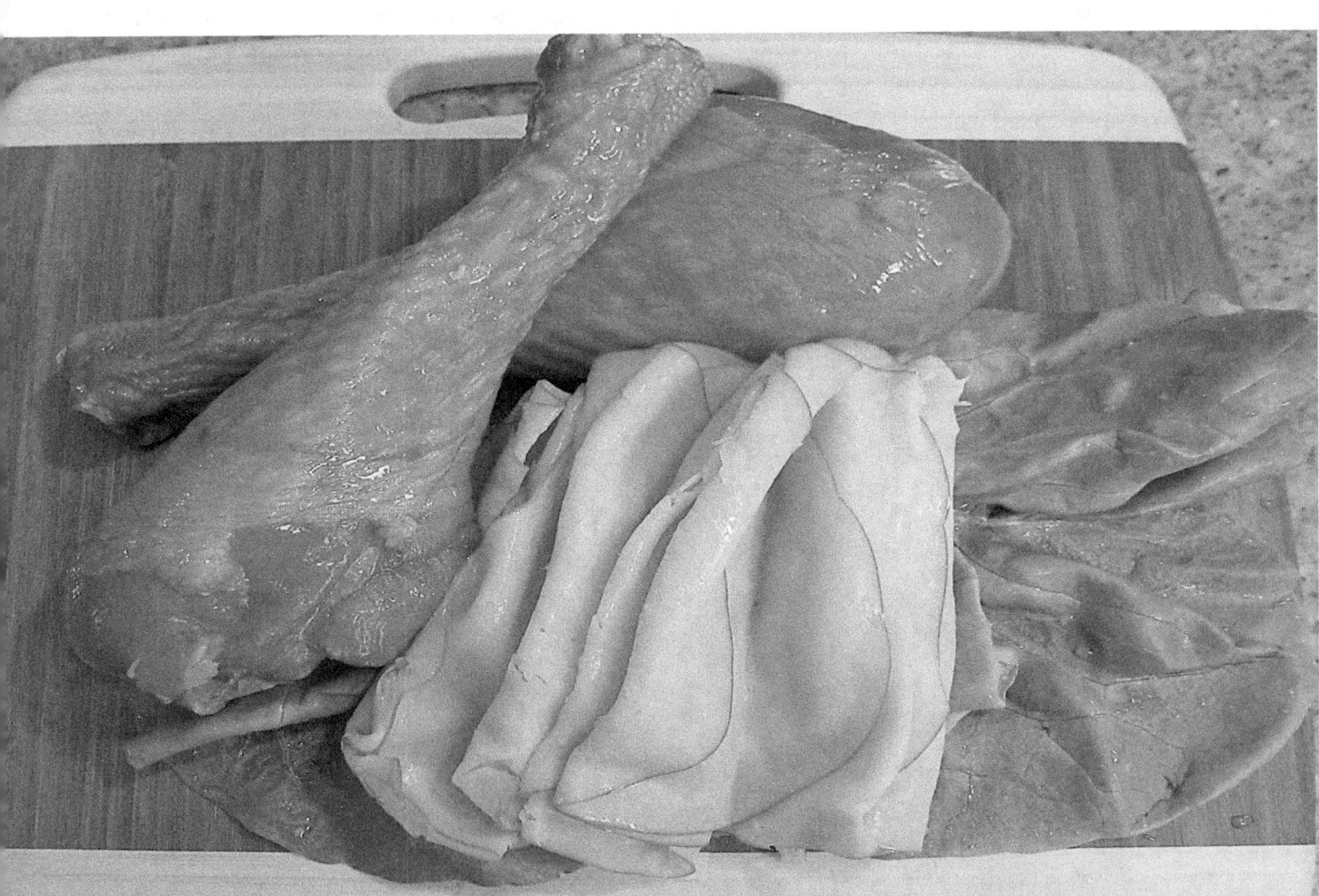

1. Carmen's Christmas Turkey Stuffing

Preparation Time: 3 - 4 hours
16 servings

Ingredients

1 turkey (12 lb.), day before: remove giblets, wash inside and out, leave submerged in pot of water overnight
Canola oil spray
6 cloves garlic, crushed
1 cup tomato sauce
1 tbsp. pepper
1 cup finely chopped white onion
1 lb. ground turkey
2 celery stalks, chopped
1 cup chopped parsley
2 apples, peeled and chopped fine
2 cups cooked brown rice
1 cup raisins
Salt and pepper to taste
½ cup green olives, pitted and sliced
½ cup chopped walnuts
1 bottle beer malt

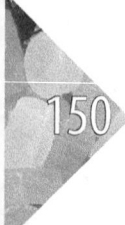

150

Preparation

Remove and dry turkey, then rub with a mix of half the garlic, pepper and tomato sauce.

Heat sprayed oil in large skillet, then brown onion and remaining garlic. Add ground turkey and cook 5 minutes, then add celery, parsley, apples, rice, raisins, salt and pepper. Stir well and simmer for 10 minutes. Add olives and walnuts then remove from heat. Stuff turkey cavity, then tie legs together to keep stuffing inside.

Preheat oven to 300°, and spray large pan with oil. Place turkey in pan and loosely cover with foil tent, halfway thru cooking (1 ½ hours) remove foil to brown skin. While cooking, baste turkey with beer and pan juice. Cook for 3 ½ hours, or until cutting with knife does not release blood.

Serve on a tray garnished with lettuce and fruits, along with other festive side dishes.

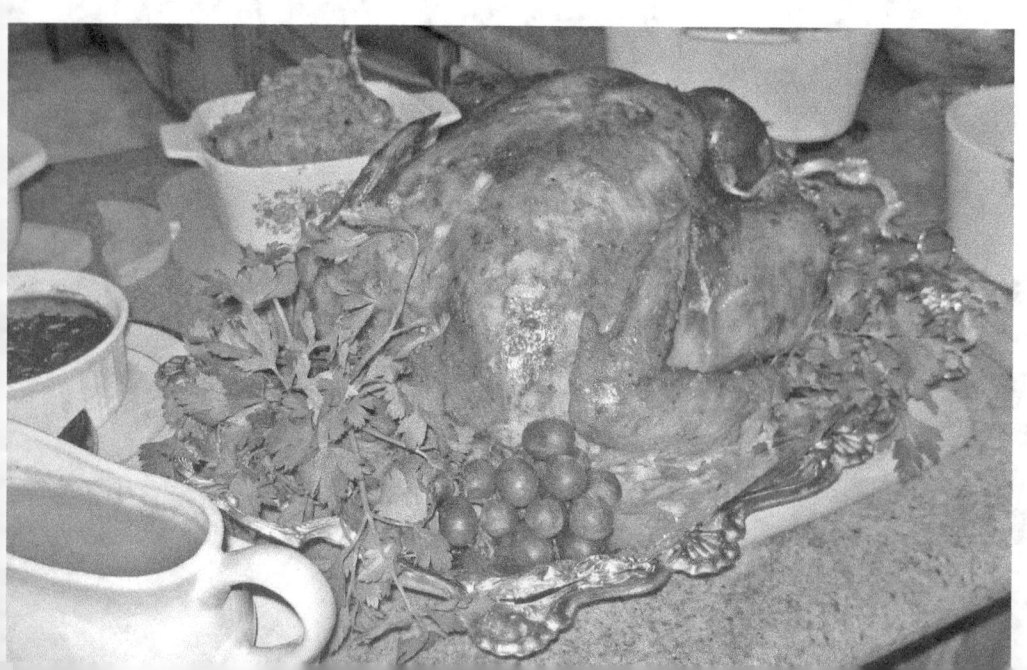

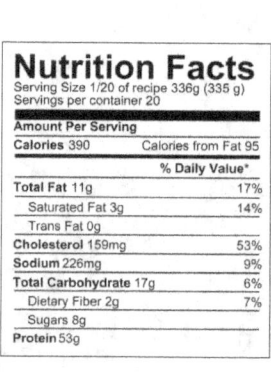

Nutrition Facts
Serving Size 1/20 of recipe 336g (335 g)
Servings per container 20

Amount Per Serving

Calories 390	Calories from Fat 95

	% Daily Value*
Total Fat 11g	17%
Saturated Fat 3g	14%
Trans Fat 0g	
Cholesterol 159mg	53%
Sodium 226mg	9%
Total Carbohydrate 17g	6%
Dietary Fiber 2g	7%
Sugars 8g	
Protein 53g	

2. Thai Turkey Burger

Preparation Time: 30 minutes
4 servings

Ingredients

1 lb. ground turkey breast
1 egg white
¼ cup breadcrumbs
2 tbsp. chopped mint leaves
2 tbsp. finely chopped cilantro
2 tbsp. finely chopped green onion
1 clove garlic, minced
½ tsp. grated fresh ginger
1 lemon, juice
½ tsp. salt
½ cup teriyaki sauce
2 tbsp. sesame seeds, toasted
Canola oil spray

Preparation

In a large bowl, mix well the turkey, egg, breadcrumbs, mint, cilantro, onion, garlic, ginger, lemon juice, salt and ¼ cup of teriyaki sauce. Divide evenly into 4 balls, then form patties and set aside.

Preheat oven to 375°. Spray bake pan with oil, then place burgers. Bake 7 minutes per side, pressing with a spatula to compact, then glaze each side with remaining teriyaki sauce.

Sprinkle each burger with toasted sesame seeds before serving.

Accompany burgers with a fruit, salad and toasted bread.

Nutrition Facts	
Serving Size 1/4 of recipe 182g (182 g)	
Servings per container 4	
Amount Per Serving	
Calories 146	Calories from Fat 14
	% Daily Value*
Total Fat 2g	2%
Saturated Fat 0g	2%
Trans Fat 0g	
Cholesterol 36mg	12%
Sodium 3023mg	126%
Total Carbohydrate 13g	4%
Dietary Fiber 1g	3%
Sugars 7g	
Protein 20g	

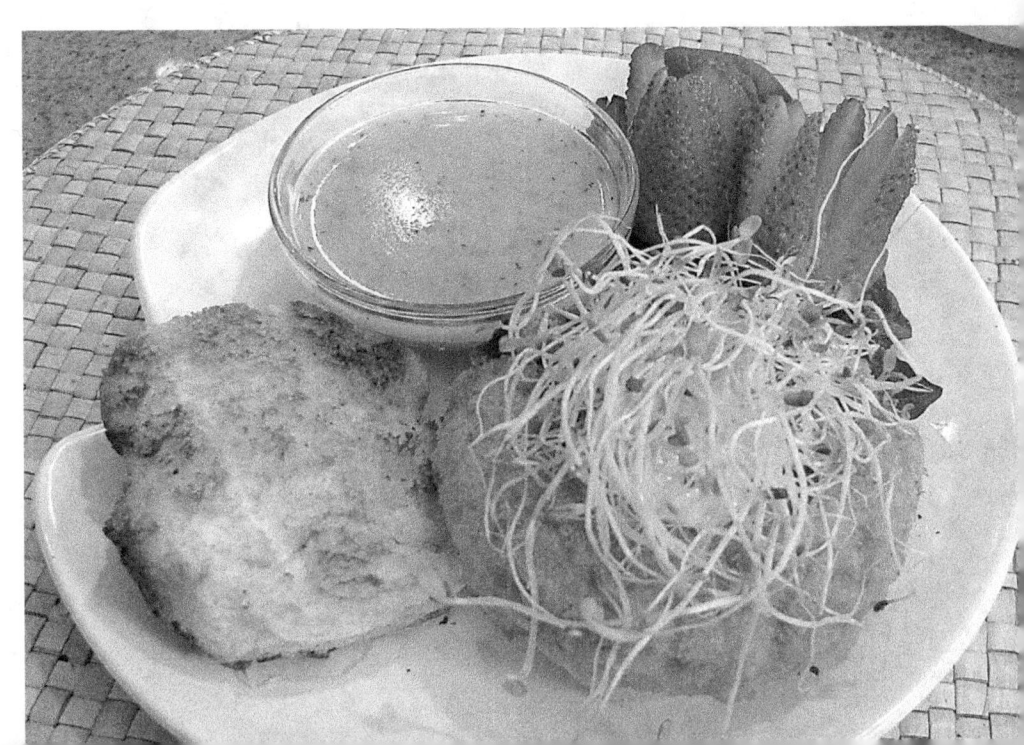

3. Turkey with Caramelized Onions

Preparation Time: 60 minutes
6 servings

Ingredients

12 seedless prunes
1 chicken broth
1 turkey breast (3 lb.), washed
6 medium sweet yellow onions, peeled and
   cut lengthwise strips
Garlic salt and pepper to taste
Canola oil spray
Finely chopped cilantro

Preparation

In a blender, puree prunes and chicken broth.

Preheat oven to 350º. Season turkey and onions with salt and pepper. Spray bake pan with oil, place breast with onions around it. Lightly spray oil on onions only, then stir them.

Bake for 45 minutes, then only cover turkey with puree. Bake another 20 minutes, or until tender with soft and golden onions.

Remove turkey and cut into thin slices. Serve with onion and sauce on side of each plate, then sprinkle with cilantro.

"Yucca" or rice is an excellent complement to this dish.

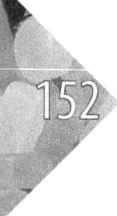

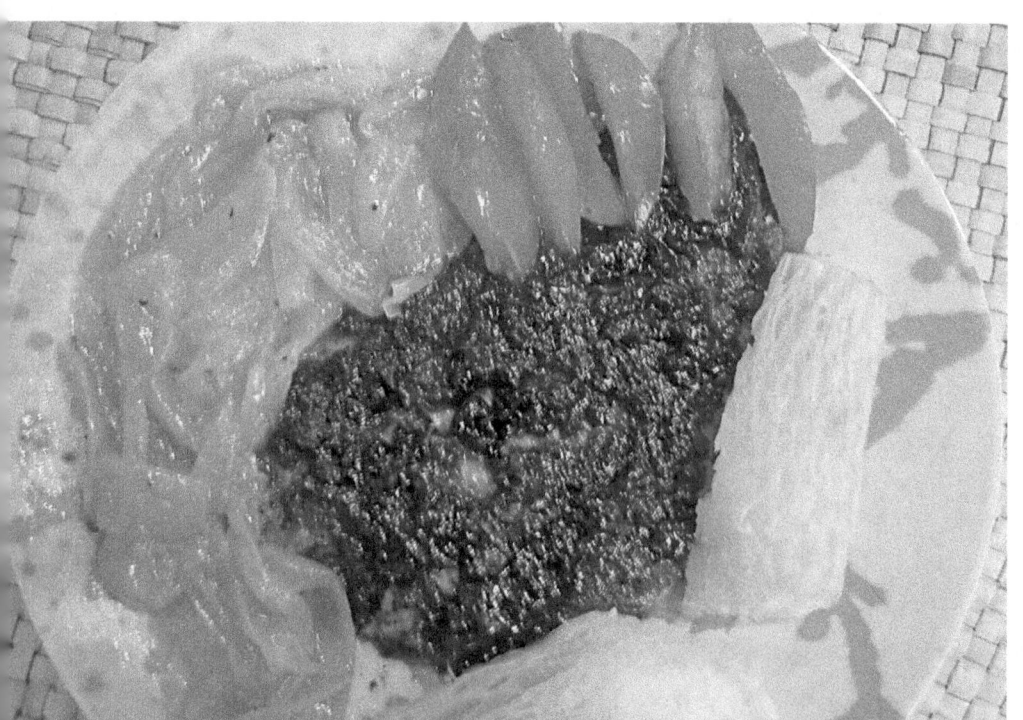

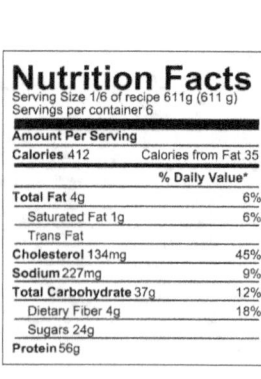

Nutrition Facts		
Serving Size 1/6 of recipe 611g (611 g)		
Servings per container 6		
Amount Per Serving		
Calories 412	Calories from Fat 35	
		% Daily Value*
Total Fat 4g		6%
Saturated Fat 1g		6%
Trans Fat		
Cholesterol 134mg		45%
Sodium 227mg		9%
Total Carbohydrate 37g		12%
Dietary Fiber 4g		18%
Sugars 24g		
Protein 56g		

4. Italian Turkey Milanese

Preparation Time: 20 minutes
4 servings

Ingredients

8 slices turkey breast, ⅛" thick
Salt and pepper to taste
1 tsp. Italian spices, ground
3 egg whites
2 tbsp. 1% milk
3 cloves garlic, minced
4 tbsp. chopped parsley
1 cup breadcrumbs
Canola oil spray
1 lemon, sliced wedges

Preparation

Preheat oven to 375º. Spray baking sheet with oil. Rub both sides of turkey breast with salt, pepper and spices.

In medium bowl, whisk egg whites and milk, with garlic and parsley. Spread breadcrumbs over wide plate. Dip each turkey slice into egg mix, then lay both side of each slice onto breadcrumbs and coat evenly.

Place turkey slices on sheet, bake until light golden brown, then turn to brown other side.

Serve slices with lemon wedges and a sprinkle of chopped parsley. Accompany with a side of steamed vegetables.

153

Nutrition Facts		
Serving Size 1/4 of recipe 133g (132 g)		
Servings per container 4		
Amount Per Serving		
Calories 192	Calories from Fat 18	
		% Daily Value*
Total Fat 2g		3%
Saturated Fat 1g		3%
Trans Fat 0g		
Cholesterol 35mg		12%
Sodium 272mg		11%
Total Carbohydrate 22g		7%
Dietary Fiber 2g		6%
Sugars 3g		
Protein 21g		

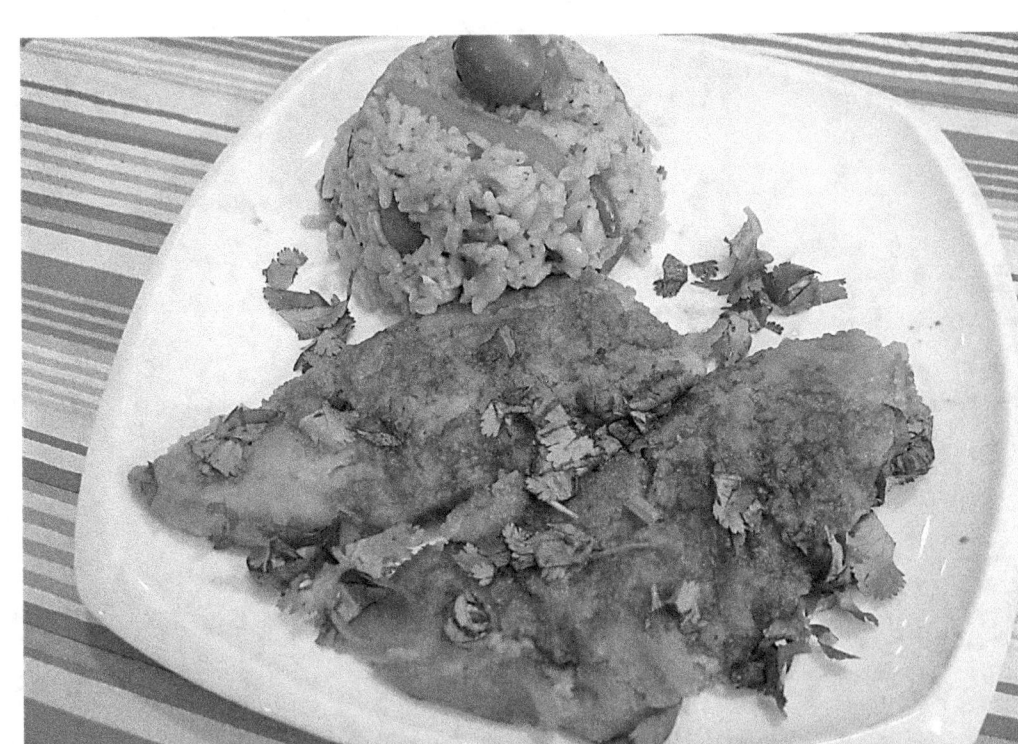

5. Creole Turkey Fillets

Preparation Time: 80 minutes
6 servings

Ingredients

1 ½ lb. of turkey breast, 92% fat
2 tbsp. canola oil
2 white onions, chopped
2 green bell peppers, chopped
1 red bell pepper, chopped
1 tsp. salt
½ tsp. each: basil, oregano, thyme, paprika, garlic powder, onion powder, chili powder
¼ tsp. each: black pepper, white pepper, cayenne pepper
1 tbsp. English black sauce
3 cups crushed tomatoes
1 cup chopped green onion
2 tbsp. chopped parsley

Preparation

Cut turkey into ¾ inch cubes.

In a large pan with oil, saute turkey, white onions, red and green peppers, until cooked through.

Reduce heat to medium, add seasonings, black sauce and tomatoes, then simmer for 30 minutes.

Add green onions and parsley and simmer for 5 minutes more.

A Louisiana favorite served with rice.

154

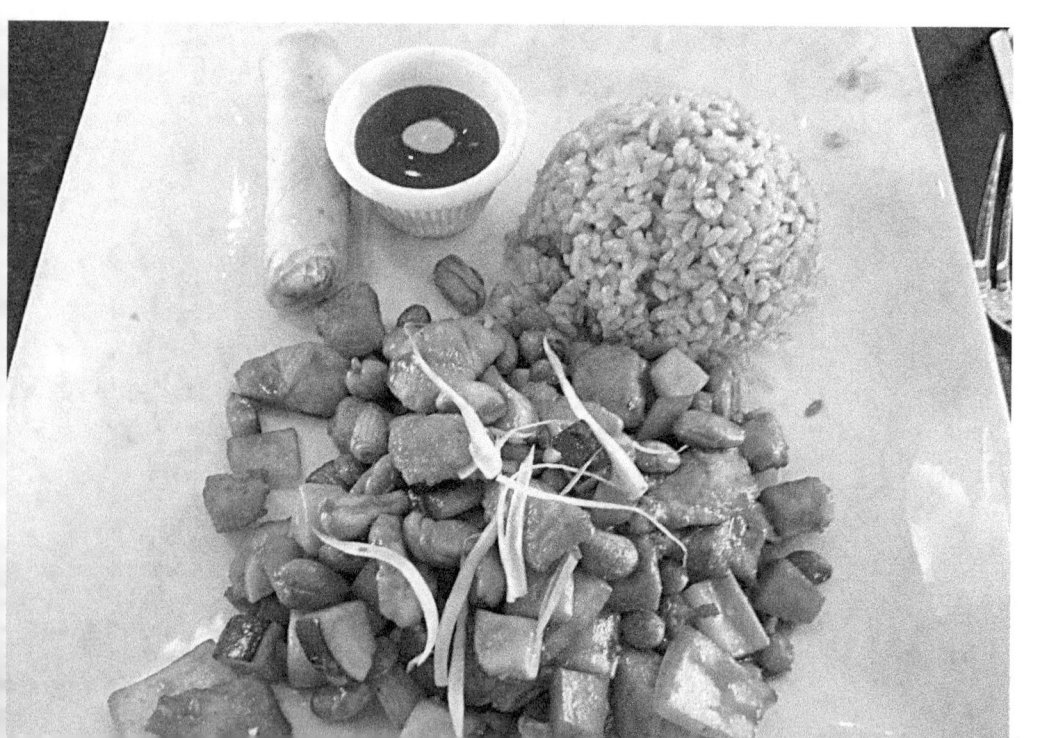

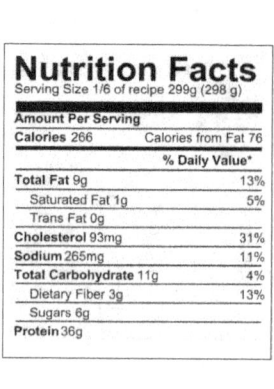

Nutrition Facts
Serving Size 1/6 of recipe 299g (298 g)

Amount Per Serving	
Calories 266	Calories from Fat 76

	% Daily Value*
Total Fat 9g	13%
Saturated Fat 1g	5%
Trans Fat 0g	
Cholesterol 93mg	31%
Sodium 265mg	11%
Total Carbohydrate 11g	4%
Dietary Fiber 3g	13%
Sugars 6g	
Protein 36g	

6. Turkey Medallions with Mango Chutney Sauce

Preparation Time: 60 minutes
8 servings

Ingredients

1 lb. turkey tenderloins, cut into ¾" medallions
1 tsp. low fat margarine
2 tsp. olive oil
2 tbsp. chopped green onions
½ cup turkey broth
1 tsp. red chili pepper flakes

Chutney

1 large mango, peeled and cubed
¼ cup distilled white vinegar
1 cup molasses
½ cup golden raisins
2 tbsp. ginger, finely grated
½ cup chopped onions
1 clove garlic, crushed

Preparation

Mix and bring to boil, molasses and vinegar. Stir in rest of chutney ingredients, then simmer uncovered 45 - 60 minutes, stirring occasionally, until syrupy and slightly thickened. Pour into clean, hot jar.

In a large skillet over medium heat, sauté medallions in margarine and 1 tsp. oil, until no pink in center. Remove medallions from pan and keep warm. Add remaining 1 tsp. oil to skillet and sauté onions for 30 seconds. Add broth and cook 1 minute to reduce liquid.

Place turkey medallions on a warm plate, then cover with chutney sauce and serve.

It's just delicious!

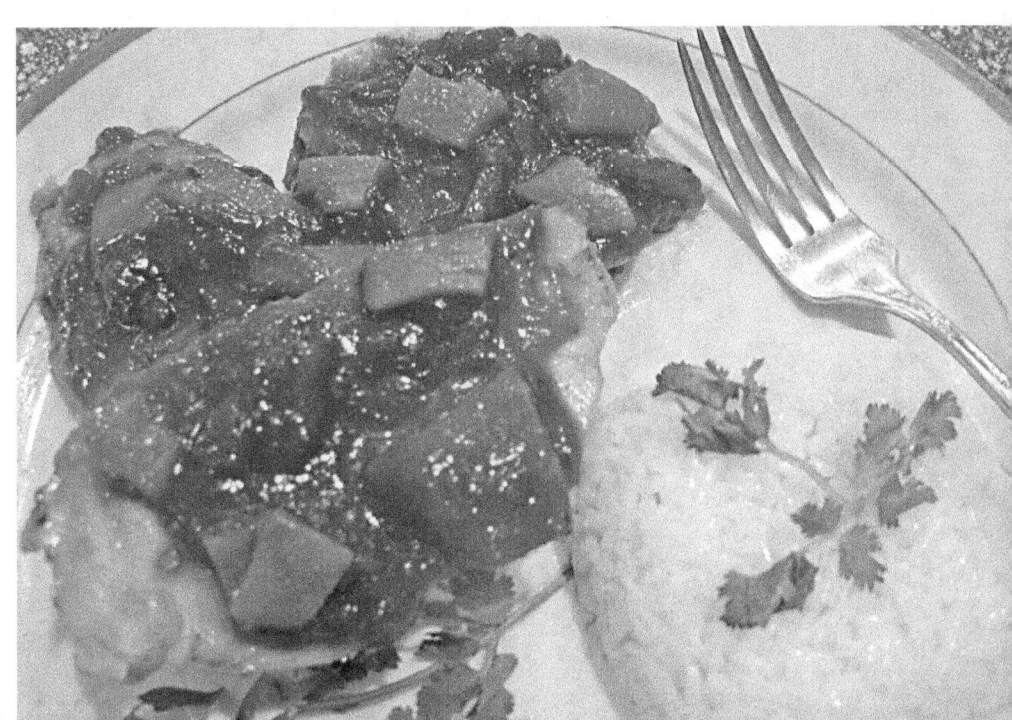

155

Nutrition Facts		
Serving Size 1/4 of recipe 299g (299 g)		
Servings per container 4		
Amount Per Serving		
Calories 372	Calories from Fat 26	
		% Daily Value*
Total Fat 3g		5%
Saturated Fat 1g		4%
Trans Fat 0g		
Cholesterol 67mg		22%
Sodium 110mg		5%
Total Carbohydrate 60g		20%
Dietary Fiber 2g		9%
Sugars 44g		
Protein 28g		

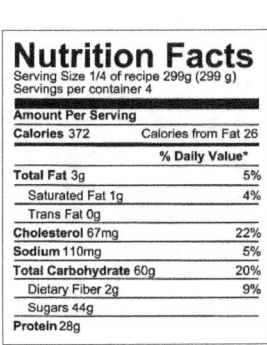

7. Onion and Cilantro Turkey

Preparation Time: 15 minutes
6 servings

Ingredients

1 ½ lb. of turkey breast, cut in finger shape
1 tbsp. salt
1 ½ tsp. molasses
Canola oil spray
1 small bunch cilantro, chopped
1 small bunch green onions, chopped
1 lemon, cut into wedges

Onion Mix

In a small bowl mix:
¼ cup finely chopped green onions,
2 tbsp. chopped cilantro
3 cloves garlic, crushed
1 tbsp. grated fresh ginger
1 tbsp. ground pepper
1 tbsp. grated lemon rind

Preparation

Wash and dry turkey, then sprinkle both sides with salt and molasses. Store in refrigerator for 2 to 3 hours, then remove, rinse lightly and pat dry.

Prepare onion mix, then rub on both sides of turkey fingers.

Preheat oven to 375º. Spray oil on bake pan. Place turkey fingers on pan then bake each side for 7 minutes, or until light brown.

Garnish with cilantro, chopped green onions and lemon slices.

Serve with brown rice or steamed vegetables on the side.

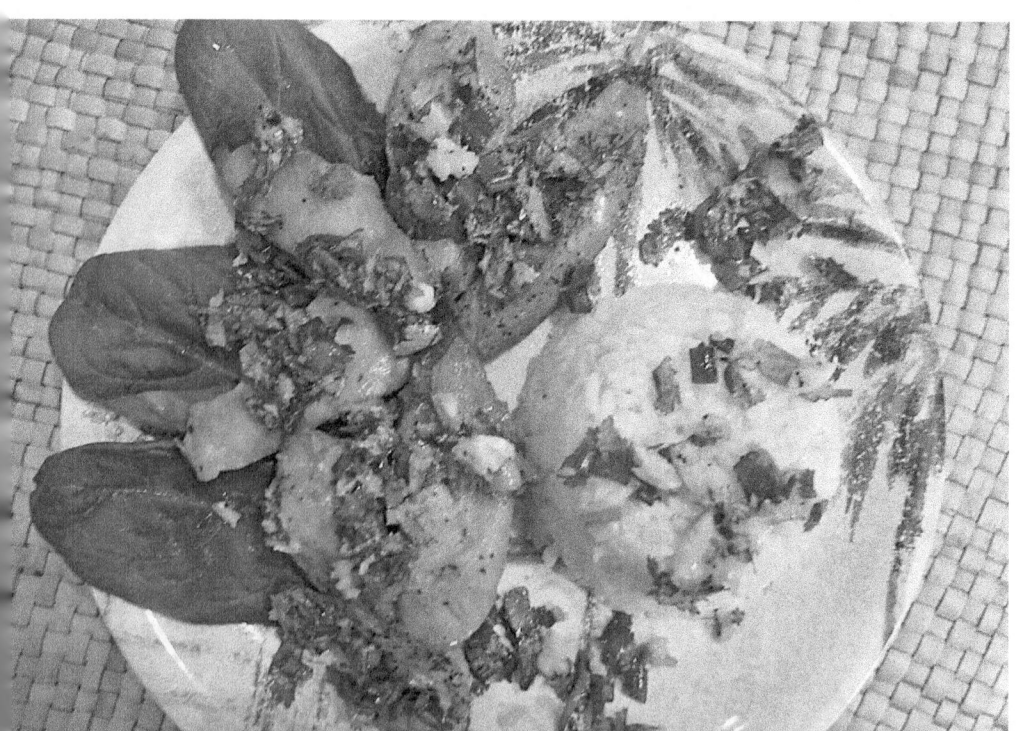

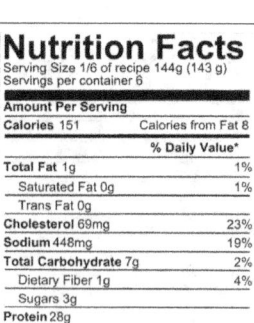

Nutrition Facts
Serving Size 1/6 of recipe 144g (143 g)
Servings per container 6

Amount Per Serving	
Calories 151	Calories from Fat 8
	% Daily Value*
Total Fat 1g	1%
Saturated Fat 0g	1%
Trans Fat 0g	
Cholesterol 69mg	23%
Sodium 448mg	19%
Total Carbohydrate 7g	2%
Dietary Fiber 1g	4%
Sugars 3g	
Protein 28g	

8. Italian Spaghetti with Turkey Meatballs

Preparation Time: 30 minutes
6 servings

Ingredients

1 ½ lb. ground turkey
½ cup milk
2 eggs, beaten
2 tbsp. grated parmesan cheese
1 tbsp. chopped parsley
1 ½ tsp. salt
½ tsp. dried oregano
¼ tsp. pepper
½ cup chopped onion

1 pack (16 oz.) spaghetti
Parmesan cheese, grated

Sauce

Canola oil spray
½ onion, chopped fine
1 clove garlic, minced
1 jar (16 oz.) whole tomatoes
1 jar (6 oz.) tomato paste
¼ cup water
¼ cup chopped parsley
1 tsp. each: sugar, salt
½ tsp. basil
¼ tsp. pepper

Preparation

Meatballs: Preheat oven to 350°. Mix turkey with milk, eggs, cheese, parsley, salt oregano, pepper and onion. Make 1 ½ inch balls and place on ungreased pan. Bake uncovered 15 - 20 minutes, or until light brown.

Sauce: Spray oil in a Dutch oven, then cook onion and garlic until tender. Add tomatoes, tomato paste, water, parsley, sugar, salt, basil and pepper. Split whole tomatoes with fork and bring to boil. Reduce heat, cover and stir occasionally for 30 minutes. Add meatballs and simmer for 15 minutes more.

Follow package directions to cook spaghetti.

Place spaghetti on large platter then top with meatballs, sauce and a sprinkle of parmesan cheese. Serve with French bread and a green salad if desired.

Nutrition Facts		
Serving Size 1/8 of recipe 270g (270 g)		
Servings per container 8		
Amount Per Serving		
Calories 390	Calories from Fat 22	
		% Daily Value*
Total Fat 2g		4%
Saturated Fat 1g		3%
Trans Fat 0g		
Cholesterol 53mg		18%
Sodium 834mg		35%
Total Carbohydrate 58g		19%
Dietary Fiber 4g		16%
Sugars 7g		
Protein 33g		

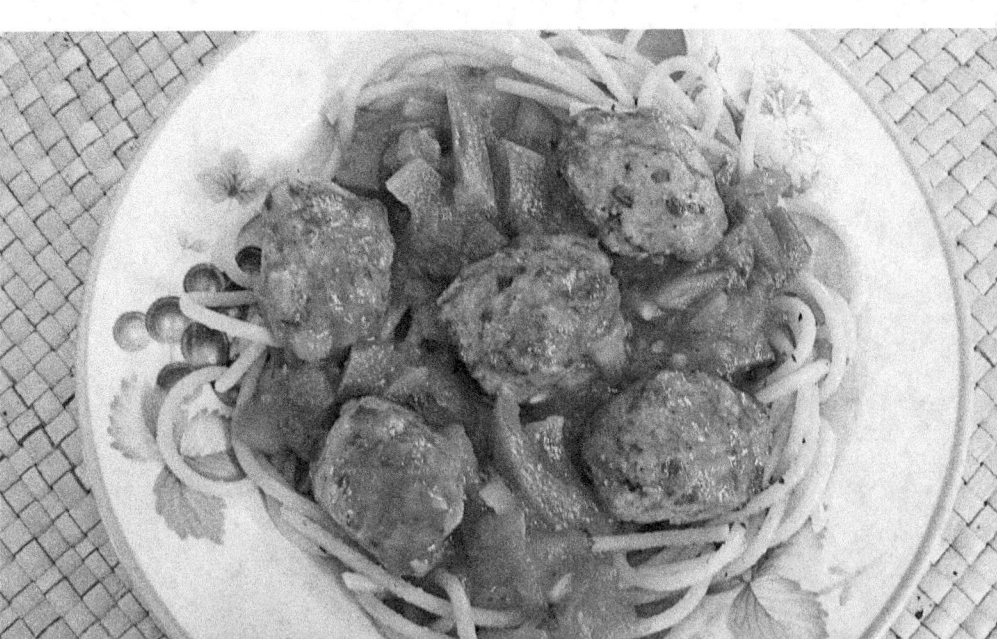

Fish Dishes
And Other Seafoods

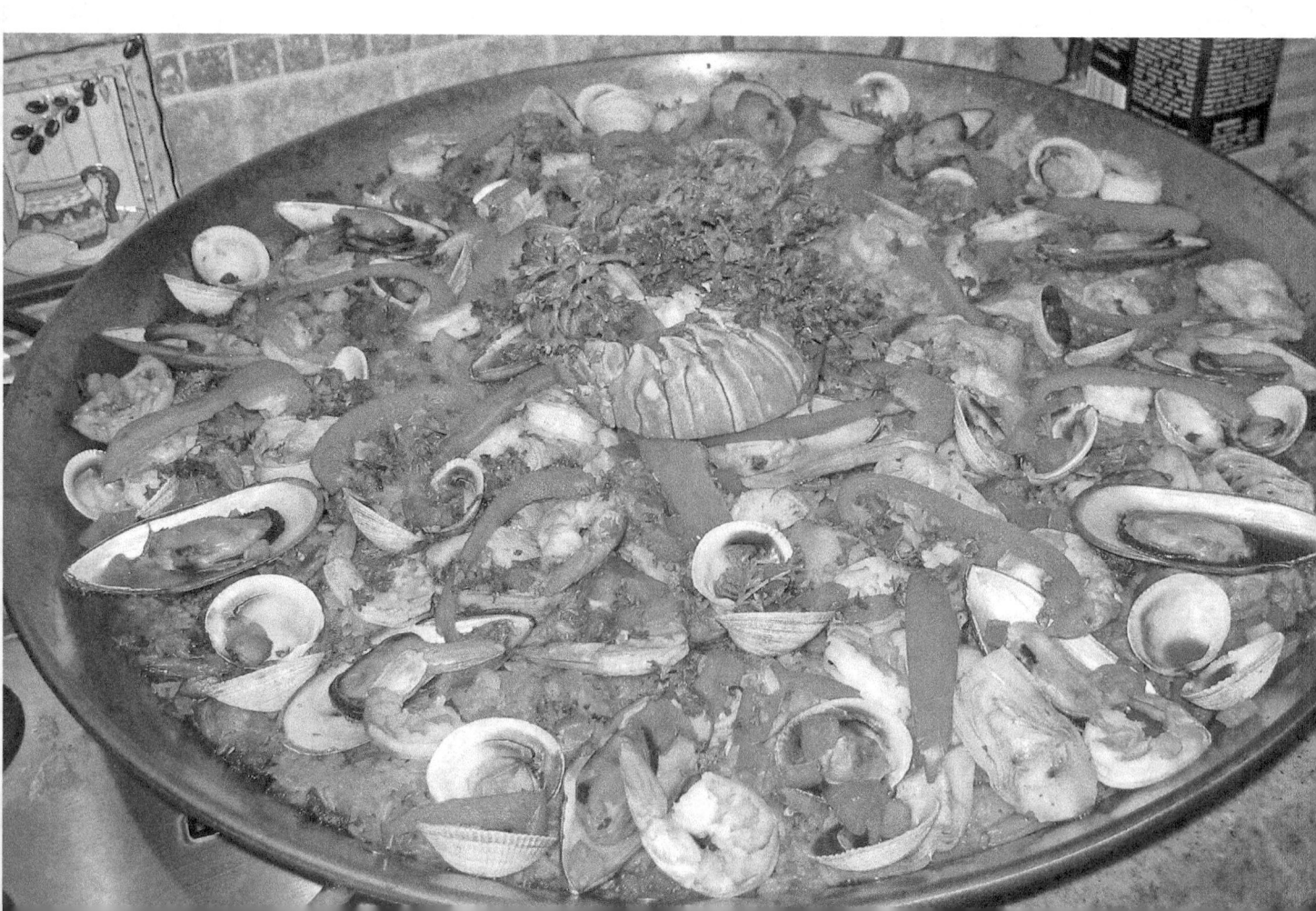

1. Chilean Shrimp with Red Pepper Sauce

Preparation Time: 35 minutes
8 servings

Ingredients

3 red bell peppers, skinned and seeded
½ cup chicken broth
1 cup wine vinegar
½ cup breadcrumbs
2 cloves garlic, minced
1 tbsp. olive oil
1 ½ cup nonfat sour cream
2 tbsp. lime juice
1 tsp. crushed red chilies
1 tsp. thyme powder
1 ½ tsp. salt
1 tsp. chili powder
½ tsp. each: paprika, black pepper,
   white pepper, cayenne, basil, oregano
2 ½ lb. large raw shrimp, shelled and deveined

Preparation

Bake red peppers at 375° until the skin blisters. Put in paper bag to cool 10 minutes, then remove skins and seeds.

In a blender mix well; red peppers, chicken broth, vinegar, breadcrumbs and garlic.

In a saucepan, heat oil then add blended sauce, sour cream, lemon juice, chilies, thyme and salt. Simmer for 10 minutes. Add rest of herbs and shrimp then mix well.

Cook or grill shrimp a few minutes each side. Then serve with remaining sauce and accompany with white rice.

159

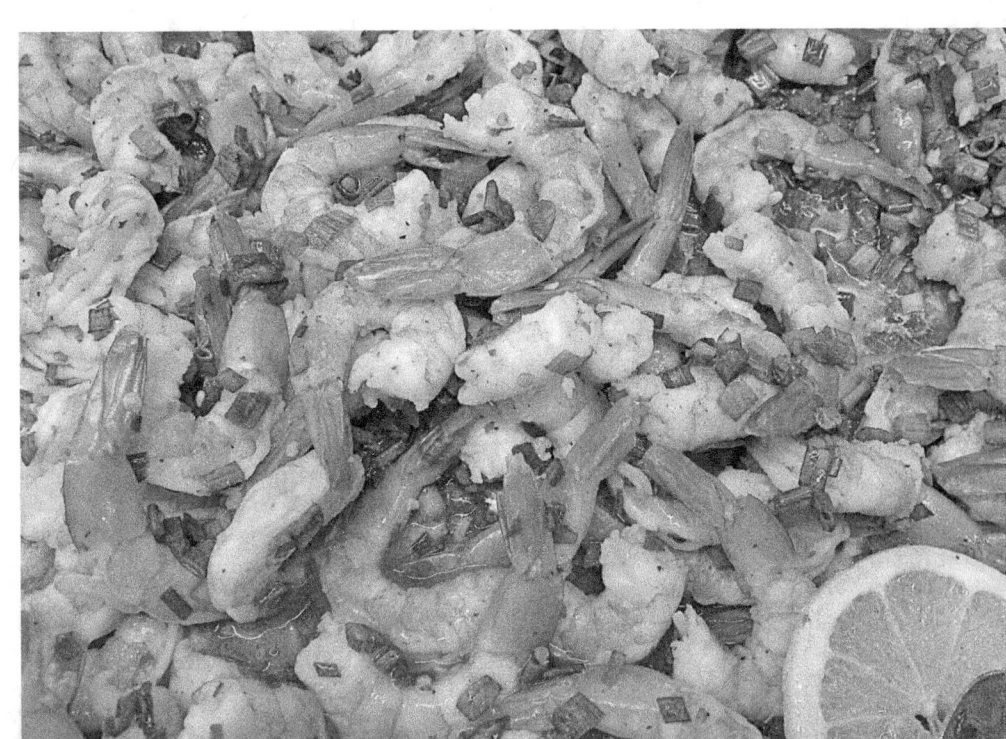

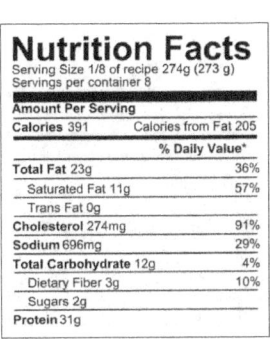

Nutrition Facts	
Serving Size 1/8 of recipe 274g (273 g)	
Servings per container 8	

Amount Per Serving	
Calories 391	Calories from Fat 205
	% Daily Value*
Total Fat 23g	36%
Saturated Fat 11g	57%
Trans Fat 0g	
Cholesterol 274mg	91%
Sodium 696mg	29%
Total Carbohydrate 12g	4%
Dietary Fiber 3g	10%
Sugars 2g	
Protein 31g	

2. Peruvian Ceviche

Preparation Time: 20 minutes
6 servings

Ingredients

- 2 ½ lb. red snapper (or tilapia or other firm white fillet), skinned and cubed
- 6 lemons, freshly squeezed and strained
- 6 limes, freshly squeezed and strained
- 2 tbsp. ginger, grated
- 3 cloves garlic, crushed
- 4 scallions or 1 red onion, thinly sliced and rinsed in warm water
- 2 tbsp. sea salt
- 1 tbsp. black pepper
- ¼ cup olive oil
- 1 sweet red pepper, seeded and cut into strips
- ¼ cup chopped cilantro
- 6 leaves of lettuce

Preparation

Remove skin from fish fillets then cut into ¼ inch cubes.

Cut lemons and limes in half, then juice them.

In a large glass bowl, combine juice, ginger, garlic, scallions (or onion), salt and pepper. Mix in fish cubes, then place in refrigerator to marinate for 2 hours.

Remove fish marinade from refrigerator, cover with oil, then toss with red pepper and cilantro.

Serve fish on top of a lettuce leaf.

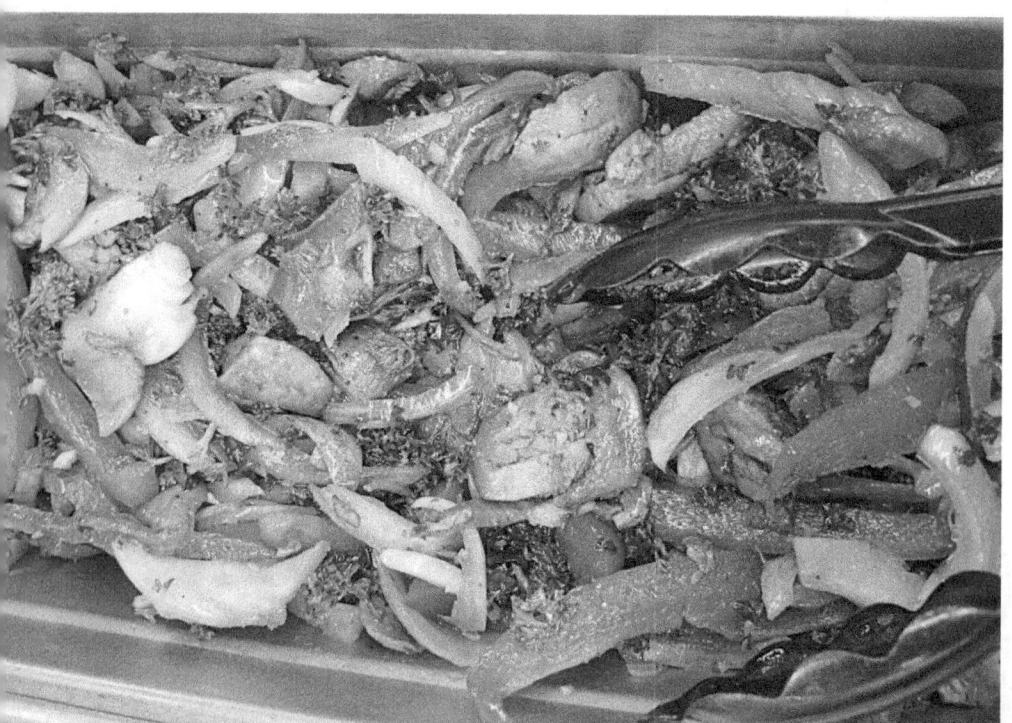

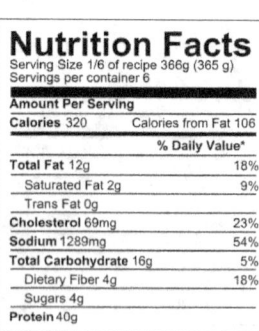

Nutrition Facts
Serving Size 1/6 of recipe 366g (365 g)
Servings per container 6

Amount Per Serving		
Calories 320		Calories from Fat 106
		% Daily Value*
Total Fat 12g		18%
Saturated Fat 2g		9%
Trans Fat 0g		
Cholesterol 69mg		23%
Sodium 1289mg		54%
Total Carbohydrate 16g		5%
Dietary Fiber 4g		18%
Sugars 4g		
Protein 40g		

3. Colombian Sea Bass with Spinach and Rice

Total time: 20 minutes
8 servings

Ingredients

2 lb. sea bass fillet
1 tsp. salt
½ tsp. ground thyme
½ tsp. ground bay leaves
¼ cup of lemon juice
3 tbsp. wheat bread crumbs
Canola oil spray
3 garlic cloves, crushed
3 tbsp. almonds, chopped
½ lb. spinach leaves, well washed
1 cup chicken broth
2 cups. white rice, cooked

Preparation

Wash fish, dry and sprinkle with salt, thyme, bay leaf, garlic, and lemon juice. Marinate in refrigerator for 1 hour.

In a large plate, spread breadcrumbs then lay fillet down on top, coating both sides.

Preheat oven to 350º. Heat oil in large pan, then bake fillet until brown, on both sides.

Heat oil in medium pan, cook almonds until golden. Add spinach and chicken broth, cook for 5 minutes. Add fish and cook for 5 more minutes.

Serve fish on top of spinach and cooked rice. You will love it!

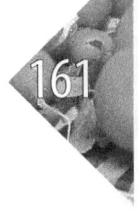

161

Nutrition Facts		
Serving Size 1/8 of recipe 196g (195 g)		
Servings per container 8		
Amount Per Serving		
Calories 200	Calories from Fat 72	
		% Daily Value*
Total Fat 8g		13%
Saturated Fat 1g		5%
Trans Fat 0g		
Cholesterol 46mg		15%
Sodium 459mg		19%
Total Carbohydrate 7g		2%
Dietary Fiber 2g		8%
Sugars 1g		
Protein 25g		

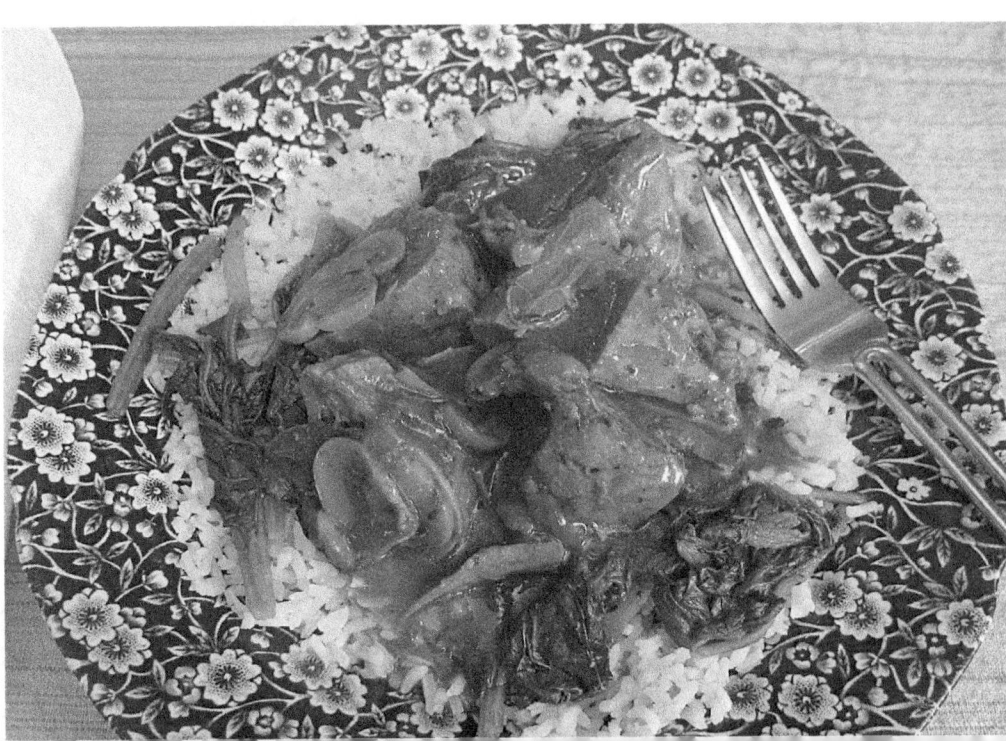

4. Alaskan Salmon Cakes

Preparation Time: 20 minutes
12 servings

Ingredients

1 ½ lb. salmon fillets, skinned and diced
1 cup 1% milk
1 bay leaf
3 ½ oz. cooked broccoli, tender
4 white potatoes, cooked and mashed
4 tbsp. chopped parsley
4 eggs (3 egg whites, 1 whole), beaten
2 cups breadcrumbs
Canola oil spray
Salt and pepper to taste

Preparation

Preheat oven to 400º. Place salmon in a pan with milk and bay leaf, bring to boil then reduce to medium heat for 2 minutes. Discard bay leaf and let cool.

In a blender, combine salmon, cooked broccoli, potatoes, parsley, salt and pepper and half the beaten eggs, then blend until smooth. Divide mix into 12 servings and form into cakes. Put remaining eggs in wide bowl and breadcrumbs in another bow. Dip each cakes into eggs then breadcrumbs, coating both sides.

Preheat oven to 400º. Spray oil on baking sheet, place salmon cakes then bake each side for 10 minutes, or until both sides are brown.

Sprinkle with parsley and serve with a side of vegetables.

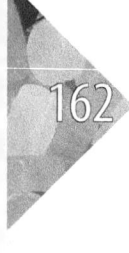
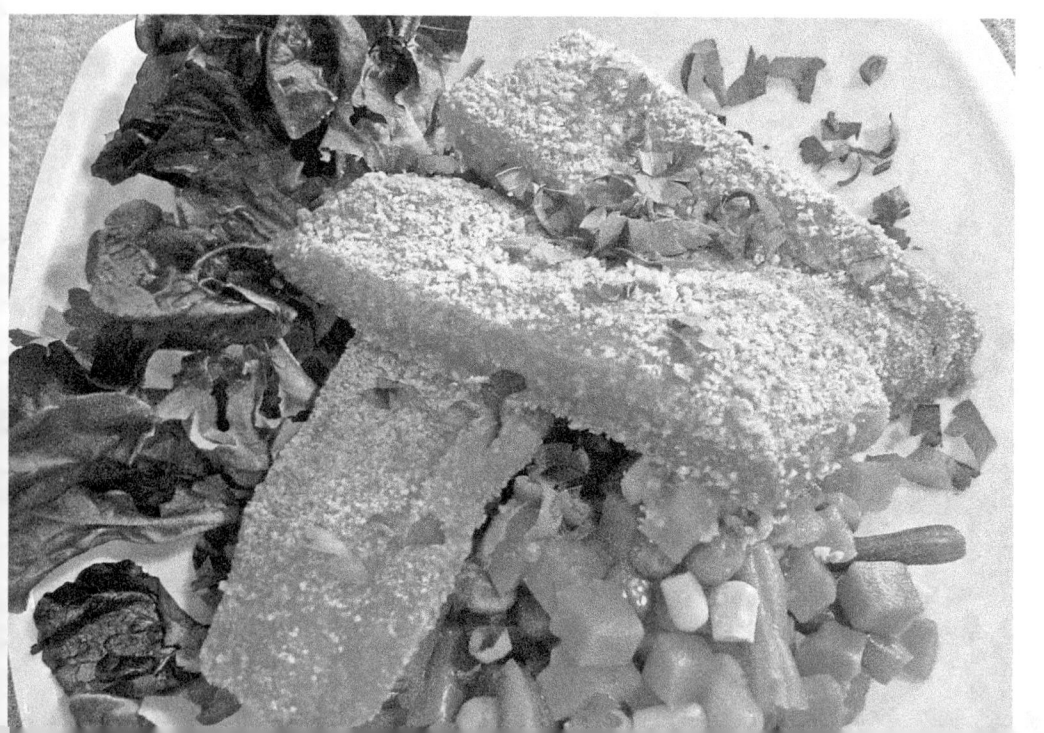

Nutrition Facts
Serving Size 1/12 of recipe 175g (174 g)
Servings per container 12

Amount Per Serving	
Calories 254	Calories from Fat 82
	% Daily Value*
Total Fat 9g	14%
Saturated Fat 2g	9%
Trans Fat	
Cholesterol 88mg	29%
Sodium 194mg	8%
Total Carbohydrate 26g	9%
Dietary Fiber 2g	8%
Sugars 3g	
Protein 17g	

5. Chinese Shrimp with Noodles

Preparation Time: 15 minutes
6 servings

Ingredients

3 (2 whites and 1 whole) eggs, beaten
½ cup water
5 tbsp. soy sauce
2 tbsp. tomato sauce
½ lb. medium shrimp, peeled and deveined, washed and pat dried
Canola oil spray
1 clove garlic, minced
½ tsp. fresh grated ginger root
1 green pepper, cut into chunks
1 medium onion, cut into chunks
2 celery stalks, cut lengthwise in thin wedges
2 tomatoes, coarsely chopped
½ tsp. grated lemon rind
1 lb. spaghetti pasta

Preparation

Mix beaten eggs with water, 2 tablespoons soy sauce, tomato sauce and shrimp.

Heat skillet sprayed with oil, add shrimp mix, fry for 1 minute then remove from pan.

Heat pan with more oil, add garlic and ginger then leave for 1 minute. Add green pepper, onion and celery then saute for 4 minutes. Add shrimp mix, lemon rind and remaining soy sauce and tomatoes, then cook while stirring until sauce boils and thickens slightly.

Cook pasta according to package directions, drain and divide servings onto plates. Top pasta serving with shrimp sauce.

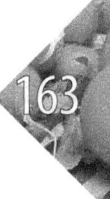

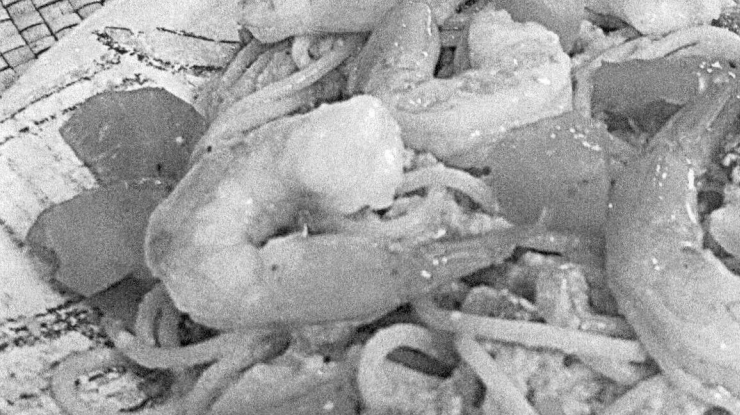

Nutrition Facts	
Serving Size 1/6 of recipe 226g (225 g)	
Servings per container 6	
Amount Per Serving	
Calories 288	Calories from Fat 26
	% Daily Value*
Total Fat 3g	5%
Saturated Fat 1g	3%
Trans Fat	
Cholesterol 118mg	39%
Sodium 987mg	41%
Total Carbohydrate 48g	16%
Dietary Fiber 1g	5%
Sugars 4g	
Protein 17g	

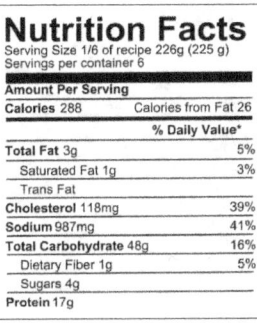

6. Baked Catfish Fillets with Almonds and Lemon

Preparation Time: 15 minutes
4 servings

Ingredients

4 catfish fillets, washed and dried
1 tsp. onion powder
½ tsp. paprika
4 tbsp. peeled and sliced almonds
2 tbsp. fresh lemon juice.
1 tbsp. finely chopped parsley
Canola oil spray
Salt and pepper to taste

Preparation

Preheat oven to 400º.

Lightly spray fillet with oil then season with salt and pepper. In a small bowl, mix onion powder and paprika then sprinkle over fillet.

Put fillet on pan sprayed with oil. Place pan in oven 4 inches from heat and bake 15 minutes or until golden brown.

In a small saucepan, brown almonds with lemon juice.

Spoon almond mixture over baked fillets and sprinkle with parsley. Accompany with a side dish of steamed vegetables.

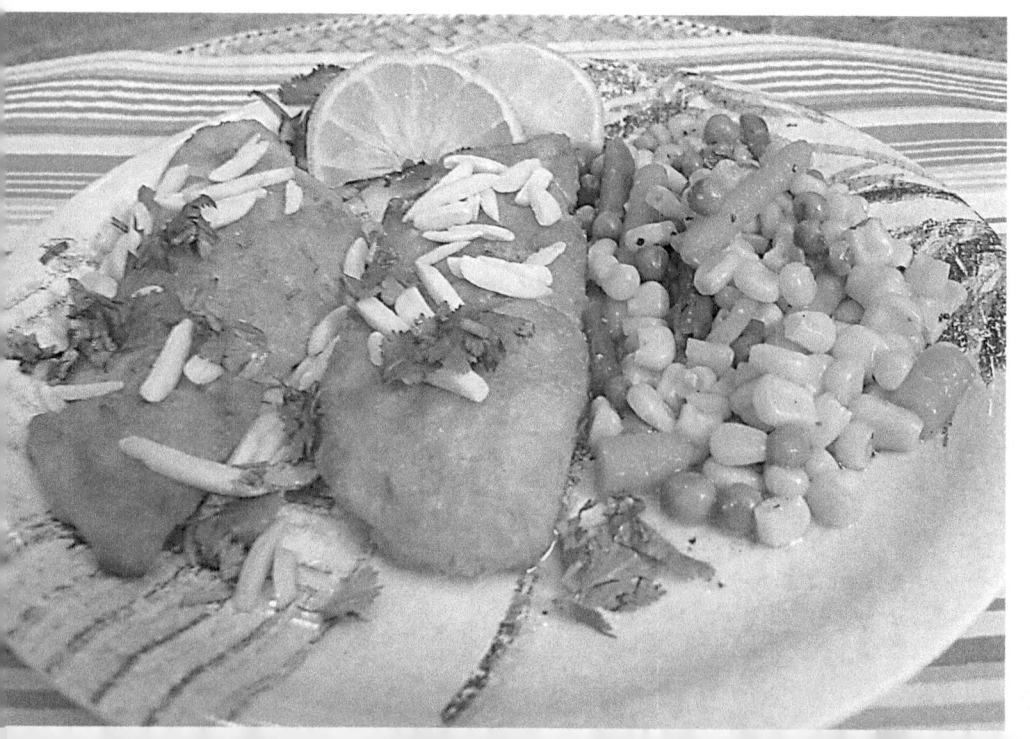

Nutrition Facts	
Serving Size 1/4 of recipe 169g (169 g)	
Servings per container 4	
Amount Per Serving	
Calories 269	Calories from Fat 147
	% Daily Value*
Total Fat 17g	26%
Saturated Fat 3g	16%
Trans Fat	
Cholesterol 75mg	25%
Sodium 85mg	4%
Total Carbohydrate 2g	1%
Dietary Fiber 1g	5%
Sugars 1g	
Protein 27g	

7. Latin American Broiled Swordfish

Preparation Time: 30 minutes
4 servings

Ingredients

4 cloves of garlic, crushed
⅓ cup white wine
¼ cup lemon juice
2 tbsp. soy sauce
2 tbsp. olive oil
1 tbsp. "Old Bay" fish spice
¼ tsp. salt
⅛ tsp. ground black pepper
4 swordfish steaks, washed and dried
1 tbsp. finely chopped fresh rosemary
1 tbsp. finely chopped cilantro
lemon wedges

Preparation

In a medium bowl, mix all ingredients (except rosemary), then put in refrigerator to marinate for 4 hours.

Heat broiler, cook fish 10 minutes each side, or until both are golden brown.

Serve swordfish with sprinkling of rosemary and cilantro with lemon wedges on the side and accompanied by a side dish of vegetables.

Nutrition Facts		
Serving Size 1/4 of recipe 173g (172 g)		
Servings per container 4		
Amount Per Serving		
Calories 241	Calories from Fat 110	
		% Daily Value*
Total Fat 12g		19%
Saturated Fat 2g		12%
Trans Fat 0g		
Cholesterol 53mg		18%
Sodium 782mg		33%
Total Carbohydrate 4g		1%
Dietary Fiber 1g		2%
Sugars 1g		
Protein 28g		

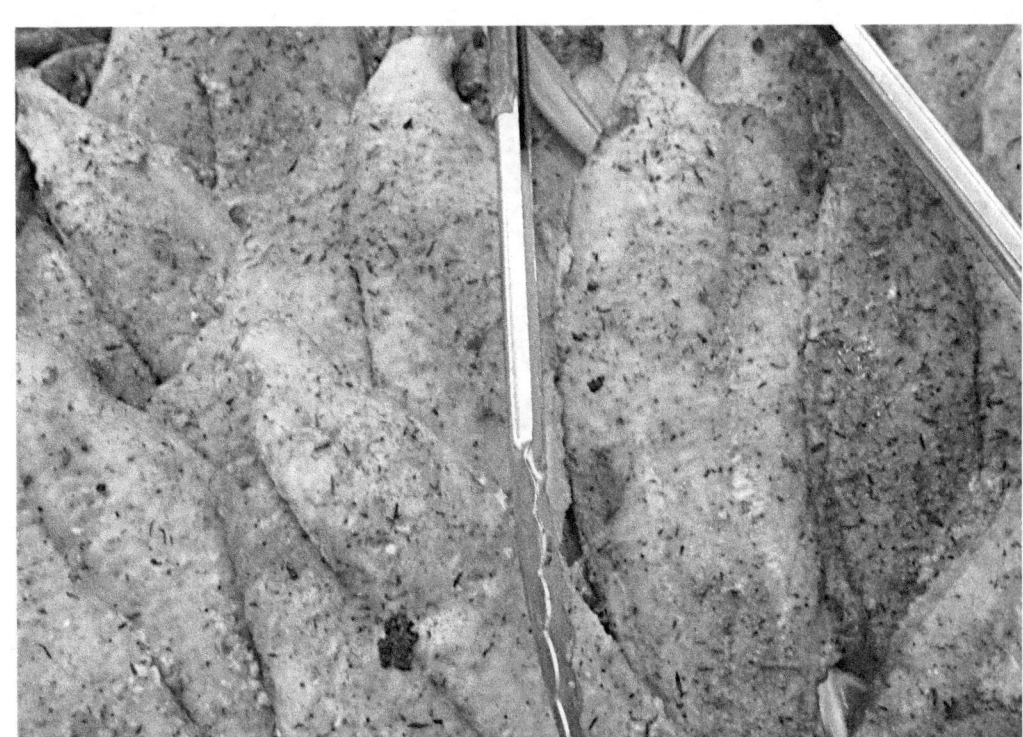

8. Skinless Poached Salmon

Preparation Time: 30 minutes
4 servings

Ingredients

1 red bell pepper, sliced round
1 green bell pepper, sliced round
Canola oil spray
1 can (8 oz.) tomatoes, peeled and chopped
1 small white onion, chopped
1 carrot, peeled and cut into 1" pieces
1 celery stalk, cut into 1" pieces
2 tbsp. balsamic vinegar
Salt and pepper to taste
1 cup chicken broth
1 lb. red salmon, skinned
2 tbsp. finely chopped parsley
1 lemon, cut into wedges

Preparation

Spray oil in large skillet, saute red and green peppers for 5 minutes. Add tomatoes and remaining ingredients and simmer 5 minutes more. Then add the chicken broth and cook for 5 minutes more.

Preheat oven to 400°. Place salmon in a baking dish, add sauted vegetable broth and bake for 20 minutes.

Serve with lemon wedges. Goes well with a side of polenta, easily prepared by following package directions.

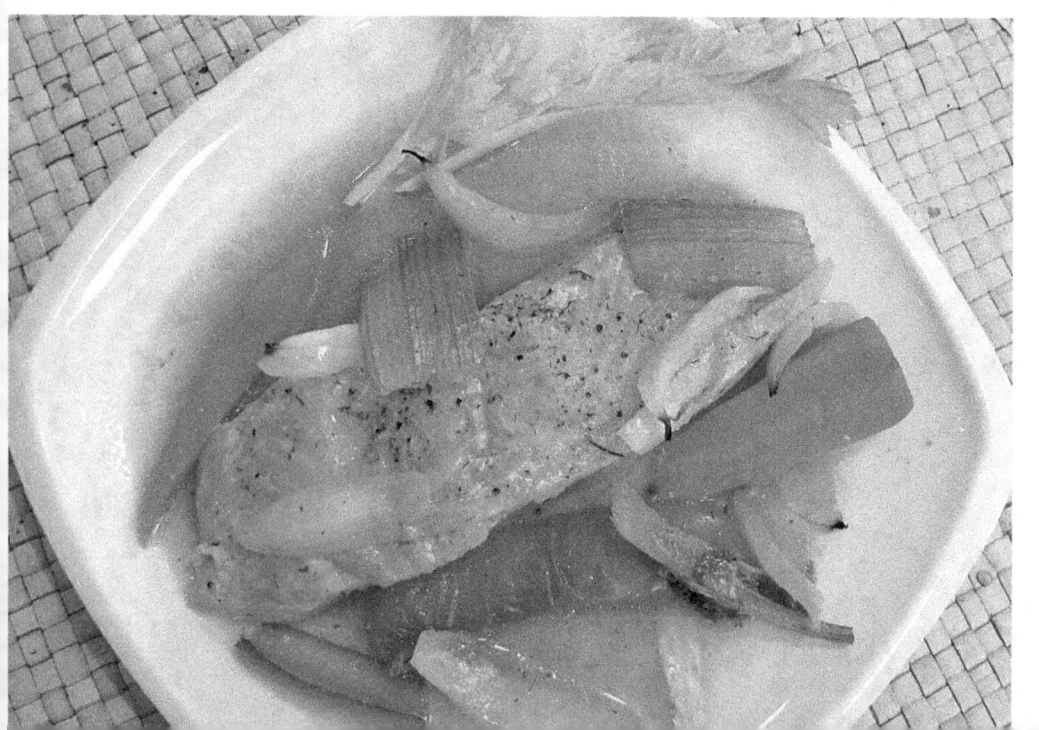

Nutrition Facts
Serving Size 1/4 of recipe 359g (359 g)
Servings per container 4

Amount Per Serving

Calories 186	Calories from Fat 39

	% Daily Value*
Total Fat 4g	7%
Saturated Fat 1g	4%
Trans Fat 0g	
Cholesterol 58mg	19%
Sodium 208mg	9%
Total Carbohydrate 12g	4%
Dietary Fiber 3g	13%
Sugars 5g	
Protein 25g	

Complementary Side Dishes

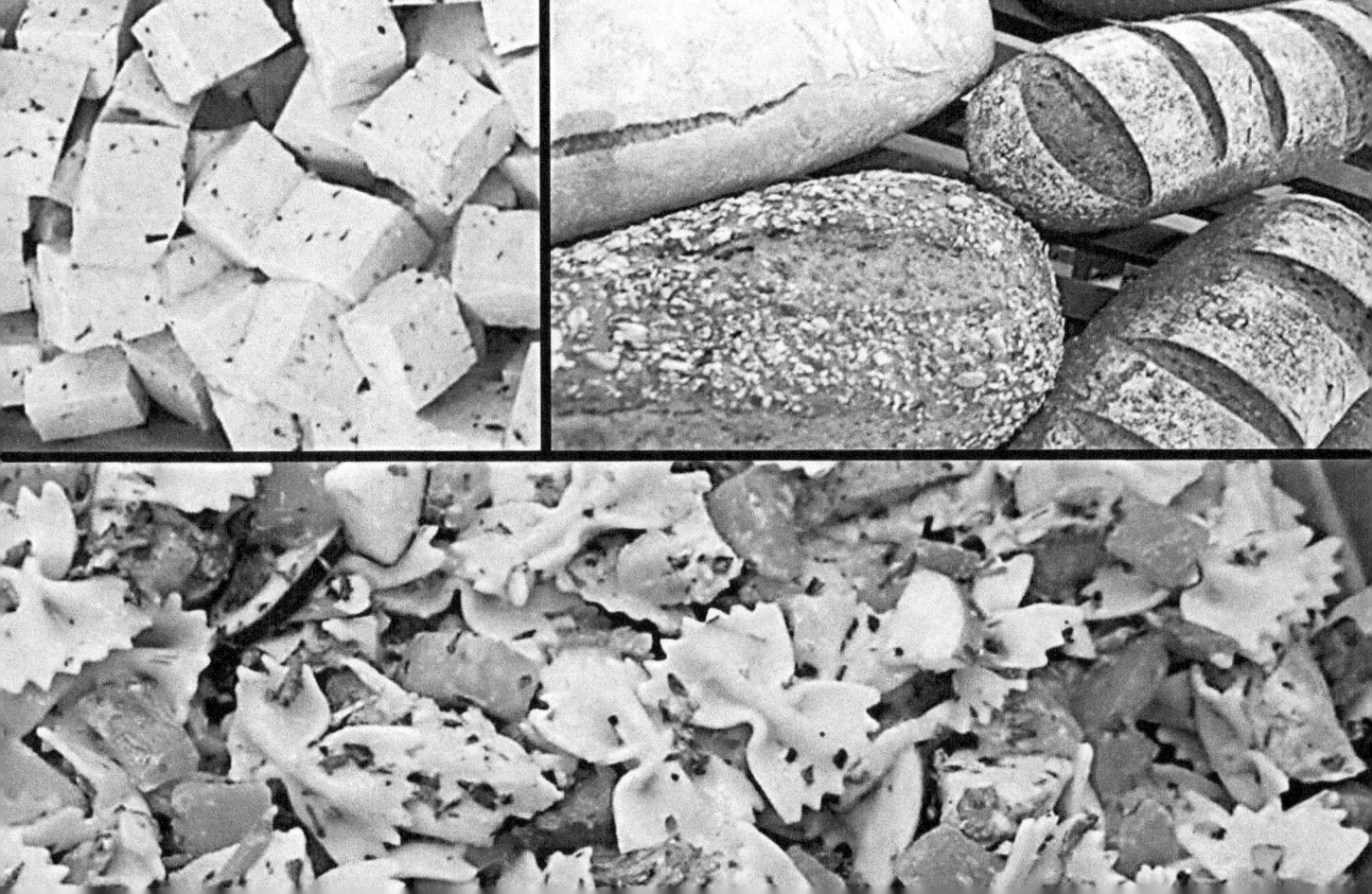

1. Spanish Bruschettas

Total time: 20 minutes
8 servings

Ingredients

1 loaf French bread (baguette), cut in half lengthwise, then in 3" pieces
2 tbsp. olive oil
2 tbsp. balsamic vinegar
¼ cup low fat sour cream
1 tsp. salt
1 tsp. oregano
1 tsp. basil
1 large tomato, chopped
1 white onion, chopped
1 cucumber, diced
½ lb. goat cheese, diced
½ lb. smoked turkey ham, diced
1 ripe pear, seeded and sliced small

Preparation

Mix olive oil, balsamic vinegar, sour cream, and salt, then spread on each 3 inch bread piece.

In a medium bowl, mix rest of ingredients. Spread in equal parts over bread pieces.

The bruschettas are a delicious dish for a light lunch, snack or as hors d'oeuvres.

168

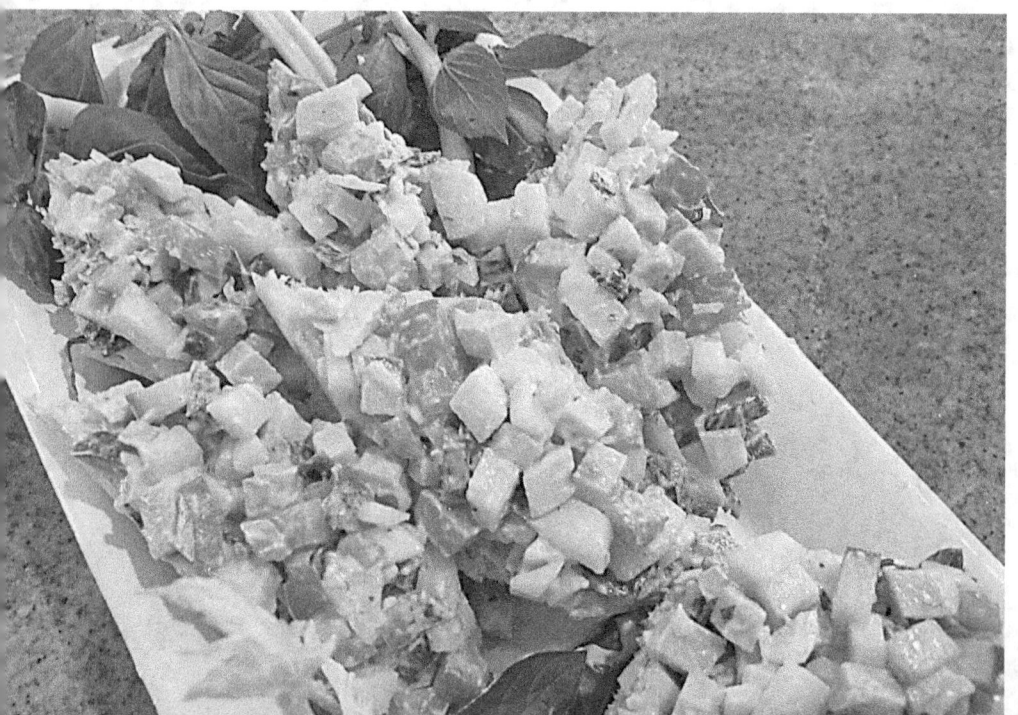

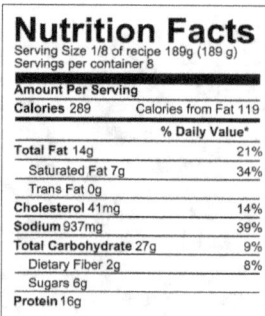

Nutrition Facts

Serving Size 1/8 of recipe 189g (189 g)
Servings per container 8

Amount Per Serving

Calories 289   Calories from Fat 119

	% Daily Value*
Total Fat 14g	21%
Saturated Fat 7g	34%
Trans Fat 0g	
Cholesterol 41mg	14%
Sodium 937mg	39%
Total Carbohydrate 27g	9%
Dietary Fiber 2g	8%
Sugars 6g	
Protein 16g	

2. Cuban Black Beans

Preparation Time: 80 minutes
4 servings

Ingredients

2 cups water
1 cup black beans
1 small green bell pepper, chopped
1 small red onion
1 clove garlic, minced
1 tbsp. canola oil
1 bay leaf
¾ tsp. oregano
½ tsp. ground cumin
½ tsp. salt
1 pinch pepper
2 cups white rice, cooked and hot

Preparation

Heat water and boil beans for 2 minutes. Remove from heat, cover pot and let stand for 1 hour.

Heat oil in a saucepan, add green pepper, onion and garlic until onion is tender. Add beans and two cups of water (more if necessary) then simmer. Add bay leaf, oregano, cumin, salt and pepper. Cover and simmer until all the beans are tender and water is absorbed.

Remove bay leaf and serve beans over hot white rice. Garnish with orange slices to enhance flavor.

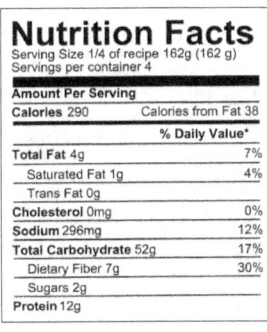

Nutrition Facts	
Serving Size 1/4 of recipe 162g (162 g)	
Servings per container 4	
Amount Per Serving	
Calories 290	Calories from Fat 38
	% Daily Value*
Total Fat 4g	7%
Saturated Fat 1g	4%
Trans Fat 0g	
Cholesterol 0mg	0%
Sodium 296mg	12%
Total Carbohydrate 52g	17%
Dietary Fiber 7g	30%
Sugars 2g	
Protein 12g	

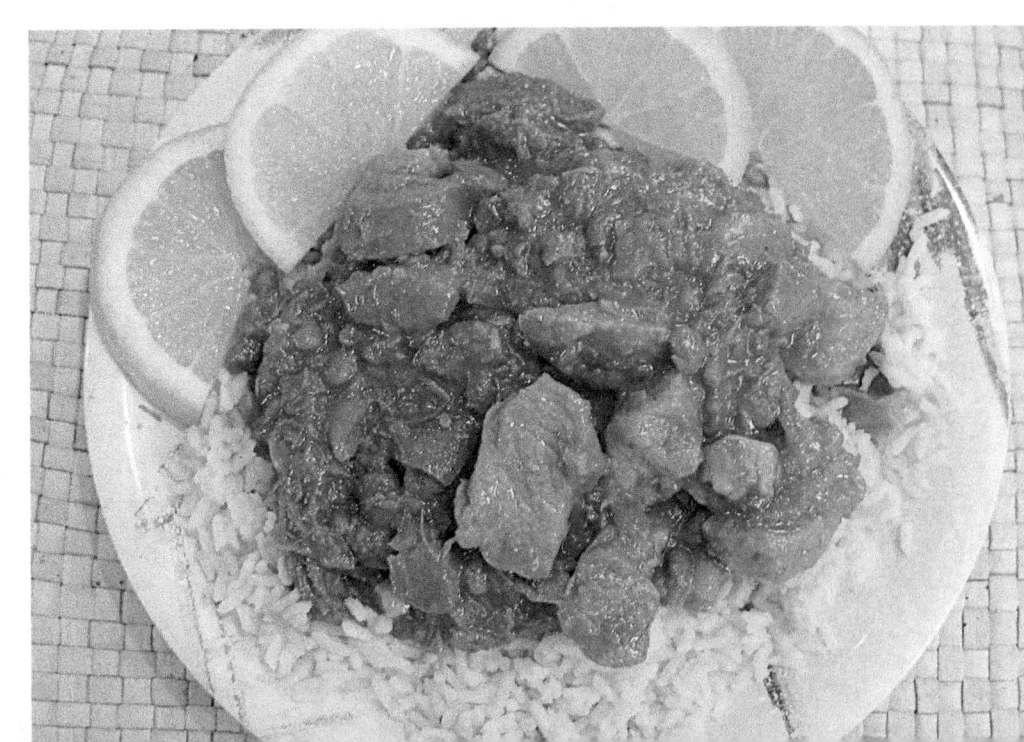

3. Chicken and Vegetable Shish Kebobs

Preparation Time: 30 minutes
8 servings

Ingredients

2 large zucchini, cut in 1" pieces
2 yellow squash, cut in 1" pieces
1 green bell pepper, cut in 1" pieces
1 red bell pepper, cut in 1" pieces
2 medium red onion, crosscut 1" pieces
16 cherry tomatoes
16 medium mushrooms (8 oz.)
1 lb. chicken breast, cut in 1" cubes
8 wooden skewers or toothpicks, washed
2 medium ears
Canola oil spray

Sauce

½ cup balsamic vinegar
2 tbsp. mustard
3 cloves garlic, minced
¼ tsp. thyme
1 tbsp. canola oil

Preparation

Wash all vegetables well and cut into
1 inch pieces, mix in bowl with tomatoes
and mushrooms.

For sauce, mix vinegar, mustard, garlic
and thyme in a small cup. Pour mixture over
vegetables then sprinkle with oil.

Thread vegetables and chicken onto
wooden skewers (previously washed), repeat
in same order until skewer full.

Preheat broiler to medium heat. Put skewer
on grill, brush with sauce and turn each as it
toasts for 20 minutes, or until soft.

Serve along with rice cooked in tomato sauce.

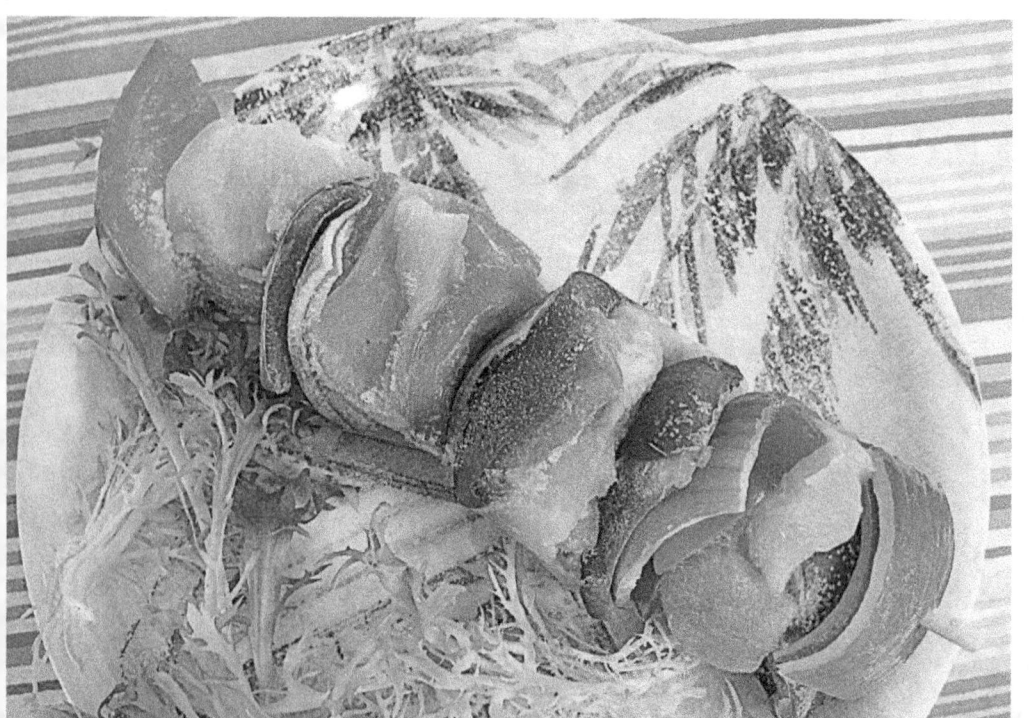

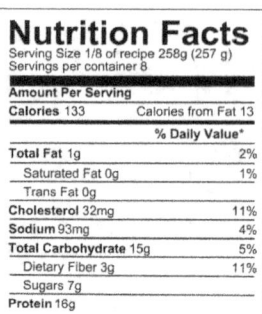

Nutrition Facts
Serving Size 1/8 of recipe 258g (257 g)
Servings per container 8

Amount Per Serving	
Calories 133	Calories from Fat 13
	% Daily Value*
Total Fat 1g	2%
Saturated Fat 0g	1%
Trans Fat 0g	
Cholesterol 32mg	11%
Sodium 93mg	4%
Total Carbohydrate 15g	5%
Dietary Fiber 3g	11%
Sugars 7g	
Protein 16g	

4. Spanish Potato Tortilla

Preparation Time: 15 minutes
4 servings

Ingredients

4 turkey sausage, cut into 1" chunks
Canola oil spray
1 large potato, peeled and cut in ½" cubes
1 medium onion, chopped
4 egg whites and 3 whole eggs, beaten
¾ tsp. salt
$\frac{1}{8}$ tsp. pepper
1 medium tomato, finely chopped
2 tbsp. parsley, chopped

Preparation

Spray small skillet with oil, then cook sausage over medium heat until browned. Remove sausage and place potatoes and onions in skillet, cook for 10 minutes or until golden brown.

Beat eggs with salt and pepper, then add to skillet along with sausage and tomatoes. Cover the pan and simmer for 10 minutes.

When browned on bottom and edges, flip over with spatula and cook 1 minute more.

Cut tortilla crosswise (4 pieces) and serve over lettuce leaves and sprinkle with parsley.

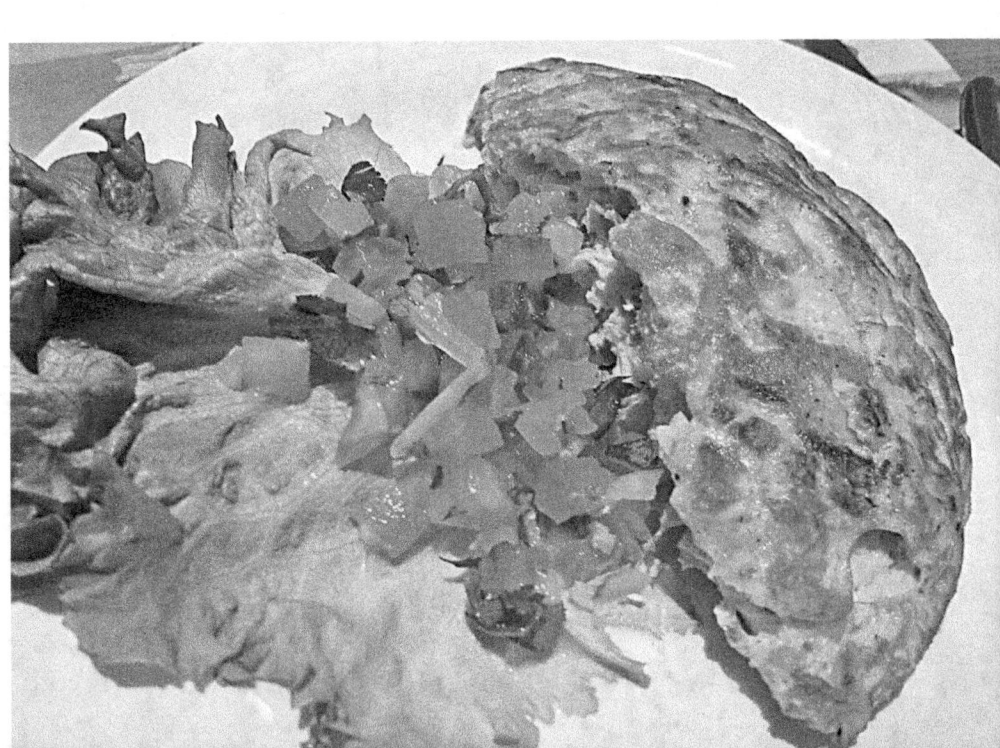

Nutrition Facts	
Serving Size 1/4 of recipe 196g (195 g)	
Servings per container 4	

Amount Per Serving

Calories 194	Calories from Fat 73

	% Daily Value*
Total Fat 8g	13%
Saturated Fat 2g	11%
Trans Fat 0g	
Cholesterol 143mg	48%
Sodium 1060mg	44%
Total Carbohydrate 15g	5%
Dietary Fiber 2g	7%
Sugars 4g	
Protein 16g	

5. Carmen's Colombian Rice "Atoyado"

Preparation Time: 30 minutes
8 servings

Ingredients

1 tbsp. olive oil
½ cup green onion, chopped
2 cloves garlic, minced
2 cups white rice
1 carrot, diced
1 cup corn
½ cup green peas
3 cups chicken broth
2 tsp. salt
4 turkey sausage, cut in ½" cubes
½ lb. roast beef, cut in ½" cubes
½ tbsp. black pepper
1 large tomato, chopped
1 banana, baked in skin and sliced in 8 pieces

Preparation

Heat oil in medium saucepan, cook onion and garlic until half browned. Stir in rice, then add carrot, corn, peas and stir. Add chicken broth and salt, then simmer until rice is dry and open.

In another pan, fry sausages until cooked through and golden brown. Drain fat, add beef and pepper, then saute 10 minutes until meat is tender.

Drain sausage and beef, then add to rice and mix together with a fork.

To serve, place each rice serving on top of lettuce, then sprinkle with chopped tomatoes and accompany with hot slice of ripe banana.

172

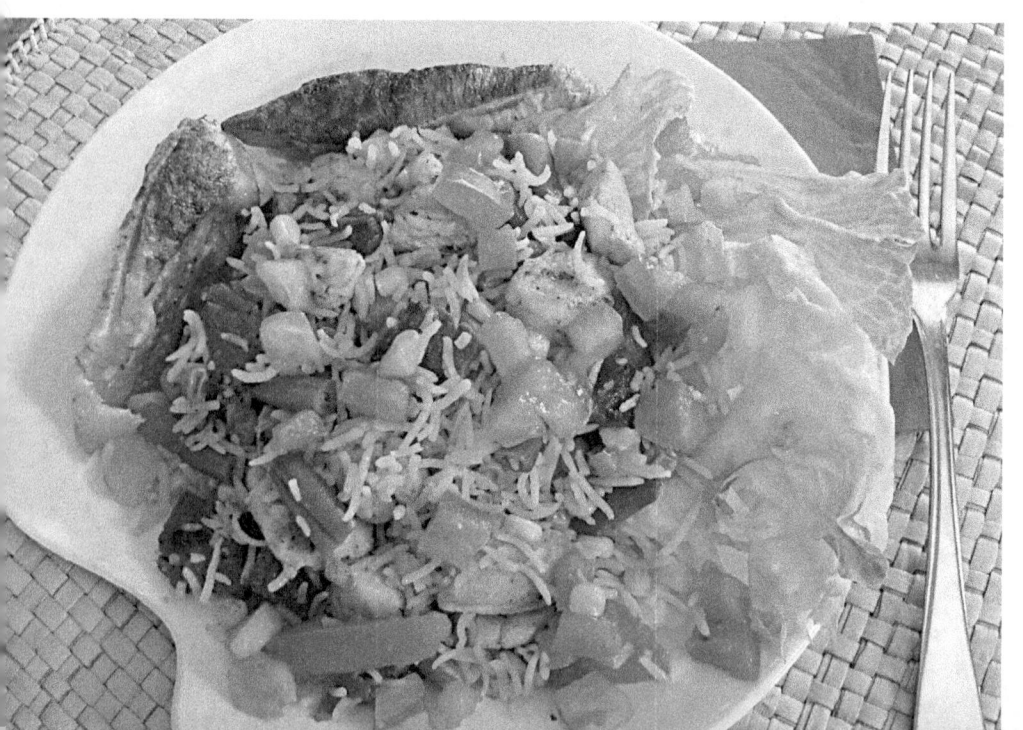

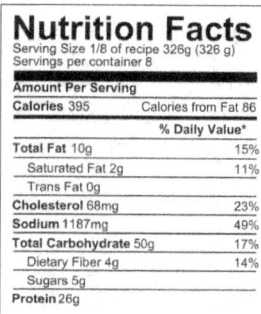

Nutrition Facts

Serving Size 1/8 of recipe 326g (326 g)
Servings per container 8

Amount Per Serving

Calories 395	Calories from Fat 86

	% Daily Value*
Total Fat 10g	15%
Saturated Fat 2g	11%
Trans Fat 0g	
Cholesterol 68mg	23%
Sodium 1187mg	49%
Total Carbohydrate 50g	17%
Dietary Fiber 4g	14%
Sugars 5g	
Protein 26g	

6. Italian Broccoli Stuffed Manicotti

Preparation Time: 30 minutes
12 rolls

Ingredients

1 box Manicotti
½ lb. broccoli, washed and finely chopped
½ lb. mushrooms, washed and finely chopped
½ lb. nonfat cheddar cheese, grated
¼ onion, minced
¼ cup egg or egg beater substitute
2 cloves garlic, minced
Canola oil spray
Parsley or cilantro, finely chopped

Sauce

1 cup 1% milk
1 cup tomato sauce
1 cup chicken broth
½ cup breadcrumbs
2 tsp. ground fresh thyme
½ cup nonfat cheddar cheese, grated
Salt and pepper to taste

Preparation

Cook pasta by box directions, drain and dry.

In medium bowl, mix egg, broccoli and mushroom. Spray oil in skillet, saute onion and garlic until brown. Add to vegetable bowl along with grated cheese, salt and pepper, mix well.

Preheat oven to 350º. Fill manicotti, and place rolls on baking sheet sprayed with oil.

Spray oil in saucepan, over medium heat, add each of the sauce ingredients in order listed, then simmer until thickened. Remove and immediately drizzle sauce over filled manicotti. Bake for 15 minutes or until hot and bubbly.

To serve, drizzle sauce over each serving and sprinkle with finely chopped parsley or cilantro.

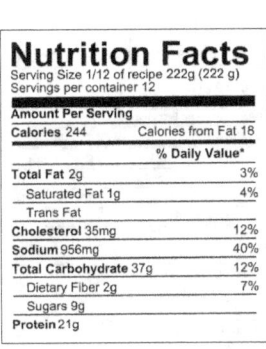

Nutrition Facts
Serving Size 1/12 of recipe 222g (222 g)
Servings per container 12

Amount Per Serving	
Calories 244	Calories from Fat 18
	% Daily Value*
Total Fat 2g	3%
Saturated Fat 1g	4%
Trans Fat	
Cholesterol 35mg	12%
Sodium 956mg	40%
Total Carbohydrate 37g	12%
Dietary Fiber 2g	7%
Sugars 9g	
Protein 21g	

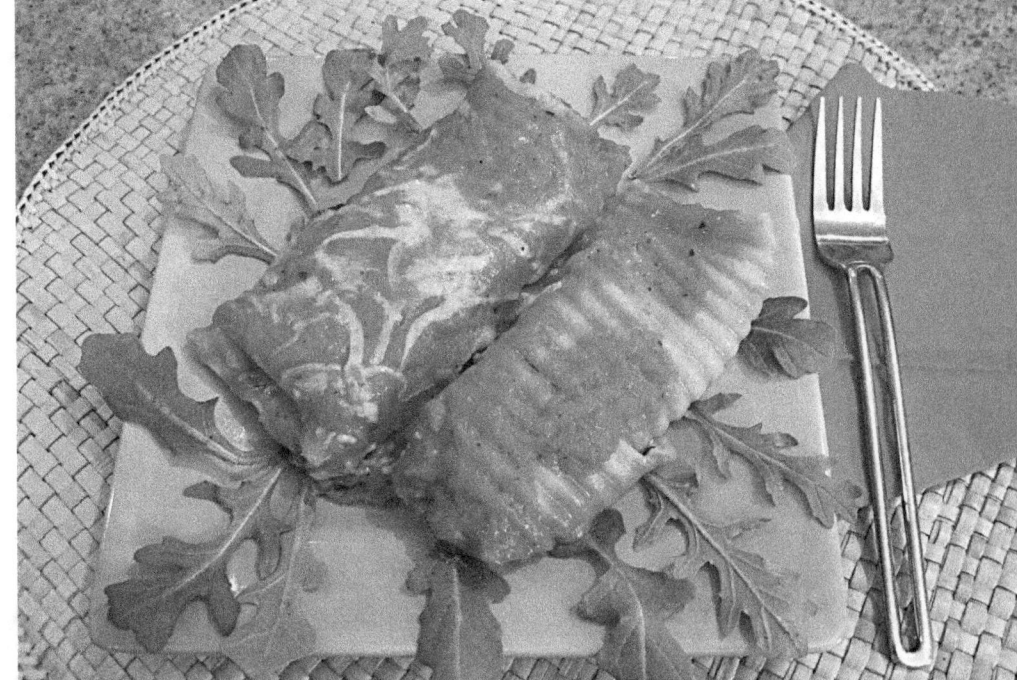

7. Roman "Peperonata"

Total Time: 20 minutes
6 servings

Ingredients

2 tbsp. olive oil
2 medium red onions, sliced
2 cloves of garlic, crushed
2 medium green bell peppers, cut into strips
2 medium red bell pepper, baked, peeled and
   cut into strips
1 tbsp. red wine vinegar
2 medium tomatoes, coarsely chopped
½ cup black olives, pitted and sliced round
1 tbsp. fresh basil leaves

Preparation

Heat oil in a large skillet, stir onions and garlic until tender.

Add remaining ingredients (except tomatoes, black olives and basil). Cover and simmer for 10 minutes.

Add tomatoes, then cover and simmer over low heat for 5 more minutes.

Mix well, then garnish with fresh basil and black olives. Great to serve with beef dish.

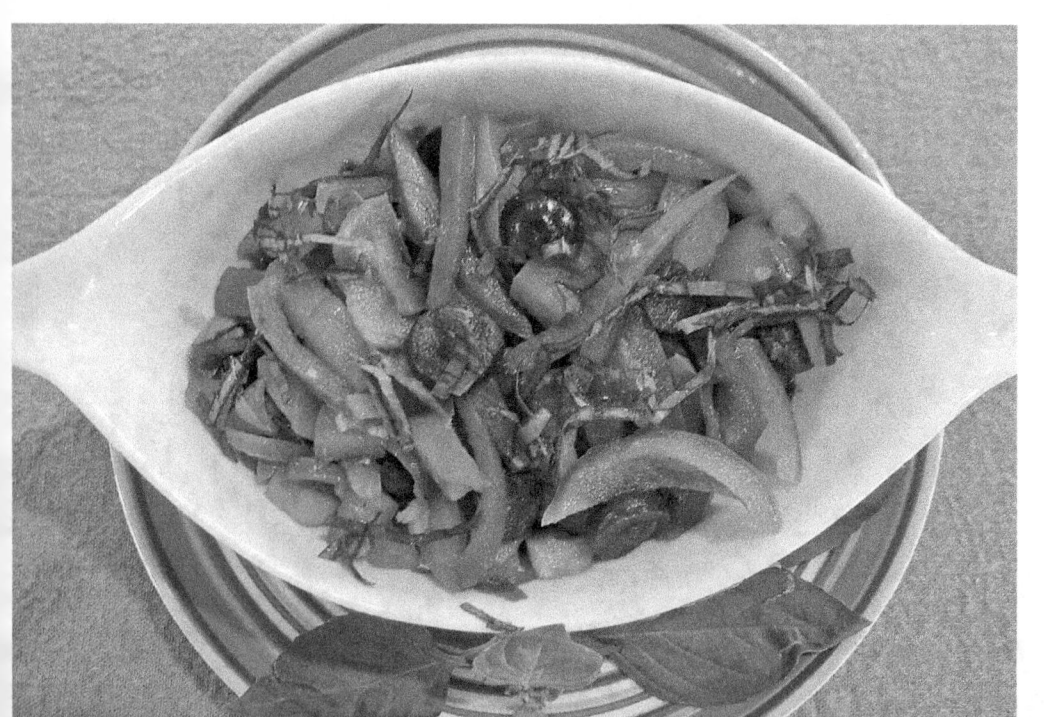

Nutrition Facts	
Serving Size 1/6 of recipe 150g (150 g)	
Servings per container 6	
Amount Per Serving	
Calories 71	Calories from Fat 32
	% Daily Value*
Total Fat 4g	6%
Saturated Fat 1g	3%
Trans Fat 0g	
Cholesterol 0mg	0%
Sodium 108mg	5%
Total Carbohydrate 9g	3%
Dietary Fiber 2g	10%
Sugars 4g	
Protein 2g	

8. French Vegetable "Ratatouille"

Preparation Time: 10 minutes
8 servings

Ingredients

1 tbsp. olive oil
1 medium onion, sliced round
1 clove garlic, minced
1 eggplant (1 lb.), cut into ½" pieces
½ cup chicken broth
4 medium tomatoes, cut in fourths
1 zucchini, sliced round
1 green bell pepper, cut in strips
¼ cup chopped parsley
1 tsp. salt
½ tsp. ground basil
¼ tsp. pepper
1 tsp. balsamic vinegar

Preparation

Heat oil in saucepan, saute onion and garlic until tender.

Add eggplant and remaining ingredients. Bring to boil, reduce heat to medium, then cover and simmer for 10 minutes. Stir occasionally until vegetables are tender but not overcooked.

Serve as a complementary supplement to any meat, poultry or fish dish.

Nutrition Facts		
Serving Size 1/8 of recipe 191g (191 g)		
Amount Per Serving		
Calories 56	Calories from Fat 18	
		% Daily Value*
Total Fat 2g		3%
Saturated Fat 0g		2%
Trans Fat 0g		
Cholesterol 0mg		0%
Sodium 314mg		13%
Total Carbohydrate 9g		3%
Dietary Fiber 4g		16%
Sugars 5g		
Protein 2g		

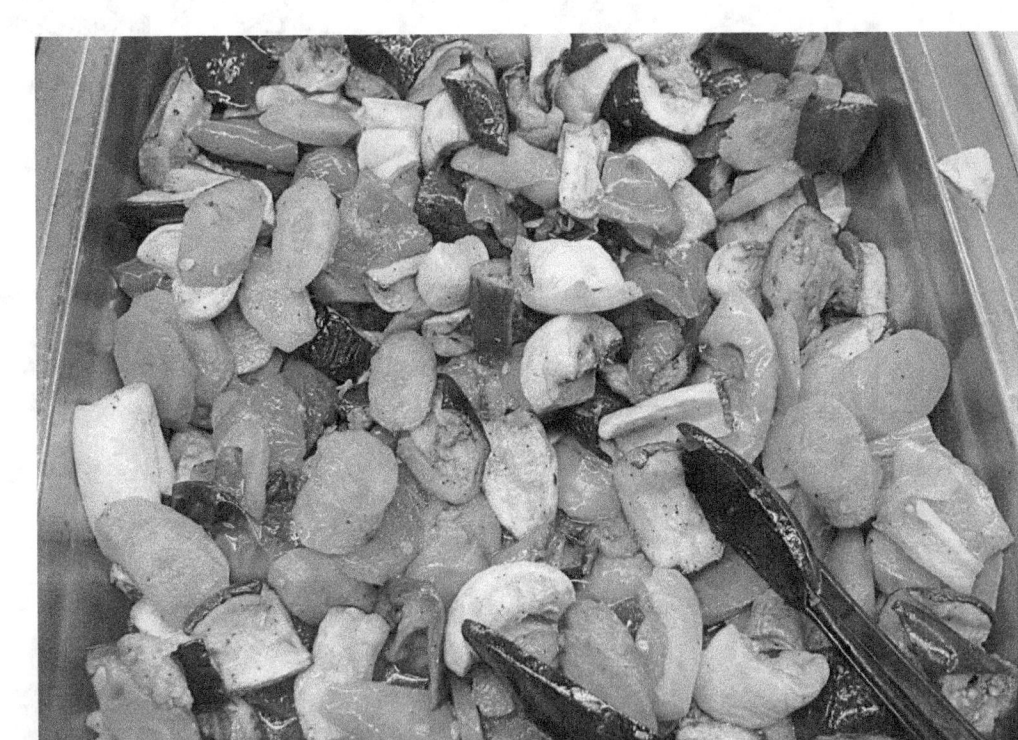

Delicious Desserts

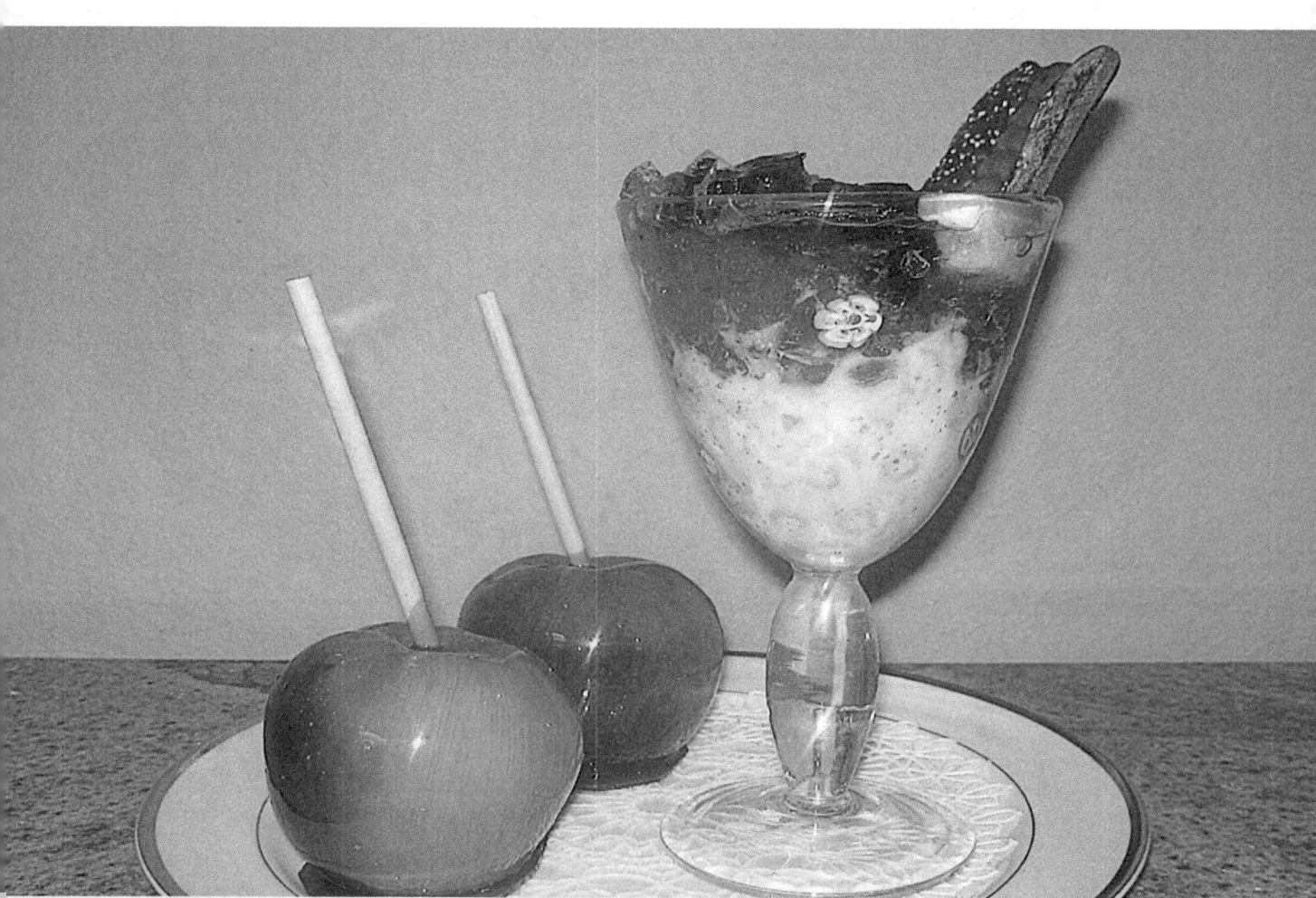

1. Cherry German Pancakes

Preparation Time: 20 minutes
4 servings

Ingredients

4 eggs
¾ cup flour
¾ cup 1% milk
½ tsp. salt
½ tsp. baking powder
2 cups pitted cherries
¼ cup molasses, maple syrup, or honey,
    diluted with water
¼ tsp. ground cinnamon
Canola oil spray

Preparation

Preheat oven to 400°. Warm 2 pancake-size pans in oven. Beat eggs in blender, add flour, milk, salt and baking powder.

Remove pans from oven and spray with oil. Add batter and cherries evenly into each pan, sprinkle with cinnamon, then return to oven. Bake uncovered until golden brown.

Cut each pancake in half and serve with more cherries or a sweetner (molasses, maple syrup or honey, diluted with water).

A deliciously good breakfast!

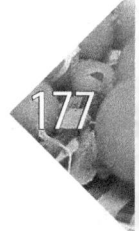

177

Nutrition Facts		
Serving Size 1/4 of recipe 223g (223 g)		
Servings per container 4		
Amount Per Serving		
Calories 283	Calories from Fat 53	
		% Daily Value*
Total Fat 6g		9%
Saturated Fat 2g		10%
Trans Fat 0g		
Cholesterol 214mg		71%
Sodium 389mg		16%
Total Carbohydrate 48g		16%
Dietary Fiber 2g		7%
Sugars 23g		
Protein 11g		

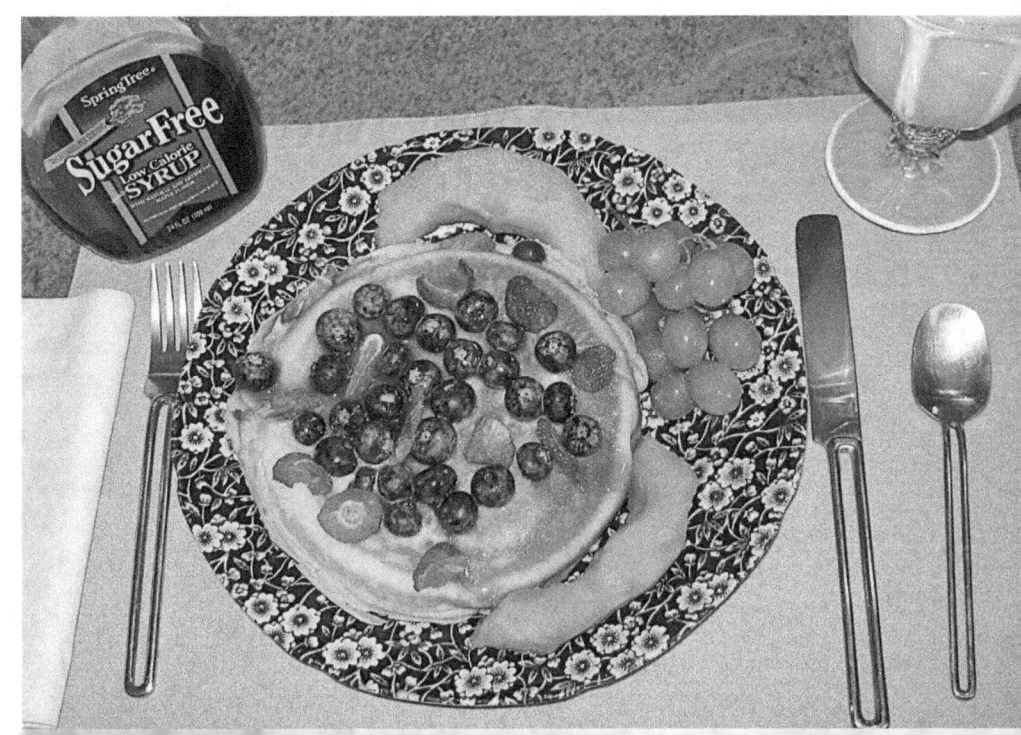

2. Spanish Flan (Caramel Custard)

Preparation Time: 1 hour
6 servings

Ingredients

1 cup brown sugar
2 cups low fat milk
2 strips lemon zest
1 tsp. ground cinnamon
1 tsp. vanilla
½ cup egg substitute
Canola oil spray

Preparation

Preheat oven to 200º.

Spray oil on bottom of baking pan, spread brown sugar, then heat until melted a golden brown. Rotate pan to spread syrup all around, then set aside.

In saucepan, mix eggs, milk, lemon zest, cinnamon and vanilla, until well blended. Pour mixture over melted sugar, but do not stir.

Place pan in center rack of oven, on the lower rack of oven place a container with cold water, (to create water bath). Bake for 1 hour, or until a thin knife poked into center of pan comes out clean. Remove, cover and refrigerate.

Before serving, run knife around inside of pan to loosen edges, then invert pan onto a dessert plate; the melted brown sugar will run over the flan.

Serve with fresh strawberries on the side of each dessert.

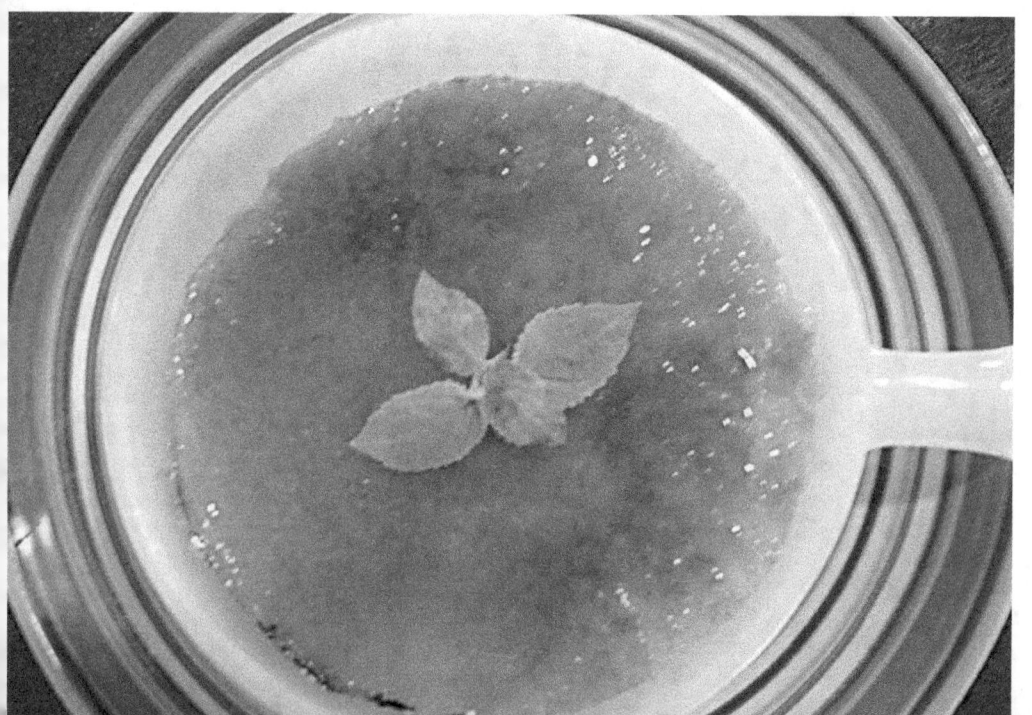

Nutrition Facts	
Serving Size 1/6 of recipe 180g (180 g)	
Servings per container 6	
Amount Per Serving	
Calories 370	Calories from Fat 34
	% Daily Value*
Total Fat 4g	6%
Saturated Fat 1g	7%
Trans Fat 0g	
Cholesterol 132mg	44%
Sodium 241mg	10%
Total Carbohydrate 70g	23%
Dietary Fiber 0g	1%
Sugars 58g	
Protein 15g	

3. Mandarin Fruit Salad

Preparation Time: 15 minutes
6 servings

Ingredients

6 ripe peaches, cut in ½" pieces
6 mandarin oranges, peeled and sectioned
6 ripe pears, cut in ½" pieces
2 ripe and hard mangoes, peeled and cut
   in ½" pieces
½ cup nonfat ricotta cheese
½ chopped almonds

Sauce

2 tbsp. almond essence
2 tbsp. honey

Preparation

Cut all fruit, then mix with mandarin orange sections. Add almonds and ricotta cheese then softly mix well.

Mix sauce ingredients.

Serve in dessert dishes with a dribble of sauce and a sprinkle almonds over each dish.

It's a fresh and deliciously easy dessert.

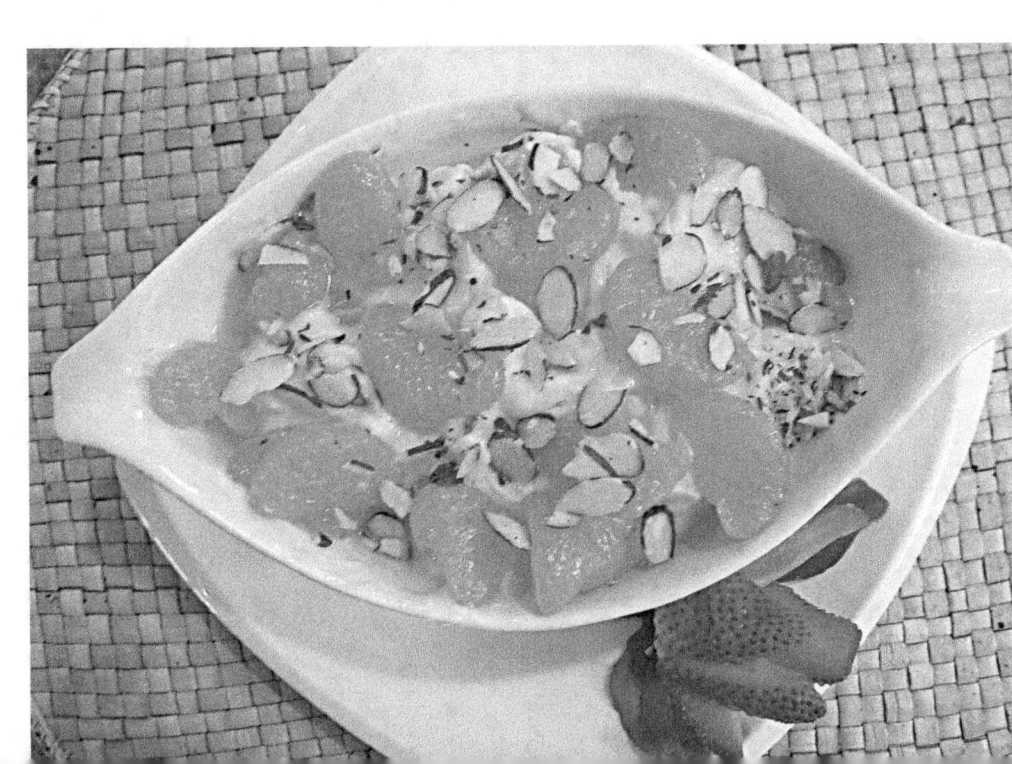

Nutrition Facts	
Serving Size 1/6 of recipe 516g (515 g)	
Servings per container 6	

Amount Per Serving	
Calories 337	Calories from Fat 55
	% Daily Value*
Total Fat 6g	10%
Saturated Fat 1g	3%
Trans Fat 0g	
Cholesterol 3mg	1%
Sodium 165mg	7%
Total Carbohydrate 66g	22%
Dietary Fiber 10g	41%
Sugars 48g	
Protein 9g	

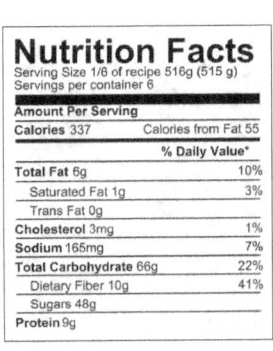

4. Strawberries with Cottage Cheese

Preparation Time: 10 minutes
4 servings

Ingredients

2 cups large fresh strawberries
1 tbsp. sugar substitute
½ cup water
4 tsp. low fat cottage cheese
2 tbsp. honey

Preparation

Wash and crush strawberries, then add sugar and water.

Mix cottage cheese and honey.

Divide crushed strawberries into 4 cups.

Drop 1 teaspoon of cottage cheese into center of each cup.

Refrigerate until cold then sprinkle with honey before serving.

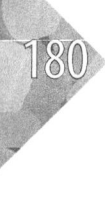

180

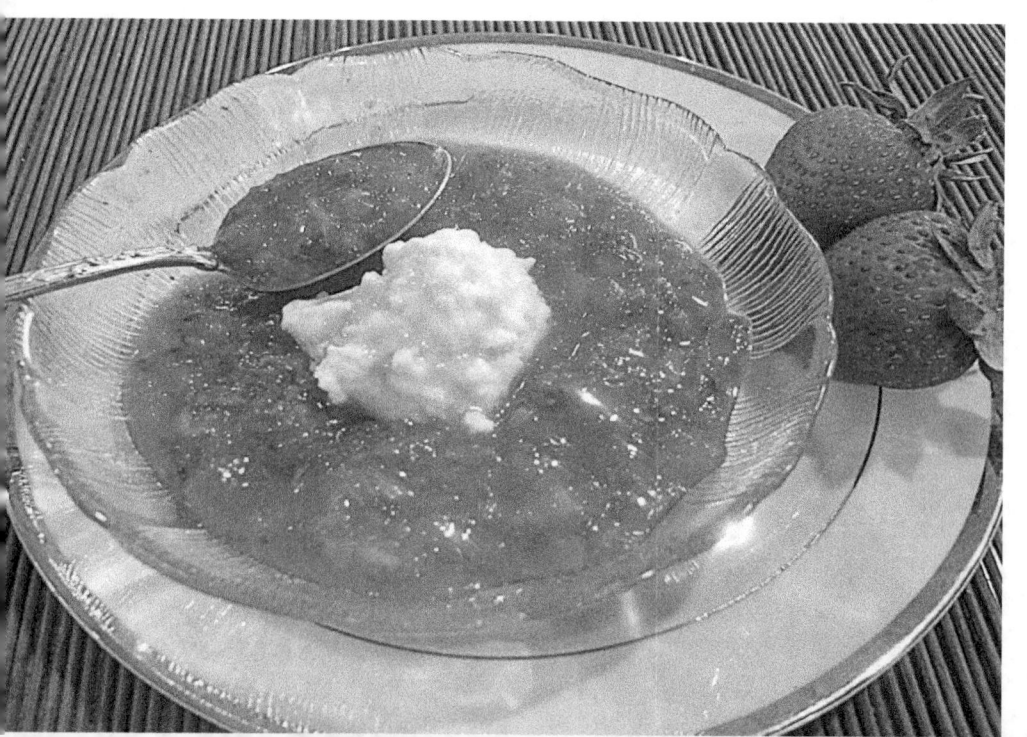

Nutrition Facts		
Serving Size 1/4 of recipe 94g (94 g)		
Servings per container 4		
Amount Per Serving		
Calories 63		Calories from Fat 3
		% Daily Value*
Total Fat 0g		0%
Saturated Fat 0g		0%
Trans Fat 0g		
Cholesterol 0mg		0%
Sodium 30mg		1%
Total Carbohydrate 15g		5%
Dietary Fiber 2g		6%
Sugars 13g		
Protein 1g		

5. Carrot and Almond Cakes

Preparation Time: 15 minutes
4 servings

Ingredients

1 egg
3 tsp. sugar substitute
3 tbsp. wheat flour
1 tsp. baking powder
1 ½ cup grated carrots
1 lemon peel, grated
¼ lb. almonds, diced
1 tsp. low fat margarine
1 tbsp. honey

Preparation

In a large bowl, mix egg and sugar substitute, then add wheat flour, baking powder, carrots, grated lemon and half the diced almonds, and mix well.

Preheat oven to 200°. Thinly coat inside of 4 small refractory molds with margarine, then fill each mold with mix. Bake for 45 minutes.

While still warm from oven, add ⅓ teaspoon of honey to each mold and sprinkle with remaining almonds to serve.

Yummmmy!!! Just Delicious!

181

Nutrition Facts		
Serving Size 1/4 of recipe 152g (152 g)		
Servings per container 4		
Amount Per Serving		
Calories 331	Calories from Fat 183	
		% Daily Value*
Total Fat 21g		33%
Saturated Fat 3g		16%
Trans Fat 0g		
Cholesterol 257mg		86%
Sodium 137mg		6%
Total Carbohydrate 24g		8%
Dietary Fiber 5g		20%
Sugars 11g		
Protein 15g		

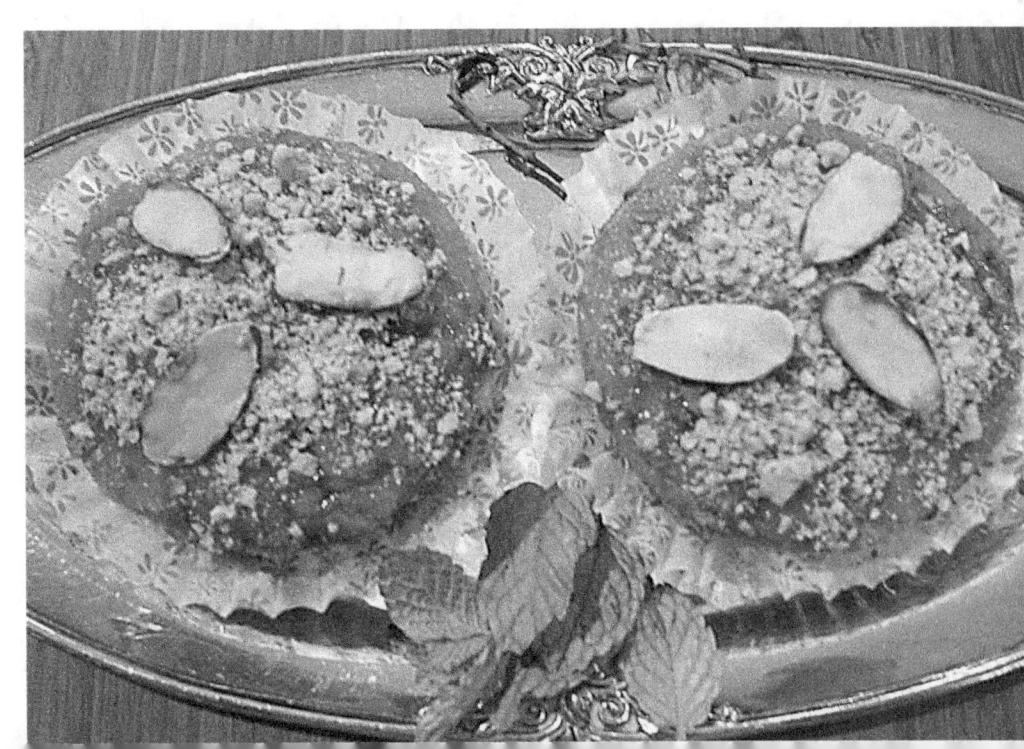

6. Carmen's Special Rice Pudding

Preparation Time: 30 minutes
8 servings

Ingredients

1 stick (4 oz.) low fat margarine
1 cup white rice (large whole grain),
   uncooked and washed
2 cups water
1 large cinnamon stick
2 cloves
2 cups apple juice
2 cups low fat milk
10 envelopes sugar substitute
   (or 1 cup molasses)
1 tbsp. vanilla extract
1 cup low fat cottage cheese
½ cup raisins
1 tbsp. cinnamon powder

Preparation

In a large pot, melt margarine, then add rice, water, cinnamon stick and clove. Cook over low heat until rice absorbs all water and is almost tender (add more water if necessary).

Add apple juice and simmer until rice is open and thick. Add milk, sugar substitute and vanilla, then stir slowly and cook for 5 minutes more. Stir in cottage cheese, then remove from heat.

Serve in dessert bowls with a decorative topping of raisins and a sprinkle of cinnamon.

Children will love this low calorie treat.

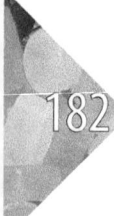

182

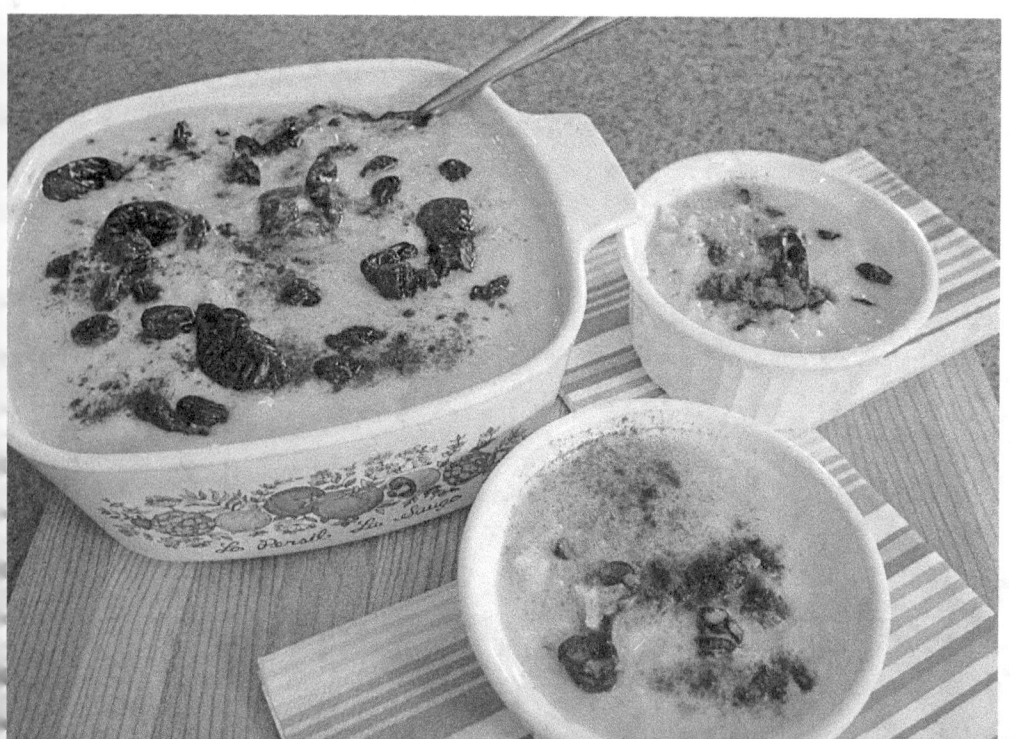

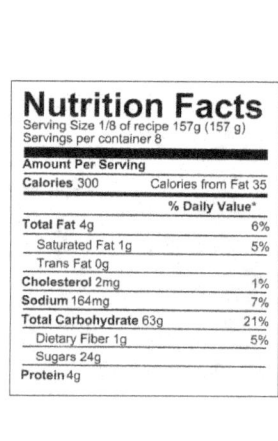

Nutrition Facts
Serving Size 1/8 of recipe 157g (157 g)
Servings per container 8

Amount Per Serving	
Calories 300	Calories from Fat 35

	% Daily Value*
Total Fat 4g	6%
Saturated Fat 1g	5%
Trans Fat 0g	
Cholesterol 2mg	1%
Sodium 164mg	7%
Total Carbohydrate 63g	21%
Dietary Fiber 1g	5%
Sugars 24g	
Protein 4g	

7. All Natural Baked Apple

Preparation Time: 30 minutes
4 servings

Ingredients

4 large red apples, washed and cored
1 cup natural apple juice, (unsweetened)
1 cup natural cranberry juice, (unsweetened)
½ tsp. cinnamon powder
1 clove
1 cinnamon stick
2 tbsp. low fat margarine

Preparation

Preheat oven to 400º.

Wash apples, then remove the center core of each with a knife.

In a baking dish, spread margarine, then place 4 apples. Add apple and cranberry juices, cinnamon and clove. Sprinkle cinnamon on top. Bake for 30 minutes, or until apples are tender and juicy.

Serve in dessert dishes with baking juice.

A wonderfully delicious, nutritious and "good for you" dessert.

Nutrition Facts	
Serving Size 1/4 of recipe 349g (348 g)	
Servings per container 4	
Amount Per Serving	
Calories 174	Calories from Fat 5
	% Daily Value*
Total Fat 1g	1%
Saturated Fat 0g	0%
Trans Fat 0g	
Cholesterol 0mg	0%
Sodium 6mg	0%
Total Carbohydrate 46g	15%
Dietary Fiber 6g	23%
Sugars 37g	
Protein 1g	

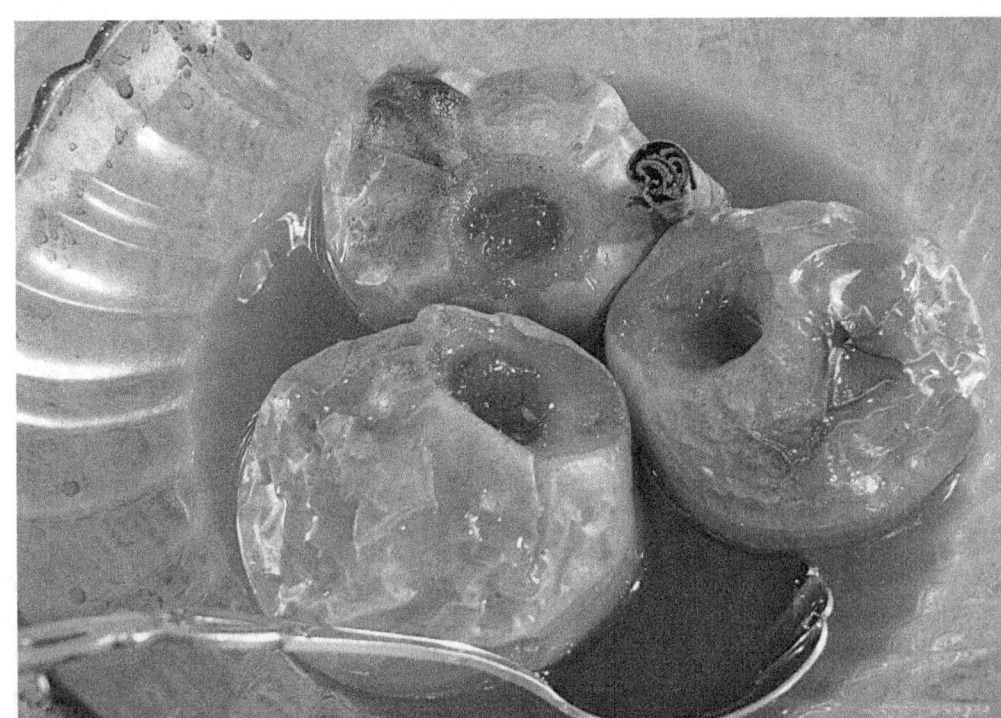

8. Crepes Suzette (Terraza Pasteur)

Preparation Time: 10 minutes
4 servings

Ingredients

2 strips lemon zest
1 tsp. vanilla extract
1 tbsp. low fat margarine
2 eggs
6 tbsp. all purpose flour
1 cup low fat milk
Canola oil spray
6 tbsp. fruit preserves (sugarless), any flavor
3 tbsp. low fat vanilla yogurt

Note

Crepes may be served hot or cold, sweet with jam or stuffed with different fillings: egg, ham, cheese, yogurt, fish, vegetables or fruits.

Preparation

In blender, mix lemon zest, vanilla, margarine, eggs, flour, and milk until a uniform mass.

Spray and heat oil in a medium skillet. Pour in ¼ of mixture and rotate skillet to form very thin layer on bottom. Cook until top is dry and bottom light brown, then flip and brown other side. Remove and repeat process for each crepe.

Place each crepe in round dessert dish, spread with fruit preserve, then carefully roll up and cover with yogurt. Garnish top with a fruit piece.

This luscious dish can be served as a dessert or for breakfast.

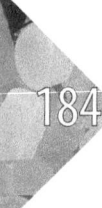

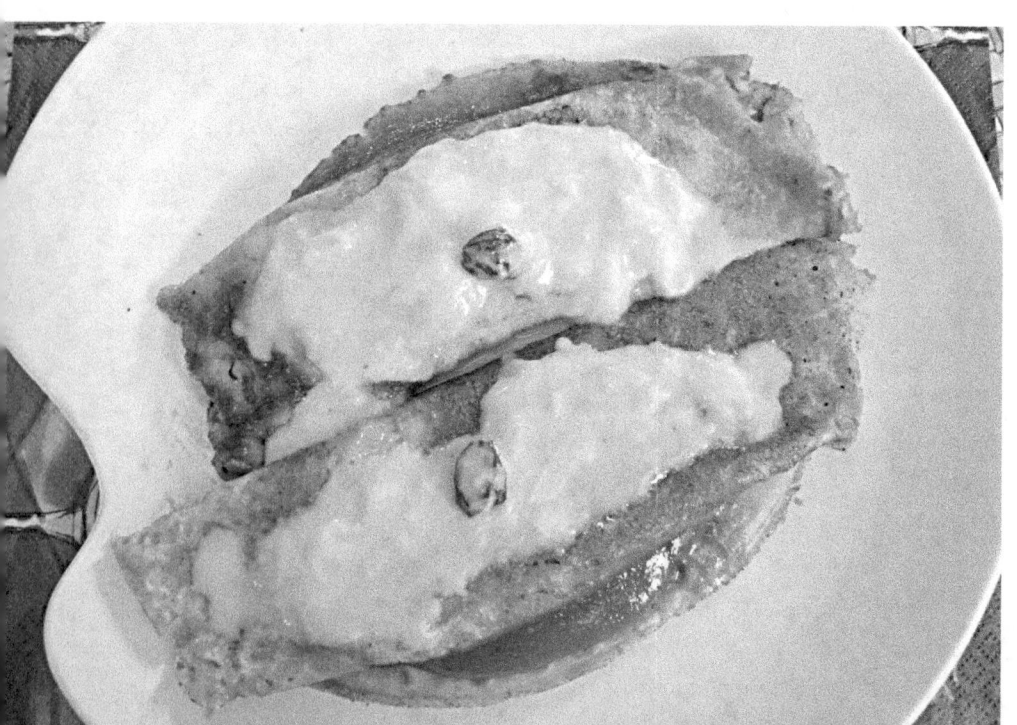

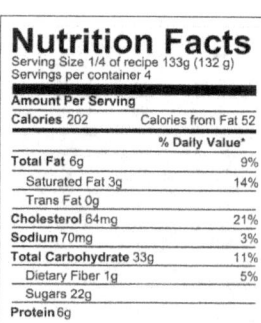

Nutrition Facts	
Serving Size 1/4 of recipe 133g (132 g)	
Servings per container 4	
Amount Per Serving	
Calories 202	Calories from Fat 52
	% Daily Value*
Total Fat 6g	9%
Saturated Fat 3g	14%
Trans Fat 0g	
Cholesterol 64mg	21%
Sodium 70mg	3%
Total Carbohydrate 33g	11%
Dietary Fiber 1g	5%
Sugars 22g	
Protein 6g	

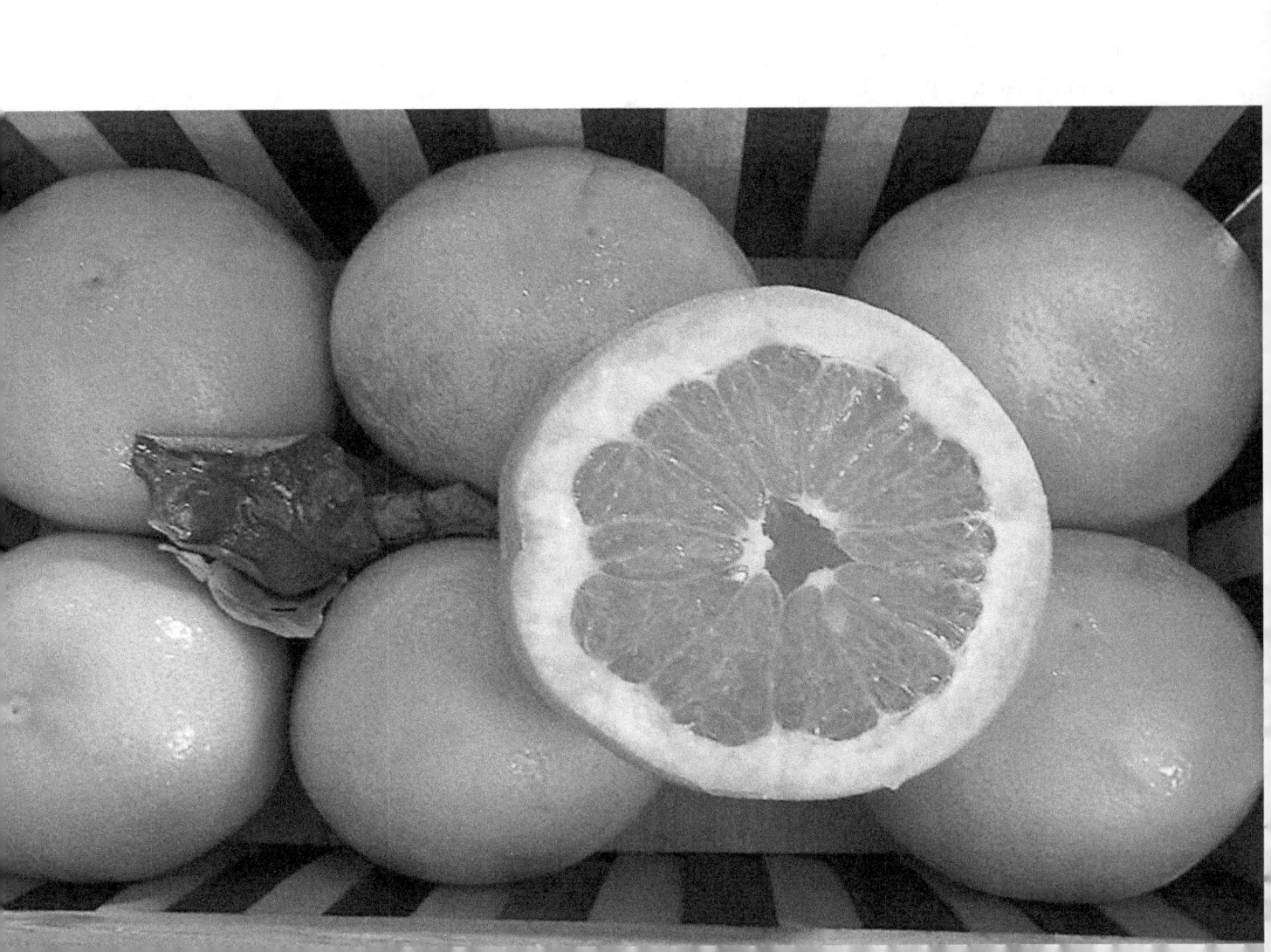

Index Of Recipes

187

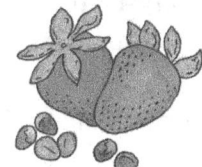

Glossary

APPETITE: is the natural desire to eat food, felt as hunger.

ANOREXIA NERVOSA (AN): is a psychiatric illness that describes an eating disorder characterized by extremely low body weight and body image distortion with an obsessive fear of gaining weight.

EATING RECORDS: detailed eating registry; includes a reminder of the previous 24 hours, questionnaires about frequency of intake and other information like weight history, changes prior to diet, supplement intake and tolerance for certain foods.

ANTHROPOMETRY: refers to measurement of the human individual for the purposes of understanding human physical variation.

BULIMIA NERVOSA (BN): is an eating disorder characterized by recurrent binge eating, followed by compensatory behaviors. The most common form is defensive vomiting, sometimes called purging; fasting, the use of laxatives, enemas, diuretics, and over exercising are also common.

EATING STUBBORNNESS: period in which foods that were previously acceptable and attractive, are now rejected or replace by a specific food type in each meal; commonly observe in children between 2 - 6 years of age.

ADEQUATE CONSUMPTION: level of daily consumption recommended based on calculations observed and determined experimentally by a group of health people. This recommendation for nutrients is used when the food requirement hasn't been determined (RDA)

DAILY FOOD CONSUMPTION CONSIDERED SAFE AND ADEQUATE (ESADDI): recommended ranges of appropriate consumption of nutrients, for which no sufficient information is available to establish a recommended eating requirement.

DAILY CONSUMPTION REFERENCE: series of eating references placed in most products, based in the requirements of 1968 for vitamins and minerals, this term replaces the nutrition requirements recommended in the United States, previously used for nutritional information in products.

EATING CONSUMPTION DATA: includes the information related to the appetite and the consumption, the patterns of nutrition and the estimate of typical nutrient consumption.

BODY FAT DEPOSITS: deposits of fat around the waist and abdomen; distribution of fat in shape of an "apple".

NUTRITION DETECTION: process used to identify nutritional problems and risk factors.

NUTRITION DIARY: registry of the quantities of foods consume during a established period, in general is 3 to 7 days; often includes information about time, place and situation while eating.

VERY LOW CALORIE DIET (VLCD): diet that provides 800 kcal or less per day.

GYNOID FAT DISTRIBUTION: fat deposit in the thighs and buttocks; distribution of fat in the shape of a "pear".

YO-YO EFFECT: process of losing and gaining weight, sometimes during a lifetime; often is characterize by a larger degree of fat on each cycle. Meaning, after losing, you gain more than you had before.

NUTRITIONAL SHAPE: degree in which the physiological nutritional needs of the individual are being met.

NUTRITIONAL CONTENT LABEL: information of nutritional contents in the food products, created to help the consumers select food to incorporate in a healthy life style, using the food pyramid and the nutritional guidelines.

NUTRITIONAL EXCESS: episode of food consumption identified by two particular patterns: 1) Quantity of food consumed is larger than what the majority of individuals consume in a similar situation. 2) Excessive consumption of food occurs in a definite time lapse, usually 2 - 3 hours, accompanied by a subjective feeling of weight loss.

FAT STORAGE: fat that is accumulating under the skin and around the internal organs.

ESSENTIAL FAT: body fat located in specific places that is required to subsist; approximately 3% to 12% of your body weight.

HYPERPHAGIA: period of excessive consumption of food.

HYPERPLASIA: increase in the size of tissue by an increment in the number of cells. In infants and adolescents that gain weight this process is present at the level of the adipose cells, making it difficult to reduce because it increases not only the size of the cells but also the quantity of fat cells.

HYPOPHAGIA: Reduced food intake.

BODY IMAGE: mental concept of you, related to the rate of growth and changes in your body proportions.

BODY MASS INDEX (BMI): weight (kg)/stature (m^2); a definition of the degree of adiposity.

NUTRITIONAL INSECURITY: limit availability or uncertain of adequate and safe nutritious food, or limited capacity to acquired acceptable foods in ways sociably acceptable.

LIFE STYLE MODIFICATION: test of prior conducts and consequences regarding eating habits, exercise and thought patterns.

MORBIDITY CONCURRENT: refers to a diseased state, disability, or poor health due to obesity, aggravating the illness as it progresses; often subsiding as the treatment works satisfactory.

TOLERABLE SUPERIOR CONSUMPTION LEVEL (UL): the maximum level of daily consumption of nutrients that has less possibilities of imposing risk of side effects to most individuals' health, in general population.

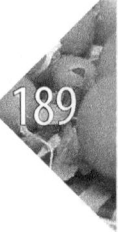

189

OBESITY: it is a condition characterized by the accumulation of excessive adiposity (body fat) in which the weight is more than 10% above the ideal, according to age and is nowadays considered a chronic disorder and is based on a predisposition that requires a high level of supervision and follow up with long term treatment.

MORBID OBESITY: estate of adiposity in which body weight exceeds 100% the ideal weight; an index of corporal mass (IMC/BMI) higher than 39 in infants and adolescents. The presence of risk factors and associated illnesses with morbid obesity are also used to establish a clinical diagnosis: Diabetes type II, Hypercholesterolemia, Hypertension. Sleep apnea among other risk factors endangers the quality of life and indicates the need for urgent clinical treatment for this type of obesity.

FOOD PYRAMID: explains the nutritional food requirements that are estimated necessary to satisfy a healthy individual in an average group.

PRESCRIPTION DIET: designated type, quantity and frequency of food consumption; can include quantities and shapes, proteins, carbohydrates, fat, liquids, vitamins and mineral.

WAIST REASON: HIP (WHR): the relation of the measurements of waist and hips; method use to access fat distribution.

ADIPOSITY REBOUND: phenomena of normal growth that occurred around six years of age, when body fat stars increasing in a child.

ESTIMATED AVERAGE REQUIRED (EAR): value of content of nutrients that is estimated satisfies the requirements of half the individuals in a group.

RECOMMENDED DIETARY ALLOWANCE: quantity of nutrients required to satisfy the needs of a healthy population (97-98%).

OVERWEIGHT: state in which weight exceeds between 5 to 10% based on height and age.

EXCESS DIETARY DISORDER (BED): disorder characterized by the excess of food consumption at least twice a week, during a period of six months.

EATING DISORDER: abnormal conducts related with the food and its ingestion, which includes fasting, binge-eating, vomiting, laxative abuse or excessive exercise accompanied by unrealistic ideas about food, distorted body image and psychological and developmental abnormalities.

DAILY VALUE (DV): reference term in the food labels to help the consumers select a healthy diet; includes two types of references, the daily consumption reference and daily value of reference.

NUTRITIONAL VALUE: science determines the nutritional state through analysis of the medical history, eating and social habits of an individual; the anthropometric data, biochemical data and the alterations of medications and nutrients.

DAILY REFERENCE VALUES (DRV): a series of food references for the labels in products that contains the nutrients (except protein), the daily values of reference establish for fat, saturated fat acids, cholesterol, total carbohydrates, protein, fiber, sodium and potassium.

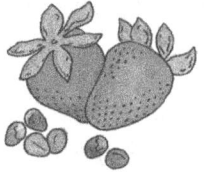

Bibliography

NUTRITION AND DIET THERAPY. Krausel Kathleen Mahan, MS, RD, CDE Sylvia Escott-Stum, MA, RD, LDN. McGraw Hill. Interamericana Editores, SA Tenth edition, ISBN 0-7216-7904-8

FOOD AND DIET THERAPY. P. Cervera, J. Clapes R. Rigolfas. McGraw Hill Interamericana Editores, SA ISBN 84-7605-427-0

TREATY OF PEDIATRICS W.E. Nelson, MD V.C. Vaughan III, MD. R.J. McKay, MD. Salvat Editores, SA ISBN 0-7216-9018-1

Articles

1. OBESE CHILDREN – Diabetic Adults. Caroline Delgado. Nexos Magazine. September 2008.

2. THE NEW YORK TIMES – Supplement. Obesity in Children. Published in January 2006 with the participation of the University of California, San Francisco (UCSF), Kaiser Permanente, University of California, Los Angeles (UCLA), together with other institutions engaged in the battle against the scourge of obesity in children.

3. THE NEW YORK TIMES. Health Section. September 2008. Discusses the different forms of surgery such as Gastric Bypass.

4. CHILDREN'S HOSPITAL OF BOSTON, UNIVERSITY OF MICHIGAN. Make Nutrition Work in Growing Children. April 2008.

5. HARVARD UNIVERSITY, USA. School of Public Health. Infant Obesity. September 30, 2008. Examines the role of parents in the prevention of obesity in their children.

6. JOHN HOPKINS CHILDREN'S CENTER, USA. Obesity in Children as a "Way to Satiate" in Spanish language television. February 2008

7. YES, WE CAN! An American government program designed to combat childhood obesity, with the participation of several organizations such as The National Heart, Lung and Blood Institute (NHLBI) and the American Academy of Pediatrics (AAP).

8. KIDSHEALTH – Overweight and Obesity. Organization of American States. First revision February 12, 2005. Second revision August 2005.

9. BRITISH MEDICAL ASSOCIATION. Report on Child Obesity. Published in 2008.

10. LE FIGARO, France. Workshop to Detect Infant Obesity. Caroline Petitnicolas. October 1, 2008.

11. McMASTER UNIVERSITY, Hamilton, Canada. Population Health Research Institute. The Predominance of Childhood Obesity and its Treatment. September 30, 2008.

Annex

12. CHILDCARE MANUAL. Spanish Association of Pediatrics. Dr. Valentin Pineda. Pediatric consultant and head of pediatric hospitalization and the Pediatric Infectious Diseases Unit of Sabadell Hospital, Spain.

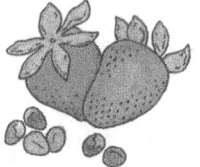

For More Information:

Email Us

dietista@obesidadtratamiento.com

recetas@obesidadtratamiento.com

Or Visit Our Website

www.ObesityTreatmentJuvenile.com

www.ingramcontent.com/pod-product-compliance
Lightning Source LLC
Chambersburg PA
CBHW081349280526
45788CB00009B/2815